Advances in Translational Medical Science

Lipids and Atherosclerosis

Advances in Translational Medical Science

Lipids and Atherosclerosis

Edited by

C.J. Packard, BSc, PhD, FRCPath, DSc

Department of Vascular Biochemistry
Glasgow Royal Infirmary
Scotland

and

D.J. Rader, MD

Department of Medicine and Institute for Translational Medicines and Therapeutics
University of Pennsylvania School of Medicine
Philadelphia, PA
USA

Foreword by

V. Fuster, MD, PhD

President, World Heart Federation
Director, Cardiovascular Institute
Mount Sinai School of Medicine
New York, NY
USA

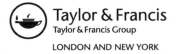
Taylor & Francis
Taylor & Francis Group

LONDON AND NEW YORK

First published in the United Kingdom in 2006
by Taylor & Francis, an imprint of the Taylor & Francis Group,
2 Park Square, Milton Park, Abingdon, Oxon OX14 4RN

Tel.:   +44 (0) 207 017 6000
Fax.:   +44 (0) 207 017 6699
E-mail: info.medicine@tandf.co.uk
Website: http://www.tandf.co.uk/medicine

A CIP record for this book is available from the British Library

Library of Congress Cataloging-in-Publication Data
Data available on application

ISBN 1-84214-229-1

Distributed in North and South America by

Taylor & Francis
2000 NW Corporate Blvd
Boca Raton, FL 33431, USA

Within Continental USA
Tel.: 800 272 7737; Fax.: 800 374 3401
Outside Continental USA
Tel.: 561 994 0555; Fax.: 561 361 6018
E-mail: orders@crcpress.com

Distributed in the rest of the world by
Thomson Publishing Services
Cheriton House
North Way
Andover, Hampshire SP10 5BE, UK
Tel.: +44 (0) 1264 332424
E-mail: salesorder.tandf@thomsonpublishingservices.co.uk

Composition by Scribe Design Ltd, Ashford, Kent, UK
Printed and bound in Spain by Grafos SA

Contents

List of contributors

L. Asp
Department of Medical Biochemistry
The Wallenberg Laboratory for
Cardiovascular Research
Göteborg University
Sweden

K.O. Badellino
Schools of Medicine and Nursing
University of Pennsylvania
Philadelphia, PA
USA

P. Barter
The Heart Research Institute
Sydney, NSW
Australia

J.T. Billheimer
The Department of Medicine
University of Pennsylvania
Philadelphia, PA
USA

T. Claudel
Center for Liver, Digestive and Metabolic
    Diseases
Laboratory of Pediatrics
Academic Hospital Groningen
Groningen
The Netherlands

J-M. Fernández-Real
Section of Diabetes, Endocrinology and
    Nutrition
University Hospital of Girona 'Dr Josep
Trueta'
Girona
Spain

J-C. Fruchart
Unité de Recherche 545
Institute National de la Santé et de la
    Recherche Médicale
Departement d'Athérosclérose
Institut Pasteur de Lille
Université de Lille 2
Lille
France

C.D. Funk
Departments of Physiology and Biochemistry
Queen's University
Kingston, ON
Canada

P. Gervois
Unité de Recherche 545
Institute National de la Santé et de la
    Recherche Médicale
Départment d'Athérosclérose
Institut Pasteur de Lille
Université de Lille 2
Lille
France

H. Gylling
Department of Clinical Nutrition
University of Kuopio
Kuopio
Finland

R.A. Heyman
Exelixis Inc.
San Diego, CA
USA

W. Jin
School of Medicine
University of Pennsylvania
Philadelphia, PA
USA

F. Karpe
Oxford Centre for Diabetes, Endocrinology
    and Metabolism
Nuffield Department of Clinical Medicine
University of Oxford
Oxford
UK

E.L. Klett
Division of Endocrinology, Diabetes and
    Medical Genetics
Medical University of South Carolina
Charleston, SC
USA

F. Kuipers
Center for Liver, Digestive and Metabolic
    Diseases
Laboratory of Pediatrics
Academic Hospital Groningen
Groningen
The Netherlands

R.G. Lee
Department of Pathology
Wake Forest University School of Medicine
Winston-Salem, NC
USA

C.H. Macphee
Department of Vascular Biology and
    Thrombosis
GlaxoSmithKline
King of Prussia
Philadelphia, PA
USA

T.A. Miettinen
Biomedicum Helsinki
Division of Internal Medicine
Helsinki
Finland

J.S. Millar
The Department of Pharmacology
University of Pennsylvania
Philadelphia, PA
USA

B. Mukhopadhyay
Department of Vascular Biochemistry and
    Diabetes
Glasgow Royal Infirmary
Glasgow
UK

S-O. Olofsson
Wallenberg Laboratory
Sahlgrenska University Hospital
Göteborg
Sweden

S.B. Patel
Division of Endocrinology and Metabolism
Medical College of Wisconsin
Milwaukee, WI
USA

J.B. Prins
Department of Diabetes and Endocrinology
Princess Alexandra Hospital
Woolloongabba, QLD
Australia

E. Puré
The Wistar Institute
Philadelphia, PA
USA

D.J. Rader
Department of Medicine and Institute for
    Translational Medicine and Therapeutics
University of Pennsylvania School of Medicine
Philadelphia, PA
USA

L.L. Rudel
Department of Pathology
Wake Forest University School of Medicine
Winston-Salem, NC
USA

N. Sattar
Department of Vascular Biochemistry
Glasgow Royal Infirmary
Glasgow
UK

I.G. Schulman
Exelixis Inc.
San Diego, CA
USA

C.C. Shoulders
MRC Clinical Sciences Centre
Hammersmith Hospital
Du Cane Road
London
UK

B. Staels
Unité de Recherche 545
Institut National de la Santé et de la
    Recherche Médicale
Department d'Athérosclérose
Institut Pasteur de Lille
Université de Lille 2
Lille
France

E. Sturm
Center for Liver, Digestive and Metabolic
    Diseases
Laboratory of Pediatrics
Academic Hospital Groningen
Groningen
The Netherlands

G.D. Tan
Oxford Centre for Diabetes, Endocrinology
    and Metabolism
Nuffield Department of Clinical Medicine
University of Oxford
Oxford
UK

L. Zhao
Department of Pharmacology and Institute for
    Translational Medicine and Therapeutics
University of Pennsylvania
Philadelphia, PA
USA

Foreword

Recent insights into the aetiology of athcrothrombosis, the leading cause of morbidity and mortality in Western society, have opened the way to a more strategic approach to treatment and prevention. It is recognised now that the composition of the plaque as well as its size is crucial in determining the propensity to rupture and to initiate a life threatening thrombotic event. Key features associated with plaque fragility are: a large lipid core, an abundance of tissue factor and inflammatory cells including macrophages, vasovasorum, and a thin fibrous cap, the structural integrity of which is compromised by the presence of matrix degrading metalloproteinases.

Atherogenic lipoproteins play a central role in the initiation and growth of atherosclerotic plaques. The 'lipid hypothesis' is now dogma with the repeated demonstration that lowering the level of plasma low density lipoprotein (LDL) cholesterol reduces the risk of onset of recurrent myocardial infarction and many other cardiovascular complications. Statins, inhibitors of the rate-limiting enzyme in cholesterol synthesis, have been shown to prevent coronary heart disease and stroke, and are one of the success stories of modern medicine. However, many patients cannot adequately reduce their levels of atherogenic lipoproteins with statins alone. Therefore, new approaches to reducing LDL and other atherogenic lipoproteins are still needed. Furthermore, even in statin treated patients there is considerable residual risk of cardiovascular disease. Therefore, it is imperative to ask what new approaches to the control of other features of atherothrombosis will ultimately yield further risk reduction. Major areas of new therapeutic targeting include intestinal and hepatic lipid metabolism, IIDL metabolism and reverse cholesterol transport, and inflammatory processes within the vascular wall and beyond. The tremendous advances in basic science will be translated into therapeutic advances. Within this context, translational research is a term that encapsulates the idea of 'bench' to 'bedside' translation of etiological concepts and therapeutic targets. The range of technologies available now, from genome searches to molecular and clinical imaging of atherothrombotic plaques permits novel insights into one arena to be tested quickly in another, thereby developing an integrated picture of the potential of new treatment modalities.

This book will be of interest to all researchers in the field of atherothrombosis, to those seeking further understanding of lipid and lipoprotein metabolism, to those seeking new targets for drug development and to those evaluating the potential of novel biomarkers for risk assessment. Packard and Rader have assembled contributions from the world's experts in lipid and lipoprotein metabolism and atherogenesis. The chapters offer up-to-date overviews of hot topics and critical appraisal of the potential of new approaches to the prevention of vascular disease.

This book on the translation of science into new therapies for atherothrombosis is timely and will be of interest to a wide variety of readers.

Valentin Fuster, MD, PhD
Past President, American Heart Association
President, World Heart Federation
Director, Cardiovascular Institute,
Mount Sinai School of Medicine

Preface

We are pleased to present a new book entitled 'Lipids and Atherosclerosis'. Over the last two decades, there have been major advances in our understanding of the molecular regulation of lipid and lipoprotein metabolism as well as of the pathogenesis of atherosclerosis. The next step is to translate that molecular knowledge into new therapeutic approaches to lipid disorders and atherosclerosis. Therefore, we felt it appropriate to focus a book on the interface between the basic science and new therapeutic development in this critically important area of biology and medicine.

Chapters 1–4 focus on the molecular pathways by which the liver assembles and secretes very low density lipoproteins (VLDL). The microsomal transfer protein, the acyl CoA: diacylglycerol acyltransferase, and the ACAT enzymes all play an important role in this process, and each is represented by a chapter written by experts in these areas. In addition, an overview on the mechanisms of VLDL assembly in the liver is provided by Professor Olofsson, an internationally recognized pioneer in this area.

The next 3 chapters examine intestinal lipid metabolism and bioacid metabolism. Chapters on ABCG5 and ABCG8 as well as on the role of FXR in bioacid metabolism are included. An overview on intestinal lipid metabolism is provided, written by Professors Miettinen and Gylling.

Then follows 4 chapters on: HDL metabolism and reverse cholesterol transport; LXR and regulation of cholesterol efflux; endothelial lipase and the regulation of HDL metabolism; and the role of CETP and its potential as a target for the development of new therapies. An overview is written by Professor Barter, internationally recognized for his work in this area.

The adipocyte and its role in energy and lipid metabolism is the basis of chapters 12–15. PPARs, the secretory products of adipocytes, and the regulation of adipocyte triglyceride storage are all discussed in depth. An overview of insulin resistance in metabolic syndrome is provided by Professor Sattar, widely known for his work in this area.

Finally, chapters 16–19 explore the role of inflammatory pathways in atherosclerosis. Topics included in these chapters are the respective roles of CD44, lipoxygenases, and Lp-PLA$_2$ in atherogenesis. An overview of the role of innate immunity in atherosclerosis is provided by Professor Real, who has long been recognized as a key opinion leader in this field.

Our goal has been to encourage authors to present evidence and to speculate on the interface between new knowledge of molecular mechanisms and the potential to translate those mechanisms into new therapeutic approaches. Several chapters specifically discuss novel therapies that are currently in clinical development or expected to enter the clinical development arena in the near future. Other contributions discuss the potential of new molecular targets. We recognize that the areas of lipid metabolism and atherosclerosis are intensively investigated and dynamic and often changing, and every effort has been made to have the information provided as up to date as possible. Our hope is that this book will be of interest to individuals interested in the developments in the areas of lipid metabolism and atherosclerosis, and the potential for new therapies that will result.

Chris J. Packard and Daniel J. Rader

Acknowledgements

The Editors would like to thank sincerely Linda Watts and Shelley Wilkie for all their help in managing the co-ordination of this book with our publishers, Taylor and Francis, and chapter authors.

The assembly of very low density lipoproteins in the liver

S-O. Olofsson and L. Asp

OVERVIEW OF THE SECRETORY PATHWAY

Secretory proteins and integral membrane proteins are synthesized on ribosomes attached to the surface of the endoplasmic reticulum (Figure 1). During the biosynthesis, the 'nascent' polypeptide is translocated through a channel starting at the site of synthesis in the ribosome and proceeding through a

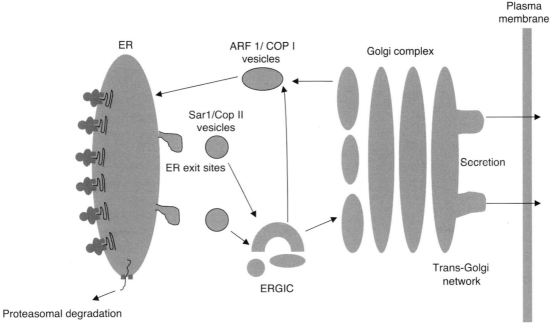

Figure 1 *Overview of the secretory pathway.* Secretory proteins are translated on ribosomes attached to the endoplasmic reticulum (ER) and translocated to the lumen of this organelle. After being folded, the proteins leave the ER at exit sites via COP II vesicles. The GTPase Sar1 is involved in the formation of these vesicles. Misfolded proteins are retracted to the cytosol and sorted for proteasomal degradation. The COP II vesicles fuse to form the ERGIC (ER-Golgi intermediate compartment; also referred to as VTC (vesicular tubular cluster)). COP I vesicles, assembled under the influence of ARF1, are involved in sorting processes in the ERGIC as well as in the next compartment, the cis-Golgi. Well-established COP I-dependent sorting processes are the return of proteins from the later part of the secretory pathway to the ER. ERGIC fuse with the cis-Golgi, and the proteins are transferred though the different levels of the Golgi apparatus to be finally sorted to secretion in the trans-Golgi network

membrane pore to the lumen of the endoplasmic reticulum (ER). In this way, the nascent chain can reach the lumen of the ER without being exposed to the cytosol. The membrane pore consists mainly of two components, the trimeric complex Sec 61 (with its α, β and γ chains) and Tram. The pore undergoes important interactions with the nascent polypeptide and influences its correct translocation, its folding and its targeting. The pore is gated in two directions: from the cytosol to the lumen and in the plane of the membrane. The first gate opens when the nascent chain starts to translocate to the ER lumen, while the second gate is involved in selectively allowing the membrane-spanning domains of membrane proteins to enter the hydrophobic portion of the membrane. (The translocon and its function have been reviewed elsewhere; see, for example, references 1, 2.)

A chaperone-aided process allows the protein to fold in the ER and the folded proteins are sorted into exit sites and allowed to leave the ER by transport vesicles (Figure 1). Misfolded proteins, on the other hand, are retained in the ER and eventually retracted through the membrane channel (i.e. Sec 61 and Tram) and sorted to proteasomal degradation (Figure 1).[1-7]

The formation of the transport vesicles and the correct transport from the ER to the Golgi apparatus are dependent on a series of proteins (these proteins and the transport processes have been reviewed extensively, and the reader is referred to such reviews for more detailed information; see, for example, references 4, 8–11). We shall restrict ourselves to a short description of SAR 1 and ARF 1 (Figure 2), as well as the coat proteins present on the transport vesicles that bud under the influence of these two proteins. ARF 1 and SAR 1 are small GTPases which function as 'switches' in intracellular processes. The proteins are activated by the exchange of GDP for GTP, a process catalysed by a GEP (guanine nucleotide exchange protein). Several such GEPs have been identified for ARF 1 (for review, see reference 8). These are soluble cytosolic proteins. SAR 1 is activated by one GEP (Sec 12p) which

is an integral membrane protein of the ER (for review, see reference 8). In the case of ARF 1, the exchange reaction targets the protein to the microsomal membrane, a process which involves a change in the structure of ARF 1 allowing an N-terminally linked myristic acid to leave a hydrophobic pocket and anchor the protein in the membrane;[12] see also reference 8 for a review (Figure 2). SAR 1 is not acylated and does not appear to contain any other lipid-anchoring structure; even so, a large portion of the SAR 1 pool is membrane associated (for review, see reference 8).

There are different so-called coat proteins which are involved in the budding of transport vesicles. The assembly of the coat is determined by SAR1 and ARF 1. Thus, after activation ARF 1 (Figure 2) triggers the assembly of the Cop I coat consisting of several proteins (α-COP, β'-COP, ε-COP, γ^1- or γ^2-COP, β-COP, δ-COP, ζ^1- or ζ^2-COP), while SAR 1 influences the assembly of the Cop II coat, which consists of the Sec23/24p and the Sec 13/31p complexes (see, for example, references 4, 8, 9, 11).

Hydrolysis of the GTP bound to ARF 1 and SAR 1 is activated by GAPs (GTPase activating proteins). The importance of this hydrolysis for the disassembly of the coat proteins and the sorting and collection of cargo to the vesicles has been reviewed elsewhere.[8,9]

Secretory proteins leave the ER at so-called exit sites, where they are sorted into COP II vesicles (Figure 1). The process is driven by SAR 1. The COP II vesicles stay close to the ER and fuse to form the ER-Golgi intermediate compartment (ERGIC; also referred to as the vesicular tubular cluster (VTC)) (Figure 1). ARF 1 and COP I are involved in important sorting processes in the ERGIC, processes which involve the sorting of proteins that should be returned to the ER. The ERGIC is transported to the cis-Golgi on microtubules and fuses with this compartment. It has been demonstrated that the activity of ARF 1 is of importance for the structure of ERGIC and for its ability to mature into the cis-Golgi. ARF 1 COP I vesicles are also involved in sorting proteins from the cis-Golgi and back to the ER (for review, see references 4, 13) (Figure 1).

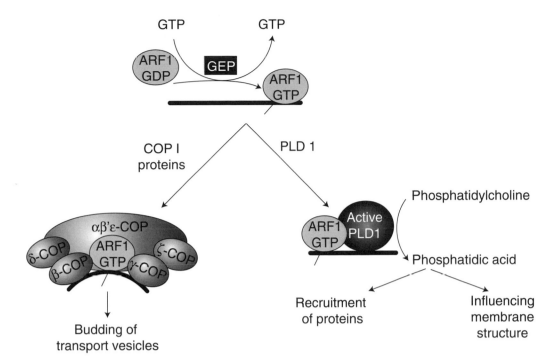

Figure 2 *The activation and functions of ARF 1.* ARF 1 is activated by a GEP which exchanges GDP for GTP. This leads to a change in the structure of ARF 1 that exposes a myristic acid, which anchors the protein to the microsomal membrane. In this position, ARF 1 can recruit COP I proteins, thus promoting the budding of transport vesicles. ARF 1 can also activate phospholipase D1 (PLD 1), which converts phosphatidylcholine to phosphatidic acid. It has been proposed that the phosphatidic acid formed recruits proteins involved in, for example, the formation of transport vesicles or influences the membrane in such a way that budding of transport vesicles is promoted

The secretory proteins are exposed to different levels of the Golgi apparatus (cis-, medial and trans-Golgi) during transfer through the secretory pathway (Figure 1). The predominant opinion seems to be that, to a large extent, this occurs through the process of maturation of the Golgi cisterns, by which the cis-Golgi cisterns mature into the medial Golgi, which in turn becomes the trans-Golgi (for review, see reference 14). The proteins are finally transported from the trans-Golgi network to the plasma membrane to be secreted (for review, see, for example, reference 4, 14). During exposure to the different Golgi cisterns, the N-linked carbohydrate (added during the translocation into the ER lumen) is processed and O-linked glycosylation occurs.

OVERVIEW OF THE BIOSYNTHESIS OF apoB-100 AND THE ASSEMBLY OF VERY LOW DENSITY LIPOPROTEINS

apoB-100 is a secretory protein and, as such, follows the secretory pathway. In order to be secreted, however, the protein must be incorporated into the Very Low Density Lipoproteins (VLDLs). These consist of a core of neutral lipids (triglycerides and cholesterol esters) surrounded by a monolayer of amphipathic structures (phospholipids, unesterified cholesterol) to which apoB-100 is bound. It is now well established that this structure is assembled in two steps (Figure 3), of which the first occurs during the translation and translocation of apoB-100 to the lumen of the endoplasmic reticulum. In the second step, which occurs outside the rough ER, apoB-100 associates with the major proportion of lipids, forming a bona fide VLDL.

The first step: a co-translational partial lipidation of apoB-100 (for reviews, see references 15–17)

The first step occurs during the biosynthesis of apoB-100 and its translocation through the translocon to the lumen of the ER (Figure 3).[18] During this process, apoB-100 is partially lipidated, forming a primordial lipoprotein – a pre-VLDL. This lipoprotein was isolated from the endoplasmic reticulum and shown to be a 100 Å particle with the density of HDL.[19–21] The primordial particle with apoB-100 is retained in the cell (for discussion, see below), while that with apoB-48 is allowed to leave the cell to be secreted.[22] The retention is dependent on the structure between aa 3266 and 4082 in apoB-100 and the interaction with chaperons (see below).[23] The pre-VLDL contains both triglycerides and phospholipids[19,21] and is relatively tightly associated with the membrane of the endoplasmic reticulum.[24]

The microsomal triglyceride transfer protein and the first step in VLDL assembly (for reviews, see references 25, 26)

The co-translational lipidation of apoB-100 is catalysed by a transfer protein which is referred to as the microsomal triglyceride transfer protein (MTP). The importance of MTP for VLDL assembly is illustrated by the observation that MTP is the gene for abeta-lipoproteinaemia,[27,28] that is, the inability to assemble apoB-containing lipoproteins.

The structure of MTP has been modelled on the structure of lamprey lipovitellin[29] and proposed to contain a hydrophobic pocket which is most likely involved in the transfer of lipids.[29] Details of the structure of MTP and its interaction with apoB-100 will be reviewed elsewhere. The protein has been demonstrated to interact with apoB, and a possible model for the role of MTP in the co-translation lipidation

of apoB-100 has been proposed.[30,31] Thus, MTP has been proposed to interact with apoB to form lipid-binding pockets which involve the amphipathic β-sheet structures in apoB-100[31] (Figure 3). These lipid-binding pockets are thought to acquire the lipids delivered by the transfer protein (details of these models are presented in references 26, 30, 31).

ApoB-100 is a very amphipathic molecule, with large regions of amphipathic β-sheet as well as regions of amphipathic α-helix (for a review of apoB structure, see reference 32). A co-translational lipidation may be necessary to allow the protein to fold in its correct position, i.e. in a lipid–water interface, when it enters the lumen of the ER.

The second step in the VLDL assembly occurs outside rough ER (for reviews, see references 15–17)

Evidence for a second step in VLDL assembly was first obtained by immuno-electron microscopy,[33] where the presence of a non-VLDL form of apoB in the rough ER and the presence of apoB free 'lipid droplets' in the smooth ER were demonstrated. ApoB-containing VLDL appeared at the junction between rough and smooth ER. Our group provided biochemical[18–21,34] and kinetic[22] evidence for a model in which a lipid-poor lipoprotein was formed during one step and converted to a lipid-rich structure in a second step. Recently, it has been possible to verify the presence of the two steps in vivo in humans by turnover studies based on stable isotopes.[35]

Very recent studies have demonstrated that the second step can be divided in two alternative steps; one leading to VLDL 2 and the other to VLDL 1.[23] The formation of VLDL 2 from pre-VLDL is due to a size dependent lipidation, i.e. the triglycerides were added in proportion to the length of apoB. Based on these observations, we concluded that the dense apoB-48 particle was an analogue to VLDL 2 rather than to the apoB-100 pre-VLDL. This explained why the apoB-48 particle could be secreted.[23] VLDL 1 was assembled from VLDL 2 by the addition of a major load of lipid. This process required

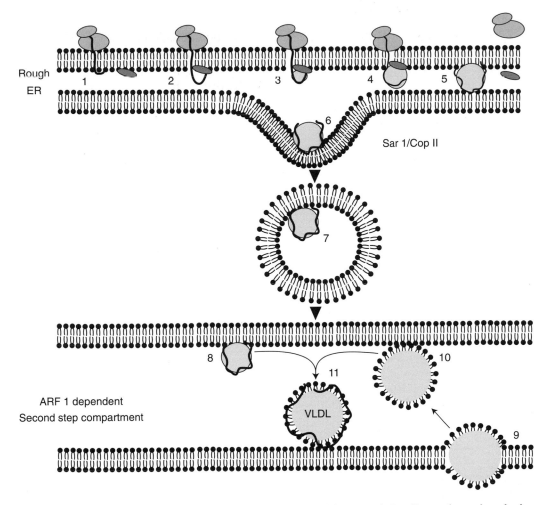

Figure 3 *Overview of the assembly of very low density lipoproteins.* ApoB is co-translationally translocated to the lumen of the endoplasmic reticulum (ER) (1). During this translocation, apoB interacts with MTP (shown in dark grey in figure) to form lipid-binding pockets (2) which accept the lipids from MTP (3). The lipid-binding pocket is thought to enlarge to accept more lipids (4). Thus, at the end of the biosynthesis of apoB a 10 nm primordial particle (a pre-VLDL) is formed (5). This pre-VLDL is relatively strongly associated with the ER membrane and leaves the ER with Sar1/Cop II vesicles (6 and 7) to eventually end up in a post-ER compartment. This compartment is dependent on ARF 1 to be intact (i.e. Golgi or ERGIC). In this 'second step compartment', lipid droplets (10) bud from the membrane (9) under the influence of a phospholipase D (see Figure 2). Pre-VLDL (8) fuses (11) with the luminal lipid droplet (10). This fusion, the second step, gives rise to the bona fide VLDL

that apoB had reached a length of apoB-48 but was otherwise independent of the length of apoB.[23]

ApoB-48 has the advantage that it is completely dependent on oleic acid for the assembly of VLDL1 in the rat hepatoma cell line McARH7777. Thus, in the absence of oleic acid the protein assembles only the dense VLDL2 analogue, while after a short incuba-tion (15 minutes) with oleic acid the cells start to produce apoB-48 VLDL1. Stillemark et al[21] took advantage of this to demonstrate that the assembly of VLDL1 occurred outside the rough ER in a smooth membrane compartment that banded with the Golgi apparatus upon subcel-lular fractionation. Localization of the second step to the Golgi apparatus has been indicated by the work of Swift and his co-workers.[36]

Moreover, an assembly of VLDL outside the rough ER is supported by results from Fisher's group[37] showing that apoB in a non-VLDL form is present in SAR 1 COP II vesicles that bud from the ER (Figure 3). As discussed above, such vesicles are known to be involved in the exit of secretory and membrane proteins from the ER.

The second step and the formation of lipid droplets

Electron microscopy studies have indicated that a fusion between pre-VLDL and a lipid-free droplet may occur in the secretory pathway (Figure 3). The mechanism for the formation of the lipid droplet has still not been elucidated in detail. We set out to investigate this process by analysing the formation of cytosolic lipid droplets. To do this, we constructed a cell-free system[38] that assembled 100–400 nm large lipid droplets with triglycerides as major lipid and caveolin, vimentin ADRP and GRP 78 as major proteins, i.e. proteins that have been reported to be on droplets in intact cells.[39–42]

We observed that the formation of the lipid droplets is dependent on a phospholipase D (PLD) activity.[38] We also identified a cytosolic activator for the formation of lipid droplets, which also activated PLD.

The formation of the droplets was also dependent on the rate of triglyceride biosynthesis;[38] however, the rate of triglyceride biosynthesis was not influenced by the assembly of lipid droplets. Thus, the assembly of lipid droplets could be inhibited by omitting the activator (see above) without any major effect on the rate of the biosynthesis of triglycerides. Instead, the triglycerides remained with the microsomes (Marchesan et al, work in progress). These observations indicate that newly formed triglycerides can be stored in association with the ER/Golgi membrane as an alternative to being released as lipid droplets. This lends support to the model for droplet formation that has been put forward by several authors.[42–44]

A model for the formation of cytosolic lipid droplets is shown in Figure 4A. According to this model, the triglycerides that are synthesized in the cytosolic leaflet of the membrane exceed its solubility in this amphipathic structure and 'oil out' as a lens in the hydrophobic portion of the membrane. There is one important prerequisite for this to happen. The concentration of triglycerides in the leaflet must become sufficiently high. This, in turn, requires a mechanism preventing the free lateral diffusion of the triglycerides in the ER membrane. Thus, there must be local foci of triglyceride accumulation, and the molecule must be prevented from leaving these foci by lateral diffusion. In this respect, it is interesting to note that caveolin is associated with the lipid droplets and that caveolin is also found in regions of membranes with modified structure. The 'oiled out' triglycerides bud from the microsomal membrane under the influence of PLD and the formation of phosphatidic acid (Figure 4A). The role of PLD and phosphatidic acid in this process remains to be elucidated. Phosphatidic acid appears to be involved in other budding

Figure 4 *A tentative model for the assembly of cytosolic (A) and luminal (B) lipid droplets.* (1) Triglycerides are synthesized from diacylglycerol and acyl CoA at regions in the microsomal membrane which limit the lateral diffusion of the formed triglyceride. We speculate that caveolin ('V' in figure) may be involved in this limitation of lateral diffusion. Due to the restriction in lateral diffusion, the concentration of triglycerides in the luminal leaflet exceeds its solubility and they oil out as a hydrophobic phase in the fatty acid portion of the membrane, forming a 'membrane-associated droplet'. Proteins that are of importance for the direction of the budding of the droplet are recruited to these 'membrane-associated droplets'. ADRP and vimentin (cytosolic droplets; Figure 4A), and also MTP (luminal droplets; Figure 4B) are tentative candidates. The size of the 'membrane-associated droplet' increases with ongoing triglyceride biosynthesis (2) and finally phospholipase D is activated by the activator PLD Act. The formation of PA triggers budding of the droplet from the membrane to the cytosol (Figure 4A) or lumen (Figure 4B). The luminal droplet fuses with pre-VLDL to form VLDL (see also Figure 3).

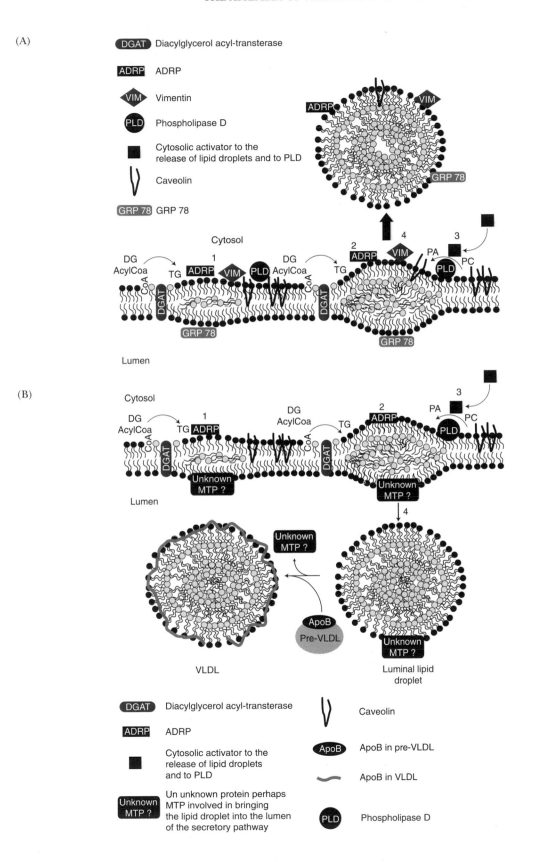

processes such as the generation of transport vesicles.[45–48] This has been questioned, however (for review, see reference 49).

More than one explanation for the role of phosphatidic acid in the budding reaction has been discussed. First, it has been proposed that the shape of the phosphatidic acid molecule could be beneficial for the bending of the membrane during the budding process (see, for example, reference 50). Second, it has been suggested that phosphatidic acid is involved in the recruitment of proteins needed for vesicular trafficking.[51] Indeed, the concept of recruitment of proteins by phosphatidic acid has been extended to other pathways that involve PLD activation.[52] It is tempting to suggest that the mechanisms discussed above are also involved in the budding of lipid droplets.

The observation that PLD is involved in the formation of lipid droplets is interesting, since we have obtained results suggesting that PLD 1 is also involved in the assembly of VLDL.[34] Since cytosolic lipid droplets have a structure very similar to that of lipoproteins (i.e. a hydrophobic core surrounded by a monolayer of amphipathic structures), it is not unlikely that the mechanism involved in the assembly of cytosolic lipid droplets is the same as that involved in the formation of lipid droplets that bud into the lumen of the secretory pathway (Figure 4B; see also references 43, 44). Indeed, the only difference may be the availability of proteins that determine to which side of the ER/Golgi membrane the droplet should bud. Another possibility is that the localization of the DGAT reaction, i.e. in the cytosolic or luminal leaflet,[53,54] is of importance for the direction of the budding.

It has been pointed out that MTP promotes the entry of triglycerides into the secretory pathway.[55,56] Thus, MTP may be a possible candidate for promoting the budding of lipid droplets into the secretory pathway. The MTP activity is required for 15–30 minutes after the translation of apoB-100 has been completed, in order for VLDL to be formed.[24] One interpretation is that the assembled pre-VLDL needs to accumulate lipid post-translationally. However, the observations would also be compatible with

a role of MTP in the second step. One prerequisite is that the second step should be rate limiting in the secretion process. This appears to be the case, since the primordial particle is produced in excess and a fusion with the lipids in the second step is a prerequisite for secretion of apoB-100 (i.e. the lipid droplets formed do not accumulate but are constantly secreted as VLDL). A role for MTP in the second step is also suggested by the observation that the protein is localized in the Golgi apparatus,[36,57,58] as well as by recent results from Björkegren and his group.[59]

The major proportion of the triglycerides found in VLDL is derived from triglycerides present in cytosolic lipid droplets. These triglycerides are hydrolysed and the fatty acids are re-esterified into new triglycerides before being incorporated into VLDL.[60–62] Interestingly, Lehner and Vance and co-workers have identified a triglyceride hydrolase[63,64] that appears to be coupled to the rate of assembly of VLDL. Thus, overexpression of the enzyme increases the assembly, while inhibition decreases it. Also, Pease and his co-workers have identified a triglyceride hydrolase that seems to influence the assembly of VLDL.[65]

The importance of small GTPases for VLDL assembly

SAR 1 appears to be the gene responsible for failure to assemble the triglyceride-rich chylomicrons in the intestine.[66] Interestingly, Fisher and his co-workers[37] demonstrated that apoB was sorted into unique SAR 1 Cop II vesicles that did not contain any other secretory proteins. Together, these results may point to the possibility that there is a unique transport system that allows apoB to leave the ER and reach the second-step compartment.

We demonstrated that ARF 1 (Figure 2) is involved in the assembly of VLDL.[34] Thus, a dominant negative mutant of ARF1 (T31N) inhibited the formation of VLDL under conditions in which the production of apoB-100 was only slightly decreased. How could ARF 1 influence the second step in the assembly? There is more than one possibility. First, ARF 1 could act as a switch to turn on enzymes of importance for the assembly process. One such enzyme that is activated by ARF 1 is PLD 1 (see above; Figure 2). Thus, one possibility is that ARF 1 influences the assembly of VLDL by activating PLD 1.[34]

Another possible role of ARF 1 in the assembly process could involve its function in sorting processes (Figure 2), processes that are essential for the integrity of organelles in the secretory pathway. Thus it is well known that the dominant negative mutant of ARF1, T31N, gives rise to disintegration of the Golgi apparatus and a redistribution of components from this organelle into the ER, ER exit sites and the cytoplasm.[67] It is therefore possible that inhibition of ARF 1 results in a loss of the compartment for the second step. Indeed recent results[68] demonstrate that the importance of ARF 1 in the assembly of VLDL 1 can be explained by the role of ARF 1 in the transport between ERGIC and cis-Golgi. Thus a decrease in the assembly coincided with a decreased transport between ERGIC and cis-Golgi. This would fit with the observation that the second step occurs in a compartment outside the rough ER[21] and that apoB in a non-VLDL form leaves the ER with COP II vesicles.[37] Thus the second step in the assembly of VLDL 1 appears to occur in the Golgi apparatus.[68]

CO- AND POST-TRANSLATIONAL DEGRADATION OF apoB-100

It has long been known that newly synthesized apoB-100 undergoes intracellular degradation (for review, see references 15, 17, 69). This is less pronounced in primary hepatocytes,[70] but is an impressive phenomenon in some hepatoma cell lines such as Hep G2 cells, where almost 80% of the newly synthesized apoB-100 can be removed by such degradation.[71] The degradation was dramatically reduced (from 80% to 20%) when oleic acid was included in the culture medium.[20,71] The intracellular degradation of apoB-100 occurs at three different levels:[72,73]

(1) Co-translationally by a mechanism that involves retraction through the translocon, ubiquitination and proteasomal degradation;[72,74–76]

(2) Post-translationally by an unknown mechanism that could be promoted by culturing the cells in the presence of polyunsaturated fatty acids.[72] This degradation seems to occur in a compartment separated from rough ER and has therefore been referred to as post-ER pre-secretory proteolysis (PERPP);[72]

(3) A reuptake from the unstirred water layer around the outside of the plasma membrane[77] via the LDL-receptor.

The LDL-receptor has been shown to have an important role in regulation of the secretion of apoB-100-containing lipoproteins.[78,79] There is even evidence that the effect of the receptor is not only due to the interaction with apoB-100 on the cell surface, but that the receptor and apoB-100 interact early in the secretory pathway and that this interaction is of importance for the post-translational degradation of apoB-100.[59,79,80]

It is well known that secretory proteins which misfold undergo proteasomal degradation (see above). Such proteins interact with chaperone proteins and are unfolded and retracted through sec 61. In the cytosol, the retracted proteins interact with cytosolic chaperones and the proteins are conjugated with ubiquitin and sorted to proteasomal degradation. In the case of apoB-100, the sorting to proteasomal degradation seems to occur co-translationally, i.e. the apoB-100 nascent chain is exposed to the cytosol, unbiquitinated and sorted to proteasomal degradation (for review, see reference 73). The co-translational degradation is influenced by the availability of lipids and the activity of MTP. Thus, when the availability of lipids or MTP activity is limiting, apoB-100 remains associated with the translocon and is sorted to proteasomal degradation.

PERPP is less well understood, thus nothing is known about the enzyme systems involved or the sorting of apoB-100 for this degradation. It appears that the process is promoted by ω-3 fatty acids. It has also been demonstrated that apoB-100 interacts with the protease/chaperone ER 60,[81,82] and that this interaction is linked to the intracellular degradation of newly synthesized apoB-100. The role of this interaction for the PERPP has not been elucidated.

Another potentially important molecule is the LDL-receptor. Thus, Attie and his co-workers have demonstrated that the LDL-receptor interacts with apoB in the secretory pathway.[79,80] In elegant studies, the ligand binding domain of the receptor was fused to a KDEL sequence that retained the construct in the ER. This construct, as well as other 'naturally occurring' mutants that retained the receptor in the ER, promoted the pre-secretory degradation of apoB-100.[80]

The apoB-100 primordial particle (pre-VLDL) is not secreted from the cell to any significant degree but appears to be retained and degraded. On the contrary, the dense apoB-48 particle is secreted from the cell as a lipoprotein within the HDL density region. The retention started when apoB reached a size between 70 and 80% of the size of apoB-100 (i.e. between apoB-70 and apoB-80).[23] This is the region of the molecule that contains the LDL-receptor binding site. However, the LDL-receptor was not involved in the retention of apoB-100 pre-VLDL. The retention of the pre-VLDL particle coincided with the binding of BiP (binding proteins) and PDI (protein disulphide isomerase) to the particle. One possibility is that the C-terminus of apoB-100 misfolds on the pre-VLDL, which leads to interaction with BiP and retention in the ER.[23]

The pre-secretory degradation of apoB-100 pre-VLDL points to the existence of a degradational pathway that can cope with both proteins and lipids. One candidate is the lysosomes, and it has been shown that lysosomal inhibitors prevent the intracellular degradation of newly formed apoB-100.[83]

In summary, there are several levels in the secretory pathway where apoB-100 and apoB-100 pre-VLDL are sorted to degradation. This degradation is important for the secretion of VLDL, but it is not yet clear whether the degradation per se is regulated or if it is a result of failure in the assembly process.

THE EFFECT OF PEROXISOME PROLIFERATOR ACTIVATED RECEPTOR ALPHA AGONIST ON THE ASSEMBLY OF VLDL: A SURPRISING MECHANISM LEADING TO SMALL VLDL

Several clinical studies have demonstrated that fibrates (i.e. proliferator activated receptor α (PPAR-α) agonists) give rise to a decrease in both the amount of large VLDL (VLDL1) and in the amount of small dense LDL (for a recent review, see reference 84). Part of the mechanism was revealed by investigating the role of PPAR-α agonists in primary rat hepatocytes.[70] The studies revealed that the agonists actually increase biosynthesis and secretion of apoB-100, while no changes were seen in the biosynthesis and secretion of apoB-48 or albumin. The mechanism behind the increased production of apoB-100 was an inhibition of the co-translational degradation. This decrease in the co-translational degradation could not be due to changes in lipid metabolism, since the agonists decreased the triglyceride biosynthesis. Instead it was due to an increase in the amount of MTP due to an increased transcription of the gene.[85]

The increased production of apoB-100 is coupled to a decreased rate of triglyceride biosynthesis induced by the PPAR-α agonist.[70] Thus, the secreted apoB-100-containing lipoproteins become smaller, and therefore have the capacity to be converted to large LDL with a much shorter residence time than small dense LDL (for reviews, see references 84, 86–88). Thus, treatment with PPAR-α agonists will lead to decreased levels of plasma apoB-100, in spite of the increased production of apoB-100. This process is accentuated by the decrease in apoC-III induced by the agonists (for reviews, see references 84, 89).

DRUG TARGETS IN VLDL ASSEMBLY

When identifying targets for drug therapy in the VLDL assembly pathway, it should be kept in mind that the assembly of VLDL is linked to the removal of triglycerides from the liver. Thus, interference may result in steatosis unless the triglyceride biosynthesis is decreased and/or the oxidation of fatty acids is increased. One example of complications due to the violation of this basic principle comes from the treatment with MTP inhibitors. Obviously, MTP is a prime drug target in the assembly process. Inhibition of MTP increases the removal of nascent apoB-100, thereby decreasing the assembly of VLDL. Moreover, it is possible that inhibition of MTP prevents the entry of lipid droplets into the secretory pathway, thereby inhibiting the second step. However, MTP inhibitors do not interfere with triglyceride biosynthesis and fatty acid oxidation and therefore the accumulation of triglycerides in the liver cell increases, leading to steatosis. This is one of the reasons why no MTP inhibitor has appeared on the market.

A more appealing strategy would be to manipulate the structure of VLDL, allowing the removal of triglycerides from the cells by small VLDLs. Such VLDLs have a more rapid turnover in plasma and give rise to large LDLs with short residence time in plasma. Thus, provided that the LDL-receptor is intact, the change from large to small VLDL decreases plasma apoB-100 and both triglycerides and LDL cholesterol. To achieve this, PPAR-α appears to be an important target (see discussion above). PPAR-α also has the advantage that it inhibits triglyceride biosynthesis and increases the β-oxidation of fatty acids.

The second step in the assembly of VLDL is an interesting target, since prevention of the lipidation of apoB-100 pre-VLDL leads to a complete retention and intracellular degradation of this primordial particle. However, steatosis is once again a threat. Moreover, a great deal of basic information will be needed before a rational approach to identifying specific drug targets can be taken. Neither Sar 1 nor ARF 1 appear to be useful targets for therapy, since both are switches in essential processes in the cell. An exception may be if a GEP or GAP that is specific for the apoB-100 related function of ARF1 or Sar 1 can be identified. Such a GEP/GAP may be a potential drug target. Also, the COP proteins and PLD carry out essential functions in the cell and are therefore unlikely drug targets for VLDL assembly. An interesting target would be the activator for the release of lipid droplets to the cytosol (and PLD) which we have identified. Inhibitors of this activator have the potential to inhibit not only the formation of cytosolic lipid droplets, but also the second step in the VLDL assembly. However, it is of course essential to first clarify the relationship between the budding of lipid droplets to the cytosol and to the lumen of the ER, and the importance of these processes for the second step. Moreover, the activator must be identified and its role in metabolism and other functions in the cell still has to be elucidated. Finally, we require more information about the fate of triglycerides and fatty acids under conditions in which lipid droplets are not formed. Interesting targets that should be explored are enzymes in triglyceride biosynthesis (such as glycerol-3-phosphate acyl-transferase (GPAT) and diacylglycerol acyltransferase (DGAT)).

In summary, we believe that PPAR-α is a well-established, but still promising drug target in the short term. In the longer term, interference with the second step in VLDL assembly should be explored.

ACKNOWLEDGEMENTS

This study was supported by grant No 7142 from the Swedish Medical Research Council and by the Swedish Heart and Lung Foundation, Novo Nordic Foundation, the Söderberg Foundation and the Swedish Strategic Funds (National Network and Graduate School for Cardiovascular Research).

References

1. Johnson AE, van Waes MA. The translocon: a dynamic gateway at the ER membrane. Annu Rev Cell Dev Biol 1999; 15:799–842

2. Johnson AE, Haigh NG. The ER translocon and retro-translocation: is the shift into reverse manual or automatic? Cell 2000; 102:709–12

3. Ellgaard L, Molinari M, Helenius A. Setting the standards: quality control in the secretory pathway. Science 1999; 286:1882–8

4. Lippincott-Schwartz J, Roberts TH, Hirschberg K. Secretory protein trafficking and organelle dynamics in living cells. Annu Rev Cell Dev Biol 2000; 16:557–89

5. Ellgaard L, Helenius A. ER quality control: towards an understanding at the molecular level. Curr Opin Cell Biol 2001; 13:431–7

6. Ellgaard L, Helenius A. Quality control in the endoplasmic reticulum. Nat Rev Mol Cell Biol 2003; 4:181–91

7. Kostova Z, Wolf DH. For whom the bell tolls: protein quality control of the endoplasmic reticulum and the ubiquitin-proteasome connection. Embo J 2003; 22:2309–17

8. Barlowe C. Traffic COPs of the early secretory pathway. Traffic 2000; 1:371–7

9. Spang A. ARF1 regulatory factors and COPI vesicle formation. Curr Opin Cell Biol 2002; 14:423–7

10. Bonifacino JS, Lippincott-Schwartz J. Coat proteins: shaping membrane transport. Nat Rev Mol Cell Biol 2003; 4:409–14

11. Haucke V. Vesicle budding: a coat for the COPs. Trends Cell Biol 2003; 13:59–60

12. Goldberg J. Structural basis for activation of ARF GTPase: mechanisms of guanine nucleotide exchange and GTP-myristoyl switching. Cell 1998; 95:237–48

13. Gorelick FS, Shugrue C. Exiting the endoplasmic reticulum. Mol Cell Endocrinol 2001; 177:13–8

14. Storrie B, Nilsson T. The Golgi apparatus: balancing new with old. Traffic 2002; 3:521–9

15. Olofsson S-O, Asp L, Borén J. The assembly and secretion of apolipoprotein B-containing lipoproteins. Curr Opin Lipidol 1999; 10:341–6

16. Olofsson S-O, Stillemark-Billton P, Asp L. The intracellular assembly of VLDL – a process that consists of two major steps that occur in separate cell compartments. Trends Cardiovasc Med 2000; 10:338–45

17. Shelness GS, Sellers JA. Very-low-density lipoprotein assembly and secretion. Curr Opin Lipidol 2001; 12:151–7

18. Borén J, Graham L, Wettesten M, et al. The assembly and secretion of apoB 100-containing lipoproteins in Hep G2 cells. ApoB 100 is cotranslationally integrated into lipoproteins. J Biol Chem 1992; 267:9858–67

19. Boström K, Borén J, Wettesten M, et al. Studies on the assembly of apo B-100-containing lipoproteins in HepG2 cells. J Biol Chem 1988; 263:4434–42

20. Borén J, Rustaeus S, Wettesten M, et al. Influence of triacylglycerol biosynthesis rate on the assembly of apoB-100-containing lipoproteins in Hep G2 cells. Arterioscler Thromb 1993; 13:1743–54

21. Stillemark P, Borén J, Andersson M, et al. The assembly and secretion of apolipoprotein-B48-containing very low density lipoproteins in McA-RH7777 cells. J Biol Chem 2000; 275:10506–13

22. Borén J, Rustaeus S, Olofsson S-O. Studies on the assembly of apolipoprotein B-100- and B-48-containing very low density lipoproteins in McA-RH7777 cells. J Biol Chem 1994; 269:25879–88

23. Stillemark-Billton P, Beck C, Boren J, et al. Relation of the size and intracellular sorting of apoB to the formation of VLDL 1 and VLDL 2. J Lipid Res 2005; 46:104–14

24. Rustaeus S, Stillemark P, Lindberg K, et al. The microsomal triglyceride transfer protein catalyzes the post-translational assembly of apolipoprotein B-100 very low density lipoprotein in McA-RH7777 cells. J Biol Chem 1998; 273:5196–203

25. Gordon DA, Jamil H. Progress towards understanding the role of microsomal triglyceride transfer protein in apolipoprotein-B lipoprotein assembly. Biochim Biophys Acta 2000; 1486:72–83

26. Hussain MM, Shi J, Dreizen P. Microsomal triglyceride transfer protein and its role in apoB-lipoprotein assembly. J Lipid Res 2003; 44:22–32

27. Wetterau JR, Aggerbeck LP, Bouma M-E, et al. Abscence of microsomal triglyceride transfer protein in indivals with abetalipoproteinemia. Nature 1992; 258:999–1001

28. Gregg RE, Wetterau JR. The molecular basis of abetalipoproteinemia. Curr Opin Lipidol 1994; 5:81–6

29. Read J, Anderson TA, Ritchie PJ, et al. A mechanism of membrane neutral lipid acquisition by the microsomal triglyceride transfer protein. J Biol Chem 2000; 275:30372–7

30. Segrest JP, Jones MK, Dashti N. N-terminal domain of apolipoproteinsB has structural homology to lipovitellin and microsomal triglyceride transfer protein: a 'lipid pocket' model for self-assembly of apoB-containing lipoprotein particles. J Lipid Res 1999; 40:1401–16

31. Dashti N, Gandhi M, Liu X, et al. The N-terminal 1000 residues of apolipoprotein B associate with microsomal triglyceride transfer protein to create a lipid transfer pocket required for lipoprotein assembly. Biochemistry 2002; 41:6978–87

32. Segrest JP, Jones MK, De Loof H, et al. Structure of apolipoprotein B-100 in low density lipoproteins. J Lipid Res 2001; 42:1346–67

33. Alexander CA, Hamilton RL, Havel RJ. Subcellular

THE ASSEMBLY OF VERY LOW DENSITY LIPOPROTEINS IN THE LIVER 13

localization of B apoprotein of plasma lipoproteins in rat liver. J Cell Biol 1976; 69:241–63

34. Asp L, Claesson C, Borén J, et al. ADP-ribosylation factor 1 and its activation of phospholipase D are important for the assembly of very low density lipoproteins. J Biol Chem 2000; 275:26285–92

35. Adiels M, Packard CJ, Caslake MJ, et al. A new combined multicompartmental model for apolipoprotein B100 and triglyceride metabolism in VLDL subfractions. Lipid Res 2005; 46:58–67

36. Valyi-Nagy K, Harris C, Swift LL. The assembly of hepatic very low density lipoproteins: evidence of a role for the Golgi apparatus. Lipids 2002; 37: 879–84

37. Gusarova V, Brodsky JL, Fisher EA. Apolipoprotein B100 exit from the ER is COPII dependent and its lipidation to very low density lipoprotein occurs post-ER. J Biol Chem 2003; 278:48051–8

38. Marchesan D, Rutberg M, Andersson L, et al. A phospholipase D-dependent process forms lipid droplets containing caveolin, adipocyte differentia-tion-related protein, and vimentin in a cell-free system. J Biol Chem 2003; 278:27293–300

39. Franke WW, Hergt M, Grund C. Rearragement of vimentin cytoskeleton durin adipose conversion: formation of an intermediate filament cage around lipid globules. Cell 1987; 49:131–41

40. Londos C, Brasaemle DL, Schultz CJ, et al. Perilipins, ADRP, and other proteins that associate with intracel-lular neutral lipid droplets in animal cells. Semin Cell Dev Biol 1999; 10:51–8

41. Prattes S, Horl G, Hammer A, et al. Intracellular distribution and mobilization of unesterified choles-terol in adipocytes: triglyceride droplets are surrounded by cholesterol-rich ER-like surface layer structures. J Cell Sci 2000; 113 (Pt 17):2977–89

42. Brown DA. Lipid droplets: Proteins floating on a pool of fat. Curr Biol 2001; 11:R446–9

43. Olofsson S-O, Bjursell G, Boström K, et al. Apolipoprotein B: structure, biosynthesis and role in the lipoprotein assembly process. Atherosclerosis 1987; 68:1–17

44. Murphy DJ, Vance J. Mechanisms of lipid-body forma-tion. Trends Biochem Sci 1999; 24:109–15

45. Bi K, Roth MG, Ktistakis T. Phosphatidic acid forma-tion by phospholipase D is required for transport from the endoplasmic reticulum to the Golgi complex. Curr Biol 1997; 7:301–7

46. Humeau Y, Vitale N, Chasserot-Golaz S, et al. A role for phospholipase D1 in neurotransmitter release. Proc Natl Acad Sci USA 2001; 98:15300–5

47. Vitale N, Caumont AS, Chasserot-Golaz S, et al. Phospholipase D1: a key factor for the exocytotic machinery in neuroendocrine cells. Embo J 2001; 20:2424–34

48. Pathre P, Shome K, Blumental-Perry A, et al. Activation of phospholipase D by the small GTPase Sar1p is required to support COPII assembly and ER export. Embo J 2003; 22:4059–69

49. Jones D, Morgan C, Cockcroft S. Phospholipase D and membrane traffic. Potential roles in regulated exocytosis, membrane delivery and vesicle budding. Biochim Biophys Acta 1999; 1439:229–44

50. Kooijman EE, Chupin V, de Kruijff B, et al. Modulation of membrane curvature by phosphatidic acid and lysophosphatidic acid. Traffic 2003; 4:162–74

51. Manifava M, Thuring JW, Lim ZY, et al. Differential binding of traffic-related proteins to phosphatidic acid- or phosphatidylinositol (4,5)- bisphosphate-coupled affinity reagents. J Biol Chem 2001; 276:8987–94

52. Ktistakis NT, Delon C, Manifava M, et al. Phospholipase D1 and potential targets of its hydroly-sis product, phosphatidic acid. Biochem Soc Trans 2003; 31:94–7

53. Owen MR, Corstorphine CC, Zammit VA. Overt and latant activities of diacylglycerol acyltransfrase in rat liver microsomes: possible roles in very-low density lipoprotein triglycerol secretion. Biochem J 1997; 323:17–21

54. Owen M, Zammit VA. Evidence for overt and latent forms of DGAT in rat liver microsomes. Implications for the pathways of triacylglycerol incorporation into VLDL. Biochem Soc Trans 1997; 25:21S

55. Raabe M, Véniant MM, Sullivan MA, et al. Analysing the role of microsomal triglyceride transfer protein in the liver with tissue-specific knockout mice. J Clin Invest 1999; 103:1287–98

56. Wang Y, Tran K, Yao Z. The activity of microsomal triglyceride transfer protein is essential for accumula-tion of triglyceride within microsomes in McA-RH7777 cells. A unified model for the assembly of very low density lipoproteins. J Biol Chem 1999; 274:27793–800

57. Levy E, Stan S, Delvin E, et al. Localization of micro-somal triglyceride transfer protein in the Golgi: possi-ble role in the assembly of chylomicrons. J Biol Chem 2002; 277:16470–7

58. Swift LL, Zhu MY, Kakkad B, et al. Subcellular local-ization of microsomal triglyceride transfer protein. J Lipid Res 2003; 44:1841–9

59. Larsson SL, Skogsberg J, Bjorkegren J. The low density lipoprotein receptor prevents secretion of dense apoB100–containing lipoproteins from the liver. J Biol Chem 2003; 279:831–6

60. Wiggins D, Gibbons GF. The lipolysis/esterification cycle of hepatic triacylglyecrol. Its role in the secre-tion of very-low-density lipoprotein and its response to hormones and sulphonylureas. Biochem J 1992; 284:457–62

61. Salter AM, Wiggins D, Sessions VA, et al. The intra-cellular triacylglycerol/fatty acid cycle: a comparison of its activity in hepatocytes which secrete exclusively apolipoprotein (apo) B100 very-low-density lipopro-tein (VLDL) and in those which secrete predomi-nantly apoB48 VLDL. Biochem J 1998; 332 (Pt 3): 667–72

62. Gibbons GF, Islam K, Pease RJ. Mobilisation of triacyl-glycerol stores. Biochim Biophys Acta 2000; 1483:37–57

63. Lehner R, Vance DE. Cloning and expression of a cDNA encoding a hepatic microsomal lipase that mobilizes stored triacylglycerol. Biochem J 1999; 343 (Pt 1):1–10

64. Gilham D, Ho S, Rasouli M, et al. Inhibitors of hepatic microsomal triacylglycerol hydrolase decrease very low density lipoprotein secretion. Faseb J 2003; 17:1685–7

65. Trickett JI, Patel DD, Knight BL, et al. Characterization of the rodent genes for arylac-etamide deacetylase, a putative microsomal lipase, and evidence for transcriptional regulation. J Biol Chem 2001; 276:39522–32

66. Jones B, Jones EL, Bonney SA, et al. Mutations in a Sar1 GTPase of COPII vesicles are associated with lipid absorption disorders. Nat Genet 2003; 34:29–31

67. Ward TH, Polishchuk RS, Caplan S, et al. Maintenance of Golgi structure and function depends on the integrity of ER export. J Cell Biol 2001; 155:557–70

68. Asp L, Magnusson B, Rutberg M, et al. Role of ADP ribosylation factor 1 in the assembly and secretion of ApoB-100-containing lipoproteins. Arterioscler Thromb Vasc Biol 2005; 25:566–70

69. Davidson NO, Shelness GS. Apolipoprotein B: mRNA editing, lipoprotein assembly, and presecretory degra-dation. Ann Rev Nutr 2000; 20:169–93

70. Lindén D, Lindberg K, Oscarsson J, et al. Influence of agonists to the peroxisome proliferator activated receptor a (PPARa) on the intracellular turnover and secretion of apoB-100 and apoB-48. J Biol Chem 2002; 277:23044–53

71. Boström K, Wettesten M, Borén J, et al. Pulse-chase studies of the synthesis and intracellular transport of apolipoprotein B-100 in Hep G2 cells. J Biol Chem 1986; 261:13800–6

72. Fisher EA, Pan M, Chen X, et al. The triple threat to nascent apolipoprotein B. Evidence for multiple, distinct degradative pathways. J Biol Chem 2001; 276:27855–63

73. Fisher EA, Ginsberg HN. Complexity in the secretory pathway: the assembly and secretion of apolipopro-tein B-containing lipoproteins. J Biol Chem 2002; 277:17377–80

74. Mitchell DM, Zhou M, Pariyarath R, et al. Apoprotein B 100 has a prolonged interaction with the translocon during which its lipidation and translocation change from dependence on the microsomal triglyceride transfer protein to independence. Proc Natl Acad Sci USA 1998; 95:14733–8

75. Liang J-S, Wu X, Fisher EA, et al. The amino-terminal domain of apolipoprotein B does not undergo retro-grade translocation from the endoplasmic reticulum to the cytosol. Proteasomal degradation of nascent apolipoprotein B begins at the carboxyl terminus of the protein, while apolipoprotein B is still in its

76. Pariyarath R, Wang H, Aitchison JD, et al. Co-transla-tional interactions of apoprotein B with the ribosome and translocon during lipoprotein assembly or targeting to the proteasome. J Biol Chem 2001; 276:541–50

77. Williams KJ, Brocia RW, Fisher EA. The unstirred water layer as a site of control of apolipoprotein B secretion. J Biol Chem 1990; 265:16741–4

78. Horton JD, Shimano H, Hamilton RL, et al. Disruption of LDL receptor gene in transgenic SREBP-1a mice unmask hyperlipidemia resulting from production of lipid-rich VLDL. J Clin Invest 1999; 103:1067–76

79. Twisk J, Gillian-Daniel DL, Tebon A, et al. The role of the LDL receptor in apolipoprotein B secretion. J Clin Invest 2000; 105:521–32

80. Gillian-Daniel DL, Bates PW, Tebon A, et al. Endoplasmic reticulum localization of the low density lipoprotein receptor mediates presecretory degrada-tion of apolipoprotein B. Proc Natl Acad Sci USA 2002; 99:4337–42

81. Adeli K, Macri J, Mohammadi A, et al. Apolipoprotein B is intracellularly associated with an ER-60 protease homologue in HepG2 cells. J Biol Chem 1997; 272:22489–94

82. Taghibiglou C, Rashid-Kolvear F, Van Iderstine SC, et al. Hepatic very low density lipoprotein-ApoB overpro-duction is associated with attenuated hepatic insulin signaling and overexpression of protein-tyrosine phosphatase 1B in a fructose-fed hamster model of insulin resistance. J Biol Chem 2002; 277:793–803

83. Fleming JF, Spitsen GM, Hui TY, et al. Chinese hamster ovary cells require the coexpression of micro-somal triglyceride transfer protein and cholesterol 7alfa hydroxylase for the assembly and secretion of apolipoprotein B-containing lipoproteins. J Biol Chem. 1999; 274:9509–14

84. Packard CJ. Triacylglycerol-rich lipoproteins and the generation of small, dense low-density lipoprotein. Biochem Soc Trans 2003; 31:1066–9

85. Kang S, Spann NJ, Hui TY, et al. ARP-1/COUP-TF II determines hepatoma phenotype by acting as both a transcriptional repressor of microsomal triglyceride transfer protein and an inducer of CYP7A1. J Biol Chem 2003; 278:30478–86

86. Berneis KK, Krauss RM. Metabolic origins and clinical significance of LDL heterogeneity. J Lipid Res 2002; 43:1363–79

87. Kwiterovich PO, Jr. Clinical relevance of the biochem-ical, metabolic, and genetic factors that influence low-density lipoprotein heterogeneity. Am J Cardiol 2002; 90:30i–47i

88. Taskinen MR. Diabetic dyslipidemia. Atheroscler Suppl 2002; 3:47–51

89. Staels B, Dallongeville J, Auwerx J, et al. Mechanism of action of fibrates on lipid and lipoprotein metabo-lism. Circulation 1998; 98:2088–93

Cardiovascular implications of partial, tissue-specific silencing of MTP

2

C.C. Shoulders

BACKGROUND

Dietary fat provides a major source of nutrition, but may in excess lead to obesity, insulin resistance, high blood lipid levels and atherosclerosis. In this chapter, I review the role of the microsomal triglyceride transfer protein (MTP) in co-ordinating whole-body lipid homeostasis, and address the prospects for reducing blood lipid levels through a tissue-specific approach that reduces MTP mass. The reason for this focus is because the past 5 years have seen remarkable progress in our understanding of the function of MTP, and of its partner protein disulphide isomerase (PDI), in the assembly of chylomicrons (Cms) in the small intestine, very low density lipoproteins (VLDLs) in the liver, and of low density lipoprotein (LDL)-like particles in cardiac myocytes. The reader is referred to Chapters 1 and 5 of this book, and other excellent reviews[1-8] for further information on apolipoprotein (apo)B, the obligatory protein component of Cm, VLDL and LDL (Figure 1).

In humans, serum cholesterol and triglyceride levels are primarily determined by a series of metabolic pathways, ligands and receptors that operate in the small intestine, liver, adipose tissue, skeletal muscle and cardiac myocytes (Figure 1). Dietary lipids initially enter the circulation in Cms, where they may provide peripheral tissues, including the heart, with an important source of energy through the β-oxidation of fatty acids. In the post-prandial period, a proportion of these dietary lipids re-enter the circulation for redistribution in VLDL particles,[9,10] which are assembled in the liver (Figure 1). VLDL also transports non-dietary lipids formed from the catabolism of dietary carbohydrate, the recycling of cellular membranes and the esterification of free fatty acids, which may derive from adipose tissue.[11-13] Similarly, the heart secretes LDL-sized lipoproteins[14,15] to remove excess lipids from this organ, which might otherwise adversely affect contractility and conductivity.[16-19]

Recognition that MTP represents a molecular target for lowering blood lipid levels arose from the discovery that this protein promotes the assembly of apoB-containing lipoproteins,[20-22] and that mutations of *MTP* are the major, if not sole, cause of abetalipoproteinaemia.[23-28] Abetalipoproteinaemia typically presents in infancy with failure to thrive due to severe fat malabsorption or, in older children, with an atypical pigmented retinopathy associated with spinocerebellar degeneration.[29] The condition is biochemically characterized by a virtual absence of apoB-containing lipoproteins in blood and deficiencies of the fat-soluble vitamins A, K and E. Once absorbed from the intestine, these vitamins are normally transported to the liver via a Cm pathway. From the liver, vitamin E is secreted on VLDL,[30,31] whereas vitamins A and K have the capacity to use different transport systems.[32,33] In the absence of treatment, patients with abetalipoproteinaemia develop a range of debilitating clinical symptoms (e.g. severe generalized

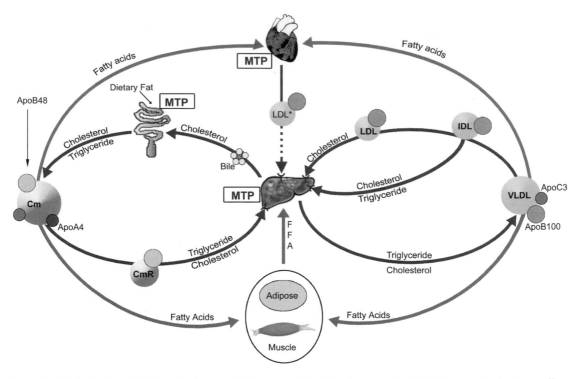

Figure 1 Cholesterol and triglyceride transport in humans, viewed in the context of MTP expression in the small intestine, liver and heart. For simplicity the transport of lipids other than cholesterol and triglyceride is not shown. CmR, chylomicron remnant particle; FFA, non-esterified fatty acids; MTP, microsomal triglyceride transfer protein. Adapted from Shoulders et al.[7]

weakness, kyphoscoliosis and lordosis), but it remains unclear whether these derive exclusively from a dependency on MTP function in affected tissues or whether they are solely due to deficiencies of fat-soluble vitamins, or a combination of both. In some patients, high doses of the fat-soluble vitamins ameliorate the neurological and ophthamological manifestations of the condition.[29,30,34–36]

THE CASE FOR PARTIAL, TISSUE-SPECIFIC SILENCING OF MTP

All of the MTP inhibitors that have been studied to date are conceptually the same: they target MTP protein, and possibly apoB, to lower the production of potentially atherogenic lipoproteins, and most probably LDL-sized lipoproteins from the heart. However, it is still not known whether long-term treatment of hyperlipidaemia with MTP inhibitors will unmask adverse side-effects related to the totality of MTP function. Such effects could include the development of pathologies in the kidney, testis, ovary and pancreas, organs in which *MTP* mRNA is present at significant levels, and therefore presumably contributing to normal function in, as yet, unknown ways.[16,24,37] *A priori*, the nature and severity of side-effects resulting from MTP inhibition may well depend on the particular class of inhibitor deployed, as each is likely to affect a different aspect of MTP functionality by virtue of binding to different sites on the MTP–PDI heterodimer. Evidence for this has already emerged from two studies.[38,39] In the first, Bakillah et al described a small (602 Da) organic molecule that blocked the secretion of apoB-containing lipoproteins from HepG2 cells, despite having no effect on MTP-mediated lipid transfer activity *in vitro*.[38]

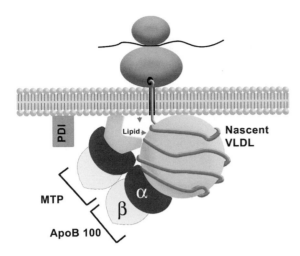

Figure 2 Model representing the Co-translational loading of ApoB with lipid. The extreme amino-terminal of apoB interacts with the amino-terminal β-barrel of MTP. This serves to align the predicted α-helical domain of apoB with the homologous domain in MTP. The figure indicates that the interaction of apoB with MTP perturbs MTP and PDI binding. Arrows indicate the transfer of lipid from their sites of synthesis in the membrane of endoplasmic reticulum to MTP and apoB, and from MTP to apoB during the initial stages of the VLDL–apoB assembly process

Instead, the inhibitor profoundly interfered with the interaction of MTP with apoB (Figure 2), and presumably subsequent loading of apoB with lipid.[22,38,40–42] In future studies, it might prove instructive to establish whether the Bakillah inhibitor actually binds to apoB, MTP or the MTP–PDI complex. In the second inhibitor study, Sellers et al compared the impact of two MTP inhibitors, BMS-200150 and BMS-197636 (Figure 3), on the secretion of apoB41-containing lipoproteins from a heterologous cell system expressing either human or Drosophila MTP.[39] MTP inhibitor BMS-200150 decreased apoB41 lipoprotein secretion from both cell systems, whereas the second (BMS-197636), and more potent, MTP inhibitor only blocked the secretion of apoB41 lipoproteins from cells expressing human MTP. Even at concentrations that were 100-fold higher than that used to inhibit human

Figure 3 Chemical structures of representative MTP inhibitors. Compounds inhibit: (1) the secretion of apoB, but not apoA1, from HepG2 cells and (2) MTP-mediated transfer of radiolabelled triolein from phospholipid donor liposomes to acceptor liposomes

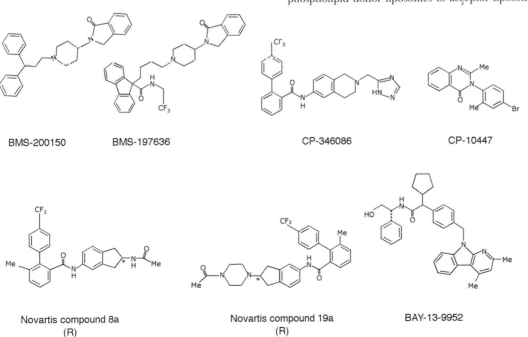

MTP, the BMS-197636 inhibitor had no impact on the secretion of apoB41-lipoproteins from cells expressing Drosophila MTP.

The totality of MTP–PDI function may rely on different lipid transport roles, but this has yet to be elucidated. The MTP–PDI heterodimer *in vitro*, has a capacity to transport a range of lipids such as triglyceride, cholesteryl ester, phosphatidylcholine and phosphatidylethanolamine,[43] all of which are needed for the production of VLDL and Cm.[1,44,45] The MTP–PDI heterodimer also has the ability to transfer diacylglycerol, lysophosphatidic acid, phosphatidic acid, squalene and phosphatidylinositol between membranes *in vitro*, but the physiological significance of this is uncertain. Read et al[46] have considered how MTP might capture triglyceride monomers from lipid membranes, the rate-limiting step of the lipid transfer process.[43,47,48] The data suggest that MTP has a fusogenic helix at the mouth of its predicted lipid-binding cavity, which interacts with a lipid membrane to perturb the arrangement of the acyl chains of phospholipid molecules. This event is envisaged to expose the acyl chains of neutral lipid and phospholipid monomers for interaction with a second helix, which acts in concert with the fusogenic helix, to ensure transfer of lipid moieties to the hydrophobic lipid-binding cavity of MTP, apoB or an acceptor membrane. Atzel and Wetterau have further suggested that MTP contains two different classes of lipid-binding sites.[49] The first is proposed to rapidly transport neutral lipid and phospholipid between membranes, while the second appears to selectively support the slow transport of phospholipid.

The structures of the MTP–PDI complex and apoB are unknown, which leaves unresolved a number of important questions regarding the mechanism of action of inhibitor compounds, such as BMS-197636 and BMS-200150 (Figure 3). From modelled structures and biochemical analyses it appears that MTP comprises three domains: an amino terminal β-barrel (amino acids 18–297), a central α-helical domain (amino acids 300–600) and a lipid-binding cavity (amino acids 601–894) that may bind up to five molecules of lipid.[48,50–52] Moreover, it appears that the major binding site on MTP for PDI is formed by a series of residues residing on the outer surface of helices 13–17 of the large central α-helical domain of MTP (Figure 2). To initiate the lipoprotein assembly process, MTP interacts with apoB through two binding sites (amino acids 22–303 and 517–603), the second of which resides close to the MTP–PDI interface.[42,50–52] The proximity of a binding site(s) on MTP for apoB and PDI suggests that apoB might displace PDI from MTP during the lipoprotein assembly process (Figure 2), only to be replaced again by PDI once the newly assembled apoB lipoprotein dissociates from MTP to exit the ER by a COPII (COat Protein)-dependent mechanism.[53,54] Indirect evidence for this mechanism may derive from a more in-depth analysis of the non-synonymous, non-truncating APOB mutation (i.e. R463W) found in an extended Christian Lebanese family with the co-dominant disorder, hypobetalipoproteinaemia.[55] *In vitro* APOB R463W interacted with MTP, but failed to support the subsequent production of apoB-containing lipoproteins. Moreover, expression of APOB R463W in a stable cell line markedly reduced the secretion of endogenous rat apoB100, leading the authors to speculate that the dominant-negative effect of APOB R463W expression on endogenous apoB secretion might be attributable to enhanced binding of the mutant APOB R463W protein to MTP.

Although inhibitors of MTP action have already produced promising reductions in blood lipid levels in phase I/II clinical trials, there is a real concern that blockage of intestinal fat absorption and hepatic lipid secretion could compromise their long-term usage in some cases, as discussed in the excellent review of Harwood and colleagues.[56] In the past year somewhat encouraging results have emerged for the MTP inhibitor CP-346086, which may be attributable to special properties of the drug itself (Figure 3), a novel dosing regime or a combination of both.[57] Eight healthy men receiving a nightly dose of the drug for 14 days experienced only occasional gastrointestinal symptoms, such as mild diarrhoea and flatulence, and these were self-limiting.[57] Moreover, magnetic resonance imaging of the liver at the end of the course provided no evidence of fatty infiltration. In these subjects, total cholesterol, LDL-cholesterol and apoB levels dropped steadily for 13, 13 and 8 days, respectively. Compared to pre-dose levels, plateau values were reduced by 47%, 68% and 52%. Importantly, high density lipoprotein (HDL) cholesterol levels remained within 10% of pre-dosing values at all time points. Serum triglyceride levels also fell by up to 75%, in a time-dependent manner. The maximum drop was observed 4 to 8 hours after drug administration, with serum triglyceride levels returning to baseline just prior to the next treatment. Although study participants had unchanged serum levels of vitamin A, vitamin E levels were lower by 43 ± 10% at the end of the study.

Therapeutic strategies that specifically reduce *MTP* expression in the small intestine and liver would be expected to markedly reduce the production of Cm and VLDL, without compromising the essential lipid transport function(s) of MTP in the heart.[14–19,58] As such, a tissue-specific approach promises to provide an efficacious therapeutic strategy to prevent the development of atherosclerotic cardiovascular disease attributable to increased production of Cm remnant particles, and of LDL, the main cholesterol-carrying particle in blood.[59,60] In principle, the numerically important treatment groups would include patients with prolonged and exaggerated post-prandial hyperlipidaemia,[59–64] combined hyperlipidaemia (i.e. raised serum levels of both cholesterol and triglyceride)[65–70] and the metabolic syndrome.[7,71–74] By analogy with mice, a therapeutic procedure that effectively inactivated one *MTP* allele would be expected to reduce total serum cholesterol, intermediate density lipoproteins/LDL-cholesterol and apoB100 levels.[75] For example, in mice, a 50% reduction in intestinal and hepatic *MTP* mRNA levels lowers serum cholesterol levels by around 24%.[37] This may also be the case in the heterozygote parents and siblings of patients with abetalipoproteinaemia,[25] but this has been difficult to establish definitively because of the wide range of cholesterol levels in the general population. Notwithstanding, a 24% drop in serum cholesterol levels would be expected to translate into a massive reduction in the incidence of cardiovascular disease, which is on track to become the world's most common cause of disease-related disability and death by the year 2020.[76,77]

INSIGHTS INTO THE REGULATION OF INTESTINAL MTP FROM MODEL SYSTEMS

Indirect evidence suggests that the specific inhibition of intestinal *MTP* gene expression might provide a therapeutic means for lowering blood lipid levels. An early study showed that the hamster duodenum–jejunum contained 2.5-fold higher levels of *MTP* mRNA levels than the ileum, and that in these tissues there was a monotonic relationship between *MTP* mRNA and protein levels.[78] As importantly, the study also demonstrated that a high-fat diet comprising 20% w/w hydrogenated coconut oil increased *MTP* mRNA levels by ~3-fold in the duodenum–jejunum preparations compared to ~1.5-fold in the ileum. In these animals, intestinal *MTP* mRNA levels were strongly correlated with serum levels of total cholesterol, non-HDL-cholesterol and triglyceride.

Other workers have also reported strong correlations between intestinal *MTP* mRNA levels and serum lipids in diabetic and insulin-resistant animal models,[79–81] suggesting that increased intestinal *MTP* mRNA levels in humans might causally contribute to the dyslipidaemia of the metabolic syndrome. In one streptozotocin-induced rat model of diabetes, for example, intestine preparations contained 4-fold higher levels of *MTP* mRNA than samples from non-induced animals.[79] There was a strong correlation between *MTP* mRNA levels and lymph Cm-triglyceride, and a moderate correlation with lymph Cm-cholesterol. In an alloxan monohydrate-induced rabbit model of diabetes, intestines contained 3- and 6-fold increased levels of *MTP* mRNA and MTP-mediated lipid transfer activity, respectively.[82]

Combining the diabetic and control groups, there was a positive correlation between intestinal *MTP* mRNA and both lymph apoB48- and B100-containing Cm. In the insulin-resistant Zucker rat model of obesity, intestinal *MTP* mRNA levels were also increased by ~4-fold, and the release of Cm into the lacteal vessels by ~2-fold.[80] By contrast, the fructose-fed hamster model of insulin resistance,[81] characterized by overproduction of intestinally derived apoB48-lipoproteins in both the fasting and post-prandial state, displayed a more modest 40% increase in MTP protein levels under basal conditions (Figure 4A–C). Thus, notwithstanding quantitative differences in *MTP* mRNA and protein levels, in four different animal models

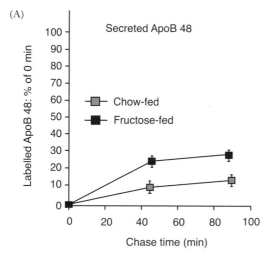

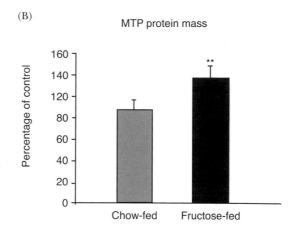

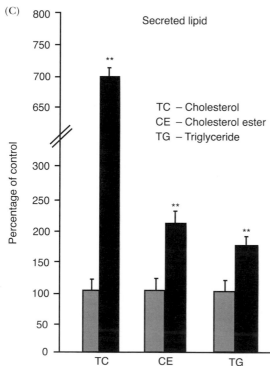

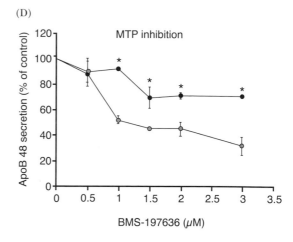

Figure 4 Intestinal apoB48 and lipid secretion from the fructose-fed model of insulin resistance, and the impact of MTP inhibition. Asterisks indicate significant differences between chow- and fructose-fed animals. Data are adapted from Haidari et al[81]

of perturbed insulin metabolism, intestinal *MTP* mRNA levels, lymph Cm concentrations and serum lipid levels varied according to the glycaemic state of the animal. Thus, by extrapolation, a capacity to develop high levels of intestinal MTP protein may contribute to the exaggerated and prolonged post-prandial hyperlipidaemia observed in insulin-resistant and/or type 2 patients.[59,60,83,84] Conversely, a reduction in MTP protein levels in the post-prandial state would be expected to reduce the risk of atherosclerotic cardiovascular disease attributable to the generation of highly atherogenic Cm remnant particles.[62,85–88]

MTP inhibitor data from the hamster model of insulin resistance suggest that in some situations MTP protein may be present in excess of that needed to support the secretion of apoB-containing lipoproteins.[81] In this animal model, for example, the MTP inhibitor, BMS-197636, had minimal impact on the secretion of Cm (Figure 4D), even at high concentrations. This finding may partly relate to higher intestinal MTP protein levels, increased lipid availability and/or differences in the composition of lipids within the membranes of the ER. In vitro, both the concentration of lipid moieties within donor membranes and specific membrane composition are major determinants influencing the rate of MTP-mediated lipid transfer.[49] For example, in one in vitro data set, the specific activity of MTP increased in proportion to the mass of triglyceride within donor membranes, and varied inversely to the concentration of negatively charged lipids (e.g. cardiolipin and phosphatidic acid). Significantly, Mensenkamp et al have also reported that the MTP inhibitor, BMS 197636, had minimal impact on the secretion of hepatic triglyceride from *Apoe*[-/-] mice.[89] These mice normally secrete around 50% less VLDL-triglyceride compared to control animals, with much of the additional triglyceride being retained within the secretory pathway of the hepatocyte. Importantly, hepatic MTP protein levels in the *Apoe*[-/-] mice are comparable to the control mice, suggesting that in conditions of neutral lipid excess, MTP may have a higher specific lipid transfer activity and/or be

prevented from binding to the MTP inhibitor, BMS 197636.

Crucially, no study has yet examined whether a reduction in intestinal *MTP* gene expression actually leads to a reduction in the number of Cms entering the circulation. Lin et al reported that fresh garlic extracts lower intestinal *MTP* mRNA,[90] and suggested that this may account for the hypolipidaemic effect attributed to this additive.[91] Additionally, Raabe et al have shown that the small intestine of *Mttp*[-/+] mice contains ~50% lower levels of *MTP* mRNA and protein than *Mttp*[+/+] mice.[37] In other words, there was no evidence that transcription from the remaining wild-type *Mttp* allele was upregulated to compensate for the inactivated allele. However, because three groups have shown that the MTP inhibitors CP-10447, BMS-200150 and an analogue of CP-10447 have remarkably little impact on the *in vitro* secretion of apoB48-containing lipoproteins (i.e. Cm in humans[92–94]), it will be important in future studies to titrate the impact of *MTP* silencing on Cm assembly. The demonstration that MTP inhibition virtually abolishes post-prandial hyperlipidaemia in rats (Novartis compound 8aR), dogs (Novartis compound 8aR and 19aR) and humans (Bay 13-9952) provides a major incentive to do so.[95–97]

INSIGHTS INTO REGULATION OF HEPATIC MTP FROM MODEL SYSTEMS

The analysis of mouse models also provides some evidence that liver-specific silencing of *MTP* might represent a useful therapeutic tool for lowering blood lipid levels, and in turn reduce the risk of atherosclerotic cardiovascular disease. In detail, in two different liver-specific (L)*Mttp*[-/-] models, mice had serum cholesterol levels that were ~50% lower than wild-type animals.[75,98] Serum triglyceride levels were also lower in both strains of L*Mttp*[-/-] mice, but to varying extents.[75,98] Pertinent to a human RNA-based therapy, liver microsomes from L*Mttp*[-/+] mice contained on average 49% lower levels of MTP-mediated lipid transfer activity than microsomes from wild-type mice,[98] again suggesting that transcription from the wild-type allele was not upregulated to compensate for the inactivated allele. These mice had 20% lower total serum cholesterol levels compared to wild-type animals.

Importantly, when Young and colleagues examined whether MTP deficiency would eliminate the heightened susceptibility of 'apoB100-only'/LDL-receptor-deficient (i.e *Apob100/100:LDLr$^{-/-}$*) mice to atherosclerosis, the answer was affirmative.[99] In outline, MTP-deficient *Apob100/100:LDLr$^{-/-}$* mice had dramatically lower serum cholesterol and triglyceride levels than *Apob100/100:LDLr$^{-/-}$* mice (i.e. 525.7 ± 32.24 mg/dl and 110.33 ± 6.45 mg/dl versus 100.6 ± 14.33 mg/dl and 23.4 ± 4.56 mg/dl). Additionally, by 20 weeks of age, atherosclerotic lesions covered 5.2 ± 0.8% of the surface of the aorta of *Apob100/100:LDLr$^{-/-}$* mice, whereas no such lesions were visible in the L*Mttp$^{-/+}$:Apob100/100:LDLr$^{-/-}$* mice. In other words, the abolition of hepatic apoB100-containing lipoprotein assembly completely prevented the development of atheroma in mice that were highly susceptible to atherosclerosis. Similarly, for *Apoe$^{-/-}$* mice, the MTP inhibitor BAY 13-9952 blocks the formation of atherosclerotic plaque in a dose-dependent manner.[100,101]

The study of genetic mouse models that produce markedly different amounts of apoB100 in the setting of half-normal levels of MTP also provides evidence that liver-specific silencing of *MTP* might provide an effective therapy for treating genetic forms of athero-genic lipoprotein profiles attributable to increased production of VLDL-apoB, such as familial combined hyperlipidaemia.[7,65,102,103] In detail, Young and colleagues compared serum apoB100 levels of wild-type and L*Mttp$^{-/+}$* mice expressing low, normal and high levels of apoB100 mRNA.[104] At each level of apoB100 expression, half-normal levels of hepatic *MTP* were associated with a reduction in serum apoB levels, average values falling by ~20–37% of control. Therefore, MTP deficiency had the largest absolute impact on lowering serum apoB levels in mice that expressed the highest

level of apoB100. In the six different groups of mice, hepatic triglyceride levels were lowest in the transgenic mice expressing high levels of apoB100 and wild-type levels of MTP, and highest in L*Mttp$^{-/+}$* mice expressing low levels of apoB100 (i.e. *apoB$^{-/+}$*). Pertinent for the human situation, the livers of L*Mttp$^{-/+}$* mice contained 3-fold lower levels of triglyceride relative to *apoB100$^{/+}$* mice, presumably because they secreted more apoB100-containing lipoproteins than *apoB100$^{/+}$* mice. Thus, in future studies it would be instructive to determine the frequency and severity of non-alcoholic fatty liver disease in the parents of patients with abetalipoproteinaemia. In the co-dominant disorder familial hypobetalipoproteinaemia, around 60% of patients have evidence of fatty liver, with the percentages of liver fat correlating positively with body mass index, waist circumference and impaired glucose tolerance.[105] Because this 'disorder' is associated with longevity and a very low risk of premature coronary disease, partial silencing of *MTP* could mimic this condition.

What is currently missing from mouse data sets is a description of the impact that insulin resistance, obesity and dietary determinants, such as alcohol and high-fat diets, would have on both hepatic and blood lipid levels in the setting of reduced hepatic MTP mass. Extrapolating from hamster models,[106,107] insulin resistance would be predicted to increase hepatic *MTP* mRNA levels, and thus the secretion of VLDL-triglyceride. Carpentier et al, for example, have shown that ameliorating insulin resistance in the fructose-fed model of insulin resistance helps normalize hepatic *MTP* mRNA levels and reduce VLDL-trigly-ceride secretion.[107] In all likelihood, the negative insulin response element within the promoter of the hamster *MTP* gene,[108] which is conserved in humans, provides a mechanism for the lowering of *MTP* mRNA levels in these animals.

In obesity, Bartel et al have shown that the livers of young leptin-deficient (i.e. ob/ob) mice contained around 12-fold higher levels of triglyceride than ob/$^+$ mice.[109] This was matched with a modest 45% increase in *MTP* mRNA levels and a 70% increase in VLDL-triglyceride secretion. However, in a second study, ob/ob and wild-type mice had comparable levels of hepatic MTP mRNA and similar production rates of VLDL-triglyceride.[110] Notwithstanding, serum cholesterol and triglyceride levels of these mice were increased by around 2-fold relative to control animals, and their livers combined, around 5- and 15-fold higher levels of hepatic triglyceride and cholesteryl ester. In a second animal model of obesity, characterized by hypertriglyceridaemia, hepatic MTP mRNA levels were raised by around 20% relative to thin animals.[111] Thus, a therapeutic strategy that reduced hepatic MTP protein levels in humans may well provide a powerful mechanism for reducing serum lipid levels in obese subjects, but this could incur a high cost in terms of promoting the initiation and/or progression of non-alcoholic fatty liver disease.[112]

Alcohol abuse would almost certainly be a contraindication for utilizing an MTP silencing approach to lower high blood triglyceride levels.[113,114] Lin et al have shown that the human MTP gene contains a negative ethanol responsive element (i.e. −612 to −142 upstream of transcription start site) and that rats gavaged with ethanol for 3 hours had 32% and 18% lower levels of hepatic and intestinal MTP mRNA levels, respectively, than control animals.[113] Moreover, these authors established that a human hepatoma cell line exposed to ethanol for 24 hours contained 50% lower levels of MTP mRNA levels than control cells. Likewise, Sugimoto et al showed that the livers of Sprague-Dawley rats fed an ethanol-containing diet for 37 days contained 60% lower levels of hepatic MTP mRNA than livers from control animals fed an isocaloric, alcohol-free diet, and rather predictably that this reduction in MTP mRNA levels was associated with dramatically increased levels of hepatic cholesterol and triglyceride.[114]

Our understanding of the potential impact of a high-fat diet on human MTP gene expression largely derives from studies performed in hamsters.[78,115,116] In one study, the feeding of these animals with increasing dietary fat concentration from 11.7 energy % to 46.8 energy % for one month increased hepatic MTP mRNA levels ($r = 0.69$, $p = 0.0023$), in a dose-dependent manner by approximately 60%.[115] At the end of the study, MTP mRNA levels were strongly correlated with total serum cholesterol ($r = 0.74$, $p < 0.001$), VLDL-cholesterol ($r = 0.60$, $p < 0.01$), LDL-cholesterol ($r = 0.55$ $p < 0.05$) and HDL-cholesterol ($r = 0.70$, $p < 0.001$), but not with fasting serum triglyceride levels. In a second dataset, Bennett et al showed that hepatic MTP gene expression may also depend on the type of fatty acid incorporated into the dietary triglyceride; diets enriched in either trimyristin or tripalmitin displayed marked increases in MTP mRNA concentrations relative to triolein, trilinolein or tristearin-rich diets.[115] Puzzlingly, in a subsequent study, modest amounts of dietary cholesterol (0.005–0.24 w/w%) abolished this effect of specific fatty acid on MTP mRNA level.[116] Irrespective of triglyceride fatty acid type, cholesterol feeding increased MTP mRNA in a dose-dependent manner, and at the end of 28 days there were significant correlations between MTP mRNA, serum VLDL-triglyceride ($r = 0.35$, $p = 0.011$) and VLDL-cholesterol levels ($r = 0.49$, $p = 0.0002$). These data accord with in vitro investigations which have established that the human MTP promoter contains a sterol responsive element (i.e. −124 to −109 upstream of transcription start site), and moreover that this element has the capacity to bind the sterol regulatory element-binding protein 2.[117]

Remarkably, an Affymetrix microarray experiment indicates that a deficiency of MTP in the liver has no major impact on the expression of most genes involved in hepatic lipid metabolism, despite the development of mild to moderate hepatic steatosis in LMttp[−/−] mice.[118] A notable exception was stearyl CoA desaturase 1 mRNA, which was reduced, a finding that led Young and colleagues to further discoveries. First, the livers of LMttp[−/−] mice contain lower levels of sterol regulatory element-binding protein 1c and the polyunsaturated fatty acid, linoleic acid, relative to control livers. Second, the animals had around 45% lower levels of plasma insulin, which may, via a transcriptional mechanism, contribute to the reduced levels of the sterol-regulatory element-binding protein 1c in these animals.[119] Consistent with histological examination, the microarray experiment also found no evidence for an active inflammatory response in the livers of LMttp[-/-] mice. Expression levels of inflammation (e.g. macrophage inflammatory proteins-1α, 1β, 2; a range of interleukins, interferon-α-β, γ and TNF-α) and apoptosis-related genes (e.g. *bax*, *bcl-2*, *c-myc*, *c-jun* and *fas*) were either comparable to control mice or below the level of detection.

INSIGHTS FROM HUMAN GENETIC AND GENE EXPRESSION STUDIES

Arguably, the best evidence that long-term tissue-specific silencing of *MTP* expression may provide a powerful mechanism for reducing the risk of cardiovascular disease derives from genetic comparisons of two types of people: those who have reached an exceptional long age and signally escaped age-associated diseases, such as cardiovascular disease, and those who have had a coronary heart disease event at an early age. For the first group, Puca and colleagues reported data showing that the much-studied *MTP*[-493T] allele[120-129] was under-represented in a group of long-lived Americans, leading them to suggest that this allele (or an allele in linkage disequilibrium) increases the risk of mortality.[130] For the second, Karpe and colleagues[58] reported that the *MTP*[-493T] allele increased the risk of a coronary heart disease event in a group of middle-aged men (i.e. 45–64 years) with serum cholesterol levels of 7.0 ± 0.6 mmol/l, and that

this was likely to be attributable to reduced transcriptional activity of this allele (or allele in linkage disequilibrium) in cardiac myocytes.[123]

CONCLUDING COMMENT

The assembly and secretion of apoB-containing lipoproteins are crucial for survival in infancy and adulthood, but the intracellular processes that regulate their production are sensitive to metabolic and genetic disease. In the future, the prevention and/or treatment of disorders attributable to increased production of Cm and VLDL should be feasible through an antisense or RNA silencing approach[131-137] that reduce hepatic and/or intestinal *MTP* mRNA levels. Partial and tissue-specific silencing of *MTP* promises to overcome a number of the potential adverse side-effects associated with long-term global inhibition of MTP.

ACKNOWLEDGEMENTS

I am grateful to the British Medical Research and the British Heart Foundation, London, UK, who have supported most of the MTP research from my group. I also thank all co-investigators, especially Professors James Scott and Maryvonne Rosseneu, Leonard Banaszak and Drs Christopher J Mann, Timothy Anderson, Arjen R Mensenkamp and Jacqueline Read, and Drs Andrew Dean and Rossi Naoumova for critical reading of the manuscript, and Rocio Lale-Montes for excellent secretarial assistance. I also thank Professor Khosrow Adeli for permission to reproduce the data in Figure 4.

References

1. Mason TM. The role of factors that regulate the synthesis and secretion of very-low-density lipoprotein by hepatocytes. Crit Rev Clin Lab Sci 1998; 35: 461–87

2. Olofsson SO, Stillemark-Billton P, Asp L. Intracellular assembly of VLDL: two major steps in separate cell compartments. Trends Cardiovasc Med 2000; 10:338–45

3. Gordon DA, Jamil H. Progress towards understanding the role of microsomal triglyceride transfer protein in apolipoprotein-B lipoprotein assembly. Biochim Biophys Acta 2000; 1486:72–83

4. Shelness GS, Sellers JA. Very-low-density lipoprotein assembly and secretion. Curr Opin Lipidol 2001; 12:151–7

5. Fisher EA, Ginsberg HN. Complexity in the secretory pathway: the assembly and secretion of apolipoprotein B-containing lipoproteins. J Biol Chem 2002; 277:17377–80

6. Hussain MM, Shi J, Dreizen P. Microsomal triglyceride transfer protein and its role in apoB-lipoprotein assembly. J Lipid Res 2003; 44:22–32

7. Shoulders CC, Jones EL, Naoumova RP. Genetics of familial combined hyperlipidemia and risk of coronary heart disease. Hum Mol Genet 2004; 13 (Suppl 1):R149–60

8. Segrest JP, Jones MK, De Loof H, et al. Structure of apolipoprotein B-100 in low density lipoproteins. J Lipid Res 2001; 42:1346–67

9. Heath RB, Karpe F, Milne RW, et al. Selective partitioning of dietary fatty acids into the VLDL-TG pool in the early postprandial period. J Lipid Res 2003; 44:2065–72

10. Teusink B, Voshol PJ, Dahlmans VE, et al. Contribution of fatty acids released from lipolysis of plasma triglycerides to total plasma fatty acid flux and tissue-specific fatty acid uptake. Diabetes 2003; 52:614–20

11. Wiggins D, Gibbons GF. Origin of hepatic very-low-density lipoprotein triacylglycerol: the contribution of cellular phospholipid. Biochem J 1996; 320 (Pt 2):673–9

12. Parks EJ, Hellerstein MK. Carbohydrate-induced hypertriacylglycerolemia: historical perspective and review of biological mechanisms. Am J Clin Nutr 2000; 71:412–33

13. Haemmerle G, Zimmermann R, Zechner R. Letting lipids go: hormone-sensitive lipase. Curr Opin Lipidol 2003; 14:289–97

14. Boren J, Veniant MM, Young SG. Apo B100-containing lipoproteins are secreted by the heart. J Clin Invest 1998; 101:1197–202

15. Nielsen LB, Veniant M, Boren J, et al. Genes for apolipoprotein B and microsomal triglyceride transfer protein are expressed in the heart: evidence that the heart has the capacity to synthesize and secrete lipoproteins. Circulation 1998; 98:13–16

16. Bjorkegren J, Veniant M, Kim SK, et al. Lipoprotein secretion and triglyceride stores in the heart. J Biol Chem 2001; 276:38511–17

17. Nielsen LB, Bartels ED, Bollano E. Overexpression of apolipoprotein B in the heart impedes cardiac triglyceride accumulation and development of cardiac dysfunction in diabetic mice. J Biol Chem 2002; 277:27014–20

18. Christoffersen C, Bollano E, Lindegaard ML, et al. Cardiac lipid accumulation associated with diastolic dysfunction in obese mice. Endocrinology 2003; 144:3483–90

19. Yokoyama M, Yagyu H, Hu Y, et al. Apolipoprotein B production reduces lipotoxic cardiomyopathy: studies in heart-specific lipoprotein lipase transgenic mouse. J Biol Chem 2004; 279:4204–11

20. Gordon DA, Jamil H, Sharp D, et al. Secretion of apolipoprotein B-containing lipoproteins from HeLa cells is dependent on expression of the microsomal triglyceride transfer protein and is regulated by lipid availability. Proc Natl Acad Sci USA 1994; 91: 7628–32

21. Leiper JM, Bayliss JD, Pease RJ, et al. Microsomal triglyceride transfer protein, the abetalipoproteinemia gene product, mediates the secretion of apolipoprotein B-containing lipoproteins from heterologous cells. J Biol Chem 1994; 269:21951–4

22. Ingram MF, Shelness GS. Folding of the amino-terminal domain of apolipoprotein B initiates microsomal triglyceride transfer protein-dependent lipid transfer to nascent very low density lipoprotein. J Biol Chem 1997; 272:10279–86

23. Sharp D, Blinderman L, Combs KA, et al. Cloning and gene defects in microsomal triglyceride transfer protein associated with abetalipoproteinaemia. Nature 1993; 365:65–9

24. Shoulders CC, Brett DJ, Bayliss JD, et al. Abetalipoproteinemia is caused by defects of the gene encoding the 97 kDa subunit of a microsomal triglyceride transfer protein. Hum Mol Genet 1993; 2:2109–16

25. Narcisi TM, Shoulders CC, Chester SA, et al. Mutations of the microsomal triglyceride-transfer-protein gene in abetalipoproteinemia. Am J Hum Genet 1995; 57:1298–310

26. Ricci B, Sharp D, O'Rourke E, et al. A 30–amino acid truncation of the microsomal triglyceride transfer protein large subunit disrupts its interaction with protein disulfide-isomerase and causes abetalipoproteinemia. J Biol Chem 1995; 270:14281–5

27. Rehberg EF, Samson-Bouma ME, Kienzle B, et al. A novel abetalipoproteinemia genotype. Identification of a missense mutation in the 97–kDa subunit of the microsomal triglyceride transfer protein that prevents complex formation with protein disulfide isomerase. J Biol Chem 1996; 271:29945–52

28. Berthier MT, Couture P, Houde A, et al. The c.419–420insA in the MTP gene is associated with abetalipoproteinemia among French-Canadians. Mol Genet Metab 2004; 81:140–3

29. Berriot-Varoqueaux N, Aggerbeck LP, Samson-Bouma M, et al. The role of the microsomal triglyceride transfer protein in abetalipoprotcinemia. Annu Rev Nutr 2000; 20:663–97

30. Rader DJ, Brewer HB, Jr. Abetalipoproteinemia. New insights into lipoprotein assembly and vitamin E metabolism from a rare genetic disease. JAMA 1993; 270:865–9

31. Wang X, Quinn PJ. Vitamin E and its function in membranes. Prog Lipid Res 1999; 38:309–36

32. Blomhoff R, Green MH, Berg T, et al. Transport and storage of vitamin A. Science 1990; 250:399–404

33. Schurgers LJ, Vermeer C. Differential lipoprotein transport pathways of K-vitamins in healthy subjects. Biochim Biophys Acta 2002; 1570:27–32

34. Illingworth DR, Connor WE, Miller RG.

Abetalipoproteinemia. Report of two cases and review of therapy. Arch Neurol 1980; 37:659–62

35. Wang J, Hegele RA. Microsomal triglyceride transfer protein (MTP) gene mutations in Canadian subjects with abetalipoproteinemia. Hum Mutat 2000; 15:294–5

36. Chowers I, Banin E, Merin S, et al. Long-term assessment of combined vitamin A and E treatment for the prevention of retinal degeneration in abetalipoproteinaemia and hypobetalipoproteinaemia patients. Eye 2001; 15(Pt 4):525–30

37. Raabe M, Kim E, Veniant M, et al. Using genetically engineered mice to understand apolipoprotein-B deficiency syndromes in humans. Proc Assoc Am Physicians 1998; 110:521–30

38. Bakillah A, Nayak N, Saxena U, et al. Decreased secretion of ApoB follows inhibition of ApoB–MTP binding by a novel antagonist. Biochemistry 2000; 39:4892–9

39. Sellers JA, Hou L, Athar H, et al. A Drosophila microsomal triglyceride transfer protein homolog promotes the assembly and secretion of human apolipoprotein B. Implications for human and insect transport and metabolism. J Biol Chem 2003; 278:20367–73

40. Hussain MM, Bakillah A, Nayak N, et al. Amino acids 430–570 in apolipoprotein B are critical for its binding to microsomal triglyceride transfer protein. J Biol Chem 1998; 273:25612–15

41. Wu DA, Bu X, Warden CH, et al. Quantitative trait locus mapping of human blood pressure to a genetic region at or near the lipoprotein lipase gene locus on chromosome 8p22. J Clin Invest 1996; 97:2111–18

42. Dashti N, Gandhi M, Liu X, et al. The N-terminal 1000 residues of apolipoprotein B associate with microsomal triglyceride transfer protein to create a lipid transfer pocket required for lipoprotein assembly. Biochemistry 2002; 41:6978–87

43. Jamil H, Dickson JK, Jr, Chu CH, et al. Microsomal triglyceride transfer protein. Specificity of lipid binding and transport. J Biol Chem 1995; 270: 6549–54

44. Nishimaki-Mogami T, Yao Z, Fujimori K. Inhibition of phosphatidylcholine synthesis via the phosphatidylethanolamine methylation pathway impairs incorporation of bulk lipids into VLDL in cultured rat hepatocytes. J Lipid Res 2002; 43:1035–45

45. Noga AA, Zhao Y, Vance DE. An unexpected requirement for phosphatidylethanolamine N-methyltransferase in the secretion of very low density lipoproteins. J Biol Chem 2002; 277:42358–65

46. Read J, Anderson TA, Ritchie PJ, et al. A mechanism of membrane neutral lipid acquisition by the microsomal triglyceride transfer protein. J Biol Chem 2000; 275:30372–7

47. Atzel A, Wetterau JR. Mechanism of microsomal triglyceride transfer protein catalyzed lipid transport. Biochemistry 1993; 32:10444–50

48. Wetterau JR, Lin MC, Jamil H. Microsomal triglyceride transfer protein. Biochim Biophys Acta 1997; 1345:136–50

49. Atzel A, Wetterau JR. Identification of two classes of lipid molecule binding sites on the microsomal triglyceride transfer protein. Biochemistry 1994; 33:15382–8

50. Mann CJ, Anderson TA, Read J, et al. The structure of vitellogenin provides a molecular model for the assembly and secretion of atherogenic lipoproteins. J Mol Biol 1999; 285:391–408

51. Bradbury P, Mann CJ, Kochl S, et al. A common binding site on the microsomal triglyceride transfer protein for apolipoprotein B and protein disulfide isomerase. J Biol Chem 1999; 274:3159–64

52. Segrest JP, Jones MK, Dashti N. N-terminal domain of apolipoprotein B has structural homology to lipovitellin and microsomal triglyceride transfer protein: a 'lipid pocket' model for self-assembly of apob-containing lipoprotein particles. J Lipid Res 1999; 40:1401–16

53. Jones B, Jones EL, Bonney SA, et al. Mutations in a Sar1 GTPase of COPII vesicles are associated with lipid absorption disorders. Nat Genet 2003; 34:29–31

54. Gusarova V, Brodsky JL, Fisher EA. Apolipoprotein B100 exit from the ER is COPII dependent and its lipidation to very low density lipoprotein occurs post-ER. J Biol Chem 2003; 278:48051–8

55. Burnett JR, Shan J, Miskie BA, et al. A novel nontruncating APOB gene mutation, R463W, causes familial hypobetalipoproteinemia. J Biol Chem 2003; 278:13442–52

56. Chang G, Ruggeri RB, Harwood HJ, Jr. Microsomal triglyceride transfer protein (MTP) inhibitors: discovery of clinically active inhibitors using high-throughput screening and parallel synthesis paradigms. Curr Opin Drug Discov Devel 2002; 5:562–70

57. Chandler CE, Wilder DE, Pettini JL, et al. CP-346086: an MTP inhibitor that lowers plasma cholesterol and triglycerides in experimental animals and in humans. J Lipid Res 2003; 44:1887–901

58. Ledmyr H, McMahon AD, Ehrenborg E, et al. The microsomal triglyceride transfer protein gene -493T variant lowers cholesterol but increases the risk of coronary heart disease. Circulation. 2004; 109:2279–84

59. Karpe F, Hellenius ML, Hamsten A. Differences in postprandial concentrations of very-low-density lipoprotein and chylomicron remnants between normotriglyceridemic and hypertriglyceridemic men with and without coronary heart disease. Metabolism 1999; 48:301–7

60. Goldberg IJ, Kako Y, Lutz EP. Responses to eating: lipoproteins, lipolytic products and atherosclerosis. Curr Opin Lipidol 2000; 11:235–41

61. Demacker PN, Hectors MP, Stalenhoef AF. Chylomicron processing in familial dysbetalipoproteinemia and familial combined hyperlipidemia studied with vitamin A and E as markers: a new physiological concept. Atherosclerosis 2000; 149:169–80

62. Mero N, Malmstrom R, Steiner G, et al. Postprandial metabolism of apolipoprotein B-48- and B-100-containing particles in type 2 diabetes mellitus:

relations to angiographically verified severity of coronary artery disease. Atherosclerosis 2000; 150: 167–77

63. Sharrett AR, Heiss G, Chambless LE, et al. Metabolic and lifestyle determinants of postprandial lipemia differ from those of fasting triglycerides: The Atherosclerosis Risk In Communities (ARIC) study. Arterioscler Thromb Vasc Biol 2001; 21:275–81

64. Castro CM. Postprandial lipaemia in familial combined hyperlipidaemia. Biochem Soc Trans 2003; 31(Pt 5):1090–3

65. Venkatesan S, Cullen P, Pacy P, et al. Stable isotopes show a direct relation between VLDL apoB overproduction and serum triglyceride levels and indicate a metabolically and biochemically coherent basis for familial combined hyperlipidemia. Arterioscler Thromb 1993; 13:1110–18

66. Austin MA, McKnight B, Edwards KL, et al. Cardiovascular disease mortality in familial forms of hypertriglyceridemia: a 20-year prospective study. Circulation 2000; 101:2777–82

67. Voors-Pette C, de Bruin TW. Excess coronary heart disease in Familial Combined Hyperlipidemia, in relation to genetic factors and central obesity. Atherosclerosis 2001; 157:481–9

68. Hopkins PN, Heiss G, Ellison RC, et al. Coronary artery disease risk in familial combined hyperlipidemia and familial hypertriglyceridemia: a case-control comparison from the National Heart, Lung, and Blood Institute Family Heart Study. Circulation 2003; 108:519–23

69. McNeely MJ, Edwards KL, Marcovina SM, et al. Lipoprotein and apolipoprotein abnormalities in familial combined hyperlipidemia: a 20-year prospective study. Atherosclerosis 2001; 159:471–81

70. Ayyobi AF, Brunzell JD. Lipoprotein distribution in the metabolic syndrome, type 2 diabetes mellitus, and familial combined hyperlipidemia. Am J Cardiol 2003; 92:27J–33J

71. World Health Organisation. Diabetes Mellitus: Report of a WHO Study Group. WHO, Geneva 1985

72. Expert Panel on Detection, Evaluation, and Treatment of High Blood Cholesterol in Adults. Executive Summary of The Third Report of The National Cholesterol Education Program (NCEP) Expert Panel on Detection, Evaluation, And Treatment of High Blood Cholesterol In Adults (Adult Treatment Panel III). JAMA 2001; 285:2486–97

73. Sattar N, Gaw A, Scherbakova O, et al. Metabolic syndrome with and without C-reactive protein as a predictor of coronary heart disease and diabetes in the West of Scotland Coronary Prevention Study. Circulation 2003; 108:414–19

74. Ninomiya JK, L'Italien G, Criqui MH, et al. Association of the metabolic syndrome with history of myocardial infarction and stroke in the third national health and nutrition examination survey. Circulation 2004; 109:42–6

75. Raabe M, Veniant MM, Sullivan MA, et al. Analysis of the role of microsomal triglyceride transfer protein in the liver of tissue-specific knockout mice. J Clin Invest 1999; 103:1287–98

76. Murray CJ, Lopez AD. Alternative projections of mortality and disability by cause 1990–2020: Global Burden of Disease Study. Lancet 1997; 349:1498–504

77. Fuster V. Epidemic of cardiovascular disease and stroke: the three main challenges. Presented at the 71st scientific sessions of the American Heart Association. Dallas, Texas. Circulation 1999; 99:1132–7

78. Lin MC, Arbeeny C, Bergquist K, et al. Cloning and regulation of hamster microsomal triglyceride transfer protein. The regulation is independent from that of other hepatic and intestinal proteins which participate in the transport of fatty acids and triglycerides. J Biol Chem 1994; 269:29138–45

79. Gleeson A, Anderton K, Owens D, et al. The role of microsomal triglyceride transfer protein and dietary cholesterol in chylomicron production in diabetes. Diabetologia 1999; 42:944–8

80. Phillips C, Owens D, Collins P, et al. Microsomal triglyceride transfer protein: does insulin resistance play a role in the regulation of chylomicron assembly? Atherosclerosis 2002; 160:355–60

81. Haidari M, Leung N, Mahbub F, et al. Fasting and postprandial overproduction of intestinally derived lipoproteins in an animal model of insulin resistance. Evidence that chronic fructose feeding in the hamster is accompanied by enhanced intestinal de novo lipogenesis and ApoB48-containing lipoprotein overproduction. J Biol Chem 2002; 277:31646–55

82. Phillips C, Bennett A, Anderton K, et al. Intestinal rather than hepatic microsomal triglyceride transfer protein as a cause of postprandial dyslipidemia in diabetes. Metabolism 2002; 51:847–52

83. Boquist S, Hamsten A, Karpe F, et al. Insulin and non-esterified fatty acid relations to alimentary lipaemia and plasma concentrations of postprandial triglyceride-rich lipoproteins in healthy middle-aged men. Diabetologia 2000; 43:185–93

84. Owens D. The extended postprandial phase in diabetes. Biochem Soc Trans 2003; 31(Pt 5):1085–9

85. Groot PH, van Stiphout WA, Krauss XH, et al. Postprandial lipoprotein metabolism in normolipidemic men with and without coronary artery disease. Arterioscler Thromb 1991; 11:653–62

86. McNamara JR, Shah PK, Nakajima K, et al. Remnant-like particle (RLP) cholesterol is an independent cardiovascular disease risk factor in women: results from the Framingham Heart Study. Atherosclerosis 2001; 154:229–36

87. Meyer E, Westerveld HT, Ruyter-Meijstek FC, et al. Abnormal postprandial apolipoprotein B-48 and triglyceride responses in normolipidemic women with greater than 70% stenotic coronary artery disease: a case-control study. Atherosclerosis 1996; 124:221–35

88. Boquist S, Ruotolo G, Tang R, et al. Alimentary lipemia, postprandial triglyceride-rich lipoproteins, and common carotid intima-media thickness in

healthy, middle-aged men. Circulation 1999; 100:723–8

89. Mensenkamp AR, Teusink B, Havinga R, et al. Involvement of apolipoprotein E in triacylglycerol incorporation into Very Low Density Lipoprotein particles. J Hepatol 2004; 40:599–606

90. Lin MC, Wang EJ, Lee C, et al. Garlic inhibits microsomal triglyceride transfer protein gene expression in human liver and intestinal cell lines and in rat intestine. J Nutr 2002; 132:1165–8

91. Ackermann RT, Mulrow CD, Ramirez G, et al. Garlic shows promise for improving some cardiovascular risk factors. Arch Intern Med 2001; 161:813–24

92. Haghpassand M, Wilder D, Moberly JB. Inhibition of apolipoprotein B and triglyceride secretion in human hepatoma cells (HepG2). J Lipid Res 1996; 37: 1468–80

93. van Greevenbroek MM, Robertus-Teunissen MG, et al. Participation of the microsomal triglyceride transfer protein in lipoprotein assembly in Caco-2 cells: interaction with saturated and unsaturated dietary fatty acids. J Lipid Res 1998; 39:173–85

94. Nicodeme E, Benoist F, McLeod R, et al. Identification of domains in apolipoprotein B100 that confer a high requirement for the microsomal triglyceride transfer protein. J Biol Chem 1999; 274:1986–93

95. Ksander GM, deJesus R, Yuan A, et al. Diaminoindanes as microsomal triglyceride transfer protein inhibitors. J Med Chem 2001; 44:4677–87

96. Sorbera LA, Martin L, Silvestre J, et al. Implitapide. Drugs of the Future 2000; 25:1138–44

97. Stein EA, Arnes SA, Moore LJ, et al. Inhibition of post-prandial fat absorption with the MTP inhibitor BAY 13–9952. Circulation 2000; 102 (Supp II):2913

98. Chang BH, Liao W, Li L, et al. Liver-specific inactivation of the abetalipoproteinemia gene completely abrogates very low density lipoprotein/low density lipoprotein production in a viable conditional knockout mouse. J Biol Chem 1999; 274:6051–5

99. Lieu HD, Withycombe SK, Walker Q, et al. Eliminating atherogenesis in mice by switching off hepatic lipoprotein secretion. Circulation 2003; 107:1315–21

100. Zaiss S, Gruetzmann R, Ullrich M. BAY 13–9952, an inhibitor of the microsomal triglyceride transfer protein (MTP) dose-dependently blocks the formation of atherosclerotic plaques and renders them more stable in apoE knockout mice. Circulation 1999; 100 (Suppl I):1343

101. Zaiss S, Sander E. BAY 13–9952 (Implitapide), an inhibitor of the microsomal triglyceride transfer protein (MTP), inhibits atherosclerosis and prolongs lifetime in apoE knockout mice. Eur Heart J 2000; 21 (Suppl):16

102. Cortner JA, Coates PM, Bennett MJ, et al. Familial combined hyperlipidaemia: use of stable isotopes to demonstrate overproduction of very low-density lipoprotein apolipoprotein B by the liver. J Inherit Metab Dis 1991; 14:915–22

103. Castro CM, de Bruin TW, de Valk HW, et al. Impaired fatty acid metabolism in familial combined hyperlipidemia. A mechanism associating hepatic apolipoprotein B overproduction and insulin resistance. J Clin Invest 1993; 92:160–8

104. Leung GK, Veniant MM, Kim SK, et al. A deficiency of microsomal triglyceride transfer protein reduces apolipoprotein B secretion. J Biol Chem 2000; 275:7515–20

105. Schonfeld G, Patterson BW, Yablonskiy DA, et al. Fatty liver in familial hypobetalipoproteinemia: triglyceride assembly into VLDL particles is affected by the extent of hepatic steatosis. J Lipid Res 2003; 44:470–8

106. Taghibiglou C, Carpentier A, Van Iderstine SC, et al. Mechanisms of hepatic very low density lipoprotein overproduction in insulin resistance. Evidence for enhanced lipoprotein assembly, reduced intracellular ApoB degradation, and increased microsomal triglyceride transfer protein in a fructose-fed hamster model. J Biol Chem 2000; 275:8416–25

107. Carpentier A, Taghibiglou C, Leung N, et al. Ameliorated hepatic insulin resistance is associated with normalization of microsomal triglyceride transfer protein expression and reduction in very low density lipoprotein assembly and secretion in the fructose-fed hamster. J Biol Chem 2002; 277: 28795–802

108. Au WS, Kung HF, Lin MC. Regulation of microsomal triglyceride transfer protein gene by insulin in HepG2 cells: roles of MAPKerk and MAPKp38. Diabetes 2003; 52:1073–80

109. Bartels ED, Lauritsen M, Nielsen LB. Hepatic expression of microsomal triglyceride transfer protein and in vivo secretion of triglyceride-rich lipoproteins are increased in obese diabetic mice. Diabetes 2002; 51:1233–9

110. Wiegman CH, Bandsma RH, Ouwens M, et al. Hepatic VLDL production in ob/ob mice is not stimulated by massive de novo lipogenesis but is less sensitive to the suppressive effects of insulin. Diabetes 2003; 52:1081–9

111. Kuriyama H, Yamashita S, Shimomura I, et al. Enhanced expression of hepatic acyl-coenzyme A synthetase and microsomal triglyceride transfer protein messenger RNAs in the obese and hypertriglyceridemic rat with visceral fat accumulation. Hepatology 1998; 27:557–62

112. Angulo P. Nonalcoholic fatty liver disease. N Engl J Med 2002; 346:1221–31

113. Lin MC, Li JJ, Wang EJ, et al. Ethanol down-regulates the transcription of microsomal triglyceride transfer protein gene. FASEB J 1997; 11:1145–52

114. Sugimoto T, Yamashita S, Ishigami M, et al. Decreased microsomal triglyceride transfer protein activity contributes to initiation of alcoholic liver steatosis in rats. J Hepatol 2002; 36:157–62

115. Bennett AJ, Billett MA, Salter AM, et al. Regulation of hamster hepatic microsomal triglyceride transfer

protein mRNA levels by dietary fats. Biochem Biophys Res Commun 1995; 212:473–8

116. Bennett AJ, Bruce JS, Salter AM, et al. Hepatic microsomal triglyceride transfer protein messenger RNA concentrations are increased by dietary cholesterol in hamsters. FEBS Lett 1996; 394:247–50

117. Sato R, Miyamoto W, Inoue J, et al. Sterol regulatory element-binding protein negatively regulates microsomal triglyceride transfer protein gene transcription. J Biol Chem 1999; 274:24714–20

118. Bjorkegren J, Beigneux A, Bergo MO, et al. Blocking the secretion of hepatic very low density lipoproteins renders the liver more susceptible to toxin-induced injury. J Biol Chem 2002; 277:5476–83

119. Shimomura I, Shimano H, Korn BS, et al. Nuclear sterol regulatory element-binding proteins activate genes responsible for the entire program of unsaturated fatty acid biosynthesis in transgenic mouse liver. J Biol Chem 1998; 273:35299–306

120. Couture P, Otvos JD, Cupples LA, et al. Absence of association between genetic variation in the promoter of the microsomal triglyceride transfer protein gene and plasma lipoproteins in the Framingham Offspring Study. Atherosclerosis 2000; 148:337–43

121. Talmud PJ, Palmen J, Miller G, et al. Effect of microsomal triglyceride transfer protein gene variants (-493G > T, Q95H and H297Q) on plasma lipid levels in healthy middle-aged UK men. Ann Hum Genet 2000; 64(Pt 4):269–76

122. Watts GF, Riches FM, Humphries SE, et al. Genotypic associations of the hepatic secretion of VLDL apolipoprotein B-100 in obesity. J Lipid Res 2000; 41:481–8

123. Ledmyr H, Karpe F, Lundahl B, et al. Variants of the microsomal triglyceride transfer protein gene are associated with plasma cholesterol levels and body mass index. J Lipid Res 2002; 43:51–8

124. Juo SH, Han Z, Smith JD, et al. Common polymorphism in promoter of microsomal triglyceride transfer protein gene influences cholesterol, ApoB, and triglyceride levels in young african american men: results from the coronary artery risk development in young adults (CARDIA) study. Arterioscler Thromb Vasc Biol 2000; 20:1316–22

125. Vincent S, Planells R, Defoort C, et al. Genetic polymorphisms and lipoprotein responses to diets. Proc Nutr Soc 2002; 61:427–34

126. Bjorn L, Leren TP, Ose L, et al. A functional polymor-phism in the promoter region of the microsomal triglyceride transfer protein (MTP -493G/T) influences lipoprotein phenotype in familial hypercholesterolemia. Arterioscler Thromb Vasc Biol 2000; 20:1784–8

127. Yanagisawa Y, Kawabata T, Tanaka O, et al. Improvement in blood lipid levels by dietary sn-1,3–diacylglycerol in young women with variants of lipid transporters 54T-FABP2 and -493g-MTP. Biochem Biophys Res Commun 2003; 302:743–50

128. Bernard S, Touzet S, Personne I, et al. Association between microsomal triglyceride transfer protein gene polymorphism and the biological features of liver steatosis in patients with type II diabetes. Diabetologia 2000; 43:995–9

129. St Pierre J, Lemieux I, Miller-Felix I, et al. Visceral obesity and hyperinsulinemia modulate the impact of the microsomal triglyceride transfer protein -493G/T polymorphism on plasma lipoprotein levels in men. Atherosclerosis 2002; 160:317–24

130. Geesaman BJ, Benson E, Brewster SJ, et al. Haplotype-based identification of a microsomal transfer protein marker associated with the human lifespan. Proc Natl Acad Sci U S A 2003; 100:14115–20

131. Bi F, Liu N, Fan D. Small interfering RNA: a new tool for gene therapy. Curr Gene Ther 2003; 3:411–17

132. Biroccio A, Leonetti C, Zupi G. The future of antisense therapy: combination with anticancer treatments. Oncogene 2003; 22:6579–88

133. Lavery KS, King TH. Antisense and RNAi: powerful tools in drug target discovery and validation. Curr Opin Drug Discov Devel 2003; 6:561–9

134. Gonzalez FM, Crooke RM, Tillman L, et al. Stability of polycationic complexes of an antisense oligonucleotide in rat small intestine homogenates. Eur J Pharm Biopharm 2003; 55:19–26

135. Xing HR, Cordon-Cardo C, Deng X, et al. Pharmacologic inactivation of kinase suppressor of ras-1 abrogates Ras-mediated pancreatic cancer. Nat Med 2003; 9:1267–8

136. Wang L, Prakash RK, Stein CA, et al. Progress in the delivery of therapeutic oligonucleotides: organ/cellular distribution and targeted delivery of oligonucleotides in vivo. Antisense Nucleic Acid Drug Dev 2003; 13:169–89

137. Wood MJ, Trulzsch B, Abdelgany A, et al. Therapeutic gene silencing in the nervous system. Hum Mol Genet 2003; 12 Spec No 2:R279–84

Acyl CoA: Diacylglycerol acyltransferases (DGATs) as therapeutic targets for cardiovascular disease

3

J.S. Millar and J.T. Billheimer

INTRODUCTION

Coronary heart disease (CHD) is a major cause of death in Westernized societies and is projected to be the leading cause of death well into the millennium.[1] Over the last 30 years the role of plasma cholesterol and hypercholesterolaemia in the development of CHD has been well established. Recently the role of a second plasma lipid, triglyceride (TG), in the development of CHD has come to prominence. Three CHD risk factors, hypertriglyceridaemia, obesity and insulin resistance, are associated with elevated tissue and plasma levels of TG and they are among the metabolic abnormalities whose co-existence defines syndrome X or the metabolic syndrome.[2]

Several recent studies have demonstrated an association of elevated plasma TG with CHD. This association has led the Adult Treatment Panel III to designate hypertriglyceridaemia as an independent risk factor for CHD.[3] Hypertriglyceridaemia can act to increase the development of CHD in at least two ways. First, increased levels of TG-rich particles in plasma frequently lead to increased production of remnant lipoproteins.[4] These remnant lipoproteins are prone to oxidation, which leads to their uptake by macrophages. Macrophages that have exceeded their capacity to process lipids transform into foam cells that initiate a series of steps, leading to the deposition of lipid in the arterial wall.[5] The second way that hypertriglyceridaemia can act to increase the development of CHD is through the exchange of TG in TG-rich apoB-containing particles for cholesteryl ester in high density lipoprotein (HDL).[6] This leads to a lowering of HDL levels and reduced reverse cholesterol transport from peripheral tissues to liver, where cholesterol is excreted into bile.[7]

In addition to the role of plasma TG in the development of CHD, TG accumulation in tissues, including adipose tissue, can have pathological consequences. According to the World Health Organization (WHO), more than 1 billion people are recognized as being clinically obese due, to a large extent, to the increased consumption of energy-dense foods and a sedentary lifestyle. This is anticipated to have adverse consequences regarding the development of CHD since obese individuals are more likely than lean individuals to develop CHD. The prevalence of CHD in males almost doubles and in women triples for individuals with a BMI >40 kg/m^2 compared to a normal BMI (<25 kg/m^2).[8]

Adipose tissue plays a direct role in mediating plasma lipid concentrations through the uptake of plasma TG and the release of adipose-derived fatty acids into plasma. Adipose tissue also plays an endocrine role and secretes a number of adipocytokines which affect food intake, energy expenditure and lipid metabolism.[9,10]

Several studies have demonstrated the association between non-adipose tissue TG levels and insulin resistance resulting from impaired insulin signalling.[11-14] While it is not known if cellular TG directly impairs insulin signalling[14] or if it is the fatty acid derived from TG,[15] it is known that improvements in insulin signalling resulting from the use of insulin-sensitizing agents reduce tissue TG levels.[16] Thus, it seems reasonable to conclude that a means of preventing tissue TG accumulation would have a beneficial effect on insulin signalling.

Pharmacological interventions designed to treat hypertriglyceridaemia, obesity or type 2 diabetes often have a specific effect on one of the above morbidities that may sometimes have undesirable consequences on another risk factor. For example, peroxisome proliferator activated receptor gamma agonists can improve insulin sensitivity but frequently increase plasma lipid levels and cause weight gain while sibutramine, a compound that promotes satiety, may also elevate blood pressure, itself a risk factor.[17,18] However, recently described enzymes, acyl CoA:diacylglycerol acyltransferase (DGAT1 and DGAT2), that catalyse the last step in triglyceride (TG) synthesis in tissues, have become attractive targets for pharmacotherapy since they have the potential to have a more generalized beneficial effect on hypertriglyceridaemia, obesity and insulin resistance.[19–21] These enzymes have been associated with a resistance to diet-induced weight gain,[19] improved insulin sensitivity[20] and lowering of plasma lipid levels, presumably resulting from reduced availability of TG for lipoprotein synthesis.[21] While there are adverse effects that need to be dealt with during the design phase, the potential to have a beneficial impact simultaneously on hyperlipidaemia, diet-induced obesity and type 2 diabetes by inhibiting a single enzymatic step makes DGAT an attractive target for drug discovery.

STRUCTURE AND PROPERTIES OF DGAT1 AND DGAT2

Phospholipids, triglycerides and glycerolipids share common biosynthetic pathways. The terminal and only committed step of the TG synthetic pathway involves the fatty acid acylation of diacylglycerol catalysed by DGAT.

DGAT activity is found intracellularly in the ER membrane where lipid synthesis occurs.[22] The first isolation of a protein with DGAT activity came from the work of Andersson et al.[23] This protein has never been fully characterized, but subsequently two mammalian enzymes with DGAT activity have been cloned (DGAT1 and DGAT2).[24,25] DGATs are membrane bound, presumably within the ER, and their activity has been detected on both the cytosolic and lumenal sides of the ER.[26] The presence of DGAT activity on both sides of the ER membrane suggests that these enzymes may be differentially involved in the synthesis of TG for storage in cytoplasm and for use in lipoprotein synthesis within the ER lumen similar to separate roles that ACAT 1 and 2 play in the synthesis of cholesteryl esters targeted for storage or secretion.[27]

DGAT1

DGAT1 is a member of the membrane-bound O-acyltransferase (MBOAT) family that includes acyl CoA: cholesterol acyltransferases 1 and 2 responsible for the intracellular synthesis of cholesterol esters.[28] Members of this enzyme family share a series of membrane-spanning regions (6–12 in the case of DGAT1) and catalyse the transfer of organic acids, such as fatty acids, onto membrane-bound hydroxylated targeted molecules, such as cholesterol and diacylglycerol.[28] The enzyme is active as a homotetramer,[29] although the significance of this is unknown. The orientation of the active site is unknown, although the role of DGAT1 in mammary and white adipose tissue[24] and apparent lack of a role in lipoprotein secretion[30] suggests the role of the enzyme is synthesizing cytoplasmic fat stores.

DGAT1 has been shown to be expressed in all tissues examined, with expression in the liver and small intestine being the greatest.[25] Since these tissues synthesize lipoproteins, it was anticipated that DGAT1 was involved in synthesizing TG for lipoprotein assembly. The *Dgat1−/−* (knockout) mouse, however, had normal plasma levels of TG, demonstrating that there was no strict requirement of *Dgat1* expression for lipoprotein production, although there was an effect of DGAT1 deficiency on the rate of intestinal fat absorption. Thus a second TG-synthesizing enzyme, presumably DGAT2, is required for TG targeted for secretion or can compensate for lack of DGAT1. We found that hepatic overexpression of DGAT1 in wild-type mice, which would be expected to increase hepatic TG synthesis, resulted in TG accumulation in liver but did not have an effect on VLDL TG or apoB production.[30] This indicates that the presence of TG is necessary but not sufficient for VLDL secretion.

In addition to decreased hepatic TG content, the *Dgat1* knockout mouse displays a decreased TG content within many other tissues, including white adipose tissue.[19] Interestingly, this mouse model of *Dgat1* deficiency has increased sensitivity to both leptin and insulin and is resistant to diet-induced obesity due to increased energy expenditure.[20] Post-partum-*Dgat1* knockout mice were defective in their lactation and unable to support pups. The lactation defect has recently been determined to be probably due to developmental defects resulting from disrupted cellular lipid signalling pathways.[31] *Dgat1* knockout mice of both sexes also displayed skin and hair follicle abnormalities, probably related to the lack of triglyceride as a component in skin oil.[32] DGAT1 overexpression in an adipocyte cell line resulted in increased cytoplasmic fat stores, consistent with a role in regulating cytoplasmic triglyceride stores.[33] DGAT1 expression is stimulated by glucose,[34] which would act to increase fat deposition in adipose tissue in response to feeding, although the specific glucose-sensitive response element has not been identified. It would be of interest to determine whether there is an inverse regulation of DGAT1 expression in hepatic and non-hepatic tissues since hepatic triglyceride levels are greatest during prolonged fasting and lowest during fed conditions. A polymorphism in the DGAT1 gene (K232A) has been reported in the bovine homologue of DGAT1.[35] This polymorphism affects enzyme activity by reducing the V_{max} and

consequently results in a lower milk yield from carriers of this polymorphism. The lysine at this position is conserved in the human enzyme and thus may influence DGAT1 activity in humans. Taken together, these results indicate a role of DGAT1 in synthesis of cytoplasmic TG for storage or export in milk with little or no role in regulating the production rate of lipoproteins in liver.

DGAT2

DGAT2, structurally unrelated to DGAT1,[25] is a second enzyme that catalyses the acylation of diacylglycerol using a fatty acyl CoA substrate. DGAT2 is also membrane-bound within the ER and has two to four putative membrane-spanning regions.[25] DGAT2 is a member of the DGAT2/monoacylglycerol: acyltransferase (MOGAT) family that includes monoacylglycerol and wax ester acyltransferase members.[36] Like members of the MBOAT family that includes DGAT1, the DGAT2-related enzymes catalyse the acylation of hydroxylated acceptor molecules using a fatty acyl CoA substrate.[25] Similar to DGAT1, DGAT2 has been shown to be expressed in all tissues examined, with the expression in liver, white adipose tissue, mammary tissue and peripheral leukocytes being the greatest.[25] Relative to DGAT1, DGAT2 is more sensitive to magnesium concentration, which allows one to estimate individual in vitro DGAT activity in tissues.[25] The high expression in liver indicated a potential role for DGAT2 in regulating lipoprotein production. DGAT2 overexpression in mouse liver increases hepatic TG content to a greater extent than DGAT1 and appears to have a small effect on VLDL TG but not apoB production (Millar, unpublished). The decreased plasma lipid levels seen in *Dgat2*-deficient mouse pups[21] indicate that plasma lipoprotein production can be lowered through DGAT2 inhibition by reducing hepatic TG levels to the extent that lipid becomes rate-limiting for VLDL production. However, increasing hepatic TG stores above normal levels has minimal impact on VLDL production. Under these conditions, there are sufficient lipid levels for lipoprotein production, indicating factors other than triglyceride (such as microsomal triglyceride transfer protein) are rate-limiting for VLDL production.[37] The *Dgat2* knockout mouse, although not viable for more than 24 hours following birth, shows a markedly decreased TG content of tissue, including liver and adipose tissue.[21] The rapid onset of death in these mice following birth appears to be, in part, a result of skin barrier abnormalities that cause rapid dehydration and energy depletion due to decreased fat stores. However, rearing in a humidified environment combined with saline injections to prevent dehydration only prolongs the lifespan by a few hours, suggesting that other factors contribute to their premature demise.

INVESTIGATIONS INVOLVING GENE KNOCKOUTS, POLYMORPHISMS AND KNOWN INHIBITORS OF DGAT1 AND DGAT2

The inhibition of one or both DGAT enzymes, and thereby the major pathway of TG synthesis, is a possible pharmacological strategy for treatment of hyperlipidaemia, obesity and diabetes. Much of the evidence supporting DGAT1 as a therapeutic target was learned from the disruption of the *Dgat1* gene.[19] Unexpectedly, on a chow diet, the DGAT1 knockout mouse had normal plasma TG levels and near-normal tissue TG levels, indicating other pathways of TG synthesis. The normal plasma TG led investigators to search for and find a second TG synthesizing enzyme, DGAT2,[25] to be integral for supplying TG for lipoprotein production (see below). However, the *Dgat1⁻/⁻* mice, when fed a high-fat diet, were resistant to dietary-induced obesity.[19] A 40% decrease in total body TG accounted for the weight loss with no reduction in total body protein mass. This effect did not appear to be due to fat malabsorption but due, in part, to an increase in metabolic rate resulting from increased activity. It should be noted that subsequent studies revealed a delayed fat absorption, such that a decrease in post-prandial triglyceride response

was observed in the *Dgat1⁻/⁻* mice.[38] Elevated levels of chylomicron remnants in plasma are known to be highly atherogenic and DGAT1 inhibition may therefore be expected to decrease the peak plasma concentration of chylomicrons and their remnants.[4]

In addition to observations regarding the lack of changes in lipoprotein levels, the *Dgat1* knockout mouse was reported to have a low TG content of the adipose tissue due to a decrease in adipocyte size, not reduced number.[19] Increased adipocyte size has been associated with insulin resistance and, indeed, the *Dgat1* knockout mice demonstrate an increase in insulin sensitivity.[20] Recent studies suggest that the endocrine function of white adipose tissue plays a role in the increased insulin sensitivity as well as the increased energy expenditure.[39] The transplantation of *Dgat1*-deficient white adipose tissue into wild-type mice enhances glucose disposal.[40] A two-fold increase in adiponectin, an adipokine that increases fatty acid oxidation and insulin sensitivity, was observed in these mice.[40] In contrast, overexpression of DGAT1 in rat pancreatic cells resulted in an increase in cellular TG content and reduced insulin secretion in response to glucose.[41] The *Dgat1⁻/⁻* mice also show an increase in leptin sensitivity.[20] Leptin, an adipokine synthesized by adipose tissue, interacts with satiety centres in the brain and is involved in the maintenance of whole-body TG stores[42] and, hence, body weight. Much of the overall effect on whole-body TG metabolism observed in *Dgat1⁻/⁻* mice appears to relate to changes in adipose metabolism.

While DGAT1 deficiency has not been described in humans, polymorphisms of the *DGAT1* gene and promoter have been identified.[43–45] As previously mentioned, one such polymorphism (K232A) has been shown to reduce the V_{max} of the enzyme and has a significant effect on milk fat yield in dairy cattle,[43] with carriers having a relatively low content of milk fat. Comparison of the bovine sequence to the human sequence shows the wild-type residue in the human sequence as lysine. This makes this an attractive polymorphism to test for in human studies. Ludwig et al identified a

DGAT1 promoter polymorphism (C→T at base −79) in the Turkish population which showed reduced promoter activity in cultured cells.[44] In Turkish women (but not men) this polymorphism was associated with lower body mass index (BMI). However, when obese French subjects were analysed in a similar study, there was no association with body weight.[45]

While reduced DGAT1 activity has the potential benefit of reducing body weight, a total absence of DGAT1 activity has some undesirable consequences. Female *Dgat1* knockout mice do not produce milk and subsequent studies have demonstrated that DGAT1 activity is necessary for normal development of mammary tissue.[24,31] Also, starting at puberty, the hair of the *Dgat1* knockout animals has a dry appearance and subsequently falls out, beginning on the dorsal surface of the neck.[24] Similarly, the skin of older knockout mice has atrophied sebaceous glands, oil-producing glands within hair follicles, and abnormal lipid composition of fur oils.

The fact that the *Dgat1* knockout mice maintained normal plasma TG levels led to the discovery of a second enzyme, DGAT2, capable of synthesizing TG from diacylglycerol. Recently, a *Dgat2* knockout mouse was described.[21] The knockout of the DGAT2 gene led to more severe consequences than did knocking out *Dgat1*. The *Dgat2*[−/−] mice are lipopenic, have severe skin abnormalities and die within 24 hours of birth. The plasma TG and FA content in the newborn *Dgat2* knockout mice was decreased by 70–90%. Total carcass and hepatic TG was also decreased by 90%, indicating that DGAT1 is unable to compensate for DGAT2 deficiency. TG is a normal component of skin and is one of the lipids which act as permeability barrier. DGAT2 activity is required for proper barrier function because there was a rapid loss of weight in the newborn mice that suggested dehydration due to increased transdermal water loss. It is worth noting that DGAT1 is undetectable in dermis and epidermis of neonatal *Dgat2* knockout mice. The *Dgat2* knockout newborns are much smaller than their litter mates and knockout embryos had an 86% decrease in tissue TG, suggesting that one cause of death may be related to improper fetal development. Studies with liver-specific knockout or knockdown of *Dgat2* would clarify the picture as to the role of hepatic DGAT2 in the adult animal. The role of DGAT2 in skin is also evident in humans; a recent study found that DGAT2 mRNA was decreased by two-thirds in psoriatic skin compared to normal skin.[46] Partial liver-specific inhibition of DGAT2 may lead to a beneficial profile regarding lipoprotein metabolism, while preventing adverse effects of DGAT2 inhibition in other tissues. While single nucleotide polymorphisms of the DGAT2 gene have been reported, the effects of these polymorphisms on DGAT2 activity have not been investigated.

Several naturally occurring compounds, including chalcone,[47] roselipins,[48] prenylflavonoids,[49] polyacetylenes,[50] amidepsines[51] and tashinones,[52] and synthetic compounds, benzoxiperones[53] and N-(7,10-dimethyl-11-oxo-10,11-dihydro-dibenzo[b,f][1,4]oxazepin-2-yl-4-hydroxy-benzamide,[54] have been shown to be non-specific inhibitors of DGAT activity. None are very active, having IC_{50}s in the micromolar range. One of these, xanthumol, has been associated with a reduction in TG and apoB secretion in HepG2 cells,[55] although microsomal triglyceride transfer protein levels, which were also reduced, may be responsible for this change. Most compounds were identified in microsomal systems containing both DGAT1 and DGAT2 isozymes and specificity towards individual isotypes has not been tested. Because the two isozymes are from different gene families, some specificity is expected. A 96-well plate assay has been developed which may aid in the identification of the potent and specific inhibitors needed for proof of principle studies.[54]

CURRENT THERAPY

There are three compound classes (niacin, fibrates and statins) for the treatment of hyper-triglyceridaemia. Niacin (nicotinic acid) has been shown to lower plasma TG levels 20 to 50% in several clinical trials (see review 56). Niacin is not well tolerated but the newer extended-release formulation, Niaspan®, may result in fewer side-effects and better compliance. The exact mechanism of action of niacin is not well understood but is thought to involve, in part, a decrease in TG synthesis. A recent article demonstrates that niacin is an inhibitor (albeit a weak one) of DGAT2, which could explain the decrease in TG synthesis.[57]

The fibrate class of therapeutic agents, which act to reduce plasma TG and increase HDL-C with minimal effect on LDL-C, have been shown to decrease disease progression.[58] Fibrates are ligands of peroxisome proliferator activated receptor alpha (PPAR-α) whose activation induces enzymes in fatty acid oxidation. Oxidation of fatty acids would decrease their availability for TG synthesis and secretion.[59]

The recently available, more potent statins have been shown to reduce plasma TG levels. The extent of plasma TG lowering is dependent on the baseline TG level and the % LDL cholesterol lowering achieved.[60] Statin therapy de-represses/induces the LDL-R which recognizes both apoB- and apoE-containing lipoproteins. This could result in increased removal of TG-containing VLDL remnants through binding of apoE to LDL-R. The three classes of TG-lowering compounds have individual side-effects and may be more beneficial for specific patient populations.

Presently there are two types of anti-obesity drugs, those that affect fat absorption (pancreatic lipase inhibitors) and centrally acting appetite suppressants such as sibutramine. Neither is especially effective and the uses of both are limited by side-effects.[61]

THE THERAPEUTIC POTENTIAL OF DGAT INHIBITION

The potential of therapeutic agents that can inhibit or reduce the expression of DGAT1 and DGAT2 is promising. These compounds have the potential to simultaneously reduce diet-induced obesity, increase insulin sensitivity and normalize plasma lipid levels (summarized in Table 1). An additional potential benefit that might be observed is a reduction of hepatic lipotoxicity observed in steatosis. Treatment of patients with hepatic steatosis may reduce their risk of developing hepatitis resulting from

Table 1 The cytotoxic effects of triglyceride (TG) excess in various tissues and the expected benefits or adverse effects of decreasing the tissue TG content through DGAT1 and DGAT2 inhibition

Tissue	Role of TG	Effect of excess triglyceride	Expected effect of DGAT inhibition
Liver	Lipoprotein synthesis Energy storage	Lipotoxicity Insulin resistance Inflammation	Reduced VLDL production
Adipose	Energy storage	Obesity Secondary insulin resistance	Decreased obesity and secondary sequelae
Intestine	Lipoprotein synthesis	Increased chylomicron production	Reduced chylomicron production Decreased post-prandial triglyceridaemia
Pancreas	Energy source Source of lipid for signalling	Lipotoxicity leading to decreased insulin secretion Lipoapoptosis	Normalized insulin secretion
Muscle	Energy source	Insulin resistance	Improved insulin sensitivity
Mammary	Milk component	Fat-enriched milk?	Decreased milk fat content
Skin	Water barrier component	Cytotoxicity?	Psoriasis and other skin barrier defects

cytotoxic effects, although this remains to be tested.

Despite these likely desirable effects of DGAT1 and DGAT2 inhibition, the utility of such inhibition may be limited by adverse effects of reducing activity and/or expression of these enzymes. Obviously, decreasing the synthesis of total TG to the extent that the supply of energy to tissues for basal metabolism is compromised, similar to that observed in the *Dgat2* knockout mice, would be deleterious. The extent of DGAT inhibition required for a beneficial effect versus that which shows toxicity (therapeutic index) is not known. Little is known about the potential harmful effects which may occur due to increased levels of the TG precursors, diacylglycerol (DAG) and fatty acid due to DGAT inhibition. DAG is an activator of protein kinase C (PKC) and PKC activation has been associated with the development of diabetic complications.[62] The accumulation of intracellular saturated fatty acids in several cell lines has been shown to be lipotoxic and, in fact, under these conditions increasing TG synthesis would reduce the level of saturated fatty acid and improve tissue function.[63] Whether DAG or fatty acids would accumulate or be shunted into other pathways such as phospholipid synthesis and fatty acid oxidation is unknown. Interestingly, in the *Dgat1* knockout mouse, the concentration of DAG in white adipose tissue and skeletal muscle is unchanged and the level is actually decreased in liver.[20] While much has been learned about DGAT1 and DGAT2 since their initial descriptions less than 5 years ago, some basic questions remain to be answered. Do DGAT1 and DGAT2 have separate and/or overlapping functions? Are there tissue-specific functions? Is the triglyceride produced by DGAT1 metabolically distinct from that produced by DGAT2? Can the two DGATs compensate for each other? Are potential adverse effects specific to the individual DGAT or seen with inhibition of either enzyme? The answer to this final question would determine whether a general DGAT inhibitor is sufficient or if there is a need for specific inhibitors. Answering these questions will probably require tissue-specific knockout or knockdown of DGAT1 and DGAT2 and/or the identification of a potent specific DGAT inhibitor. While DGAT inhibition looks promising, additional research is needed.

References

1. Murray D, Lopez A. Alternative projections of mortality and disability by cause 1990–2020: global burden of disease study. Lancet 1997; 349:1498–504

2. Grundy S. Hypertriglyceridemia, insulin resistance and the metabolic syndrome. Am J Cardiol 1999; 83:25F–9F

3. Expert Panel on Detection, Evaluation, and Treatment of High Blood Cholesterol in Adults, Executive Summary of the Third Report of the National Cholesterol Education Program (NCEP) Expert Panel on Detection, Evaluation, and Treatment of High Blood Cholesterol in Adults (Adult Treatment Panel III). JAMA 2001; 285:2486–97

4. Zilversmit DB. Atherogenic nature of triglycerides, postprandial lipidemia, and triglyceride-rich remnant lipoproteins. Clin Chem 1995; 41:153–8

5. Gianturco SH, Bradley WA. Pathophysiology of triglyceride-rich lipoproteins in atherothrombosis: cellular aspects. Clin Cardiol 1999; 22:117–14

6. Tall A. Plasma lipid transfer proteins. Ann Rev Biochem 1995; 64:235–57

7. Rader DJ. Regulation of reverse cholesterol transport and clinical Implications. Am J Cardiol 2003; 92:42J–9J

8. Must A, Spadno J, Coakley, et al. The disease burden associated with overweight and obesity. JAMA 1999; 282:1523–9

9. Shirai K. Obesity as the core of the metabolic syndrome and the management of coronary heart disease. Curr Med Res Opin 2004; 20:295–304

10. Spiegelman B, Choy L, Hotamisligil G, et al. Regulation of adipocyte gene expression in differentiation and syndromes of obesity/diabetes. J Biol Chem 1993; 268:6823–6

11. Perseghin G, Scifo P, De Cobelli F, et al. Intramyocellular triglyceride content is a determinant of in vivo insulin resistance in humans: a 1H–13C nuclear magnetic resonance spectroscopy assessment in offspring of type 2 diabetic parents. Diabetes 1999; 48:1600–6

12. Finck BN, Han X, Courtois M, et al. A critical role for PPARalpha-mediated lipotoxicity in the pathogenesis of diabetic cardiomyopathy: modulation by dietary fat content. Proc Natl Acad Sci USA 2003; 100:1226–31

13. Lupi R, Del Guerra S, Fierabracci V, et al. Lipotoxicity in human pancreatic islets and the protective effect of metformin. Diabetes 2002; 51:S134–7

14. Wanless IR, Shiota K. The pathogenesis of nonalcoholic steatohepatitis and other fatty liver diseases: a four-step model including the role of lipid release and hepatic venular obstruction in the progression to cirrhosis. Semin Liver Dis 2004; 24:99–106

15. Hulver MW, Lynis Dohm G. The molecular mechanism linking muscle fat accumulation to insulin resistance. Proc Nutr Soc 2004; 63:375–80

16. Mayerson AB, Hundal RS, Dufour S, et al. The effects of rosiglitazone on insulin sensitivity, lipolysis, and hepatic and skeletal muscle triglyceride content in patients with type 2 diabetes. Diabetes 2002; 51:797–802

17. van Wijk JP, de Koning EJ, Martens EP, et al. Thiazolidinediones and blood lipids in type 2 diabetes. Arterioscler Thromb Vasc Biol 2003; 23:1744–9

18. Poston, W, Foreyt, J. Sibutramine and the management of obesity. Exp Opin Pharmacother 2004; 5:633–42

19. Smith SJ, Cases S, Jensen DR, et al. Obesity resistance and multiple mechanisms of triglyceride synthesis in mice lacking Dgat. Nat Genet 2000; 25:87–90

20. Chen HC, Smith SJ, Ladha Z, et al. Increased insulin and leptin sensitivity in mice lacking acyl CoA: diacylglycerol acyltransferase 1. J Clin Invest 2002; 109:1049–55

21. Stone SJ, Myers HM, Watkins SM, et al. Lipopenia and skin barrier abnormalities in DGAT2–deficient mice. J Biol Chem 2003; 279:11767–76

22. Hamilton RL, Moorehouse A, Lear SR, et al. A rapid calcium precipitation method of recovering large amounts of highly pure hepatocyte rough endoplasmic reticulum. J Lipid Res 1999; 40:1140–7

23. Andersson M, Wettesten M, Boren J, et al. Purification of diacylglycerol: acyltransferase from rat liver to near homogeneity. J Lipid Res 1994; 35:535–45

24. Cases S, Smith SJ, Zheng YW, et al. Identification of a gene encoding an acyl CoA:diacylglycerol acyltransferase, a key enzyme in triacylglycerol synthesis. Proc Natl Acad Sci USA 1998; 95:13018–23

25. Cases S, Stone SJ, Zhou P, et al. Cloning of DGAT2, a second mammalian diacylglycerol acyltransferase, and related family members. J Biol Chem 2001; 276:38870–6

26. Owen MR, Corstorphine CC, Zammit VA. Overt and latent activities of diacylglycerol acytransferase in rat liver microsomes: possible roles in very-low-density lipoprotein triacylglycerol secretion. Biochem J 1997; 323:17–21

27. Lee R, Willingham M, Davis M, et al. Differential expression of ACAT1 and ACAT2 among cells within liver, intestine, kidney and adrenal of nonhuman primates. J Lipid Res 2000; 41:1991–2001

28. Hofmann K. A superfamily of membrane-bound O-acyltransferases with implications for wnt signaling. Trends Biochem Sci 2000; 25:111–2

29. Cheng D, Meegalla RL, He B, et al. Human acyl-CoA:diacylglycerol acyltransferase is a tetrameric protein. Biochem J 2001; 359:707–14

30. Millar JS, Tow B, Young SG, et al. Hepatic overexpression of murine acyl CoA :diacylglycerol acyltransferase (DGAT) has no effect on VLDL triglyceride or apoB production rate in vivo. Arterioscler Thromb Vasc Biol 2001; 21:78 (abstract)

31. Cases S, Zhou P, Shillingford JM, et al. Development of the mammary gland requires DGAT1 expression in stromal and epithelial tissues. Development 2004; 113:3047–55

32. Chen HC, Smith SJ, Tow B, et al. Leptin modulates the effects of acyl CoA:diacylglycerol acyltransferase deficiency on murine fur and sebaceous glands. J Clin Invest 2002; 109:175–81

33. Yu YH, Zhang Y, Oelkers P, et al. Posttranscriptional control of the expression and function of diacylglycerol acyltransferase-1 in mouse adipocytes. J Biol Chem 2002; 277:50876–84

34. Meegalla RL, Billheimer JT, Cheng D. Concerted elevation of acyl-coenzyme A:diacylglycerol acyltransferase (DGAT) activity through independent stimulation of mRNA expression of DGAT1 and DGAT2 by carbohydrate and insulin. Biochem Biophys Res Commun 2002; 298:317–23

35. Winter A, Kramer W, Werner FA, et al. Association of a lysine-232/alanine polymorphism in a bovine gene encoding acyl-CoA:diacylglycerol acyltransferase (DGAT1) with variation at a quantitative trait locus for milk fat content. Proc Natl Acad Sci USA 2002; 99:9300–5

36. Winter A, van Eckeveld M, Bininda-Emonds OR, et al. Genomic organization of the DGAT2/MOGAT gene family in cattle (Bos taurus) and other mammals. Cytogenet Genome Res 2003; 102:42–7

37. Hussain MM, Shi J, Dreizen P. Microsomal triglyceride transfer protein and its role in apoB-lipoprotein assembly. J Lipid Res 2003; 44:22–32

38. Buhman KK, Smith SJ, Stone SJ, et al. DGAT1 is not essential for intestinal triacylglycerol absorption or chylomicron synthesis. J Biol Chem 2002; 277: 25474–9

39. Guerre-Millo M. Adipose tissue and adipokines: for better or worse. Diabetes Metab 2004; 30:13–9

40. Chen HC, Jensen DR, Myers HM, et al. Obesity resistance and enhanced glucose metabolism in mice transplanted with white adipose tissue lacking acyl CoA:diacylglycerol acyltransferase 1. J Clin Invest 2003; 111:1715–22

41. Kelpe CL, Johnson LM, Poitout V. Increasing triglyceride synthesis inhibits glucose-induced insulin secretion in isolated rat islets of langerhans: a study using

adenoviral expression of diacylglycerol acyltransferase. Endocrinology 2002; 143:3326–32

42. Ahima RS, Osei SY. Leptin signaling. Physiol Behav 2004; 81:223–41

43. Grisart B, Coppieters W, Farnir F, et al. Positional candidate cloning of a QTL in dairy cattle: identification of a missense mutation in the bovine DGAT1 gene with major effect on milk yield and composition. Genome Res 2002; 12:222–31

44. Ludwig EH, Mahley RW, Palaoglu E, et al. DGAT1 promoter polymorphism associated with alterations in body mass index, high density lipoprotein levels and blood pressure in Turkish women. Clin Genet 2002; 62:68–73

45. Coudreau SK, Tounian P, Bonhomme G, et al. Role of the DGAT gene C79T single-nucleotide polymorphism in French obese subjects. Obes Res 2003; 11:1163–7

46. Wakimoto K, Chiba H, Michibata H, et al. A novel diacylglycerol acyltransferase (DGAT2) is decreased in human psoriatic skin and increased in diabetic mice. Biochem Biophys Res Commun 2003; 310:296–302

47. Tabata N, Ito M, Tomoda H, et al. Xanthohumols, diacylglycerol acyltransferase inhibitors, form Humulus lupulus. Phytochem 1997; 46:683–7

48. Tomoda H, Ohyama Y, Abe T, et al. Roselipins, inhibitors of diacylglycerol scyltransferase, produced by *Gliocladium roseum* KF-1040. J Antibiotics 1999; 52:689–94

49. Chung M, Rho M, Ko K, et al. In vitro inhibition of diacylglycerol acyl-transferase by prenylflavonoids from *Sophora flavescens*. Planta Med 2004; 70:258–60

50. Lee SW, Kim K, Rho M, et al. New polyacetylenes, DGAT inhibitors from the roots *Panax ginseng*. Planta Med 2004; 70:197–200

51. Tomoda H, Ito M, Tabata N, et al. Amidepsines, inhibitors of diacylglycerol acyltransferase produced by *Numicola* sp. FO-2942. J Antibiotics 1995; 48:937–41

52. Ko J, Ryu S, Kim Y, et al. Inhibitory activity of diacylglycerol acyltransferase by tashinones from the root of *Salvia miltiorrhiza*. Arch Pharm Res 2002; 25: 446–8

53. Burrows J, Block M, Burckett L, et al. Novel benzoxazepinone enzyme inhibitors of diacylglycerol acyl transferase. Nat Med Chem Symp 26th Virginia C-22 1998

54. Ramharack R, Spahr M. Diacylglycerol acyltransferase (DGAT) assay. US Patents 6607893. August 19, 2003.

55. Casaschi A, Maiyoh G, Rubio B, et al. The chalcone xanthohumol inhibits triglyceride and apolipoprotein B secretion in Hep G2 cells. J Nutr 2004; 134: 1340–6

56. McKenney J. New perspectives on the use of niacin in the treatment of lipid disorders. Arch Intern Med 2004; 164:697–703

57. Ganji S, Tavintharan S, Zhu D, et al. Niacin noncompetitively inhibits diacylglycerol acyltransferase-2 (DGAT2) but not DGAT1 activity in HepG2 cells. J Lipid Res 2004; 45:1835–45

58. Ginsburg H. Hypertriglyceridemia: new insights and new approaches to pharmacologic therapy. Am J Cardiol 2001; 87:1174–9

59. Francis G, Fayrd E, Picard F, et al. Nuclear receptors and the control of metabolism. Annu Rev Physiol 2003; 65:261–311

60. Stein E, Lane M, Laskarzewski P. Comparison of statins in hypertriglyceridemia. Am J Cardiol 1998; 81:66B–9B

61. Kopelman P, Grace C. New thoughts on managing obesity. Gut 2004; 53:1044–53

62. Koya D, King G. Protein kinase C activation and the development of diabetic complications. Diabetes 1998; 47:859–66

63. Listenberger LL, Han X, Lewis SE, et al. Triglyceride accumulation protects against fatty acid-induced lipotoxicity. Proc Natl Acad Sci USA 2003; 100:3077–82

The biochemical and physiological roles of ACAT1 and ACAT2 in cholesterol homeostasis and atherosclerosis

4

R.G. Lee and L.L. Rudel

INTRODUCTION TO ACAT

Two isoforms of the enzyme known as acyl coenzyme A:cholesterol acyltransferase (ACAT, E.C. 2.3.1.26) have been identified. The official name of these enzymes is sterol *o*-acyltransferase (SOAT), but the enzymes are much more widely known as ACAT and this name will be used throughout this chapter. Both isoforms, ACAT1 and ACAT2, are integral membrane proteins localized to the endoplasmic reticulum and catalyse the reaction in which cholesterol and long-chain fatty acyl CoA molecules are converted into a cholesteryl ester molecule.[1] This conversion to cholesteryl ester limits the solubility of cholesterol in a phospholipid bilayer from a 1:1 molar ratio to a 1:50 cholesteryl ester to phospholipid molar ratio.[2,3] This decrease in solubility facilitates the storage of cholesteryl esters in lipid droplets and prevents cytotoxicity due to build up of cholesterol in membranes, making the ACAT reaction essential in maintaining intracellular cholesterol balance.[4] A key event in the pathology of atherosclerosis is the accumulation of cholesteryl esters in the arterial intima, often first appearing in macrophage-derived foam cells. Accordingly, the inhibition of ACAT, particularly in arterial macrophages, has long been considered a pharmaceutical target. However, the following discussion will provide evidence that the most effective ACAT inhibition to prevent atherosclerosis is probably not in the macrophage, a site of ACAT1. Rather, the gene deletion of ACAT2, the isoform primarily expressed in hepatocytes and enterocytes, has been found to be more effective in limiting atherogenesis in mouse models, a finding recommending ACAT2 as a preferred target.

IDENTIFICATION OF THE ACYLTRANSFERASE GENE FAMILY

While the ACAT reaction was first described in liver in 1957,[5] the inability to purify an active form of ACAT from membranes has been a major hurdle for studies of the enzyme for over 35 years.[6] This obstacle was partially alleviated in 1993 when TY Chang and colleagues used somatic cell genetics to clone ACAT1 by transfecting human macrophage genomic DNA into ACAT-deficient CHO (AC29) cells.[7] Cells were then screened for cholesterol esterification activity, and the source DNA for the enzymatic activity was identified. The Chang group was able to isolate a 4 kb gene that, when transfected into AC29 cells, increased cholesterol esterification activity by 20-fold.[8] This seminal work in the Chang laboratory provided the essential tool, the ACAT1 cDNA sequence, for the many subsequent molecular studies that have contributed to our understanding of the structure and function of ACAT enzymes.

After the identification of ACAT1, Robert Farese Jr and colleagues[9,10] generated and characterized an ACAT1 knockout mouse, and unexpectedly found that while cholesterol esterification was ablated in the adrenal of the ACAT$^{-/-}$ mice, it was essentially unchanged in the liver and small intestine, suggesting that at least one additional ACAT enzyme was present in these tissues.[9,10] The cloning of two ACAT isoforms from the yeast genome at about the same time by Yang et al[11] further supported the possibility that more than one ACAT isoform existed. To follow up on the experiments done in yeast, these workers identified two expressed sequence tags that exhibited sequence similarity to regions within the human ACAT1 gene. The first sequence was subsequently identified as a part of the acyl coenzyme A:diacylglycerol acyltransferase (DGAT) gene, an enzyme that catalyses the reaction in which an acyl CoA is esterified to a diacylglcyerol molecule, resulting in a triacylglycerol product.[12] The second sequence was later identified as a part of the ACAT2 gene in monkeys, mice and humans.[13-15] The ACAT2 gene product increased cholesterol esterification activity by almost 200-fold when transfected into AC29 cells.[13] A key difference between the ACAT1 and ACAT2 isoforms was discovered when Northern blots from 17 non-human primate tissues were probed with isoform-specific radioprobes. ACAT1 mRNA was present in all tissues examined, but ACAT2 mRNA was present primarily in the liver and small intestine.[13] Despite the sequence differences in the three enzymes, the shared ability to transfer acyl chains from coenzyme A to an acceptor substrate permitted the ACAT1, ACAT2 and DGAT1 enzymes to be identified collectively as members of the acyltransferase gene family.[16]

CHROMOSOMAL LOCATION AND GENE STRUCTURE OF ACAT1 AND ACAT2

Chang and colleagues mapped the human ACAT1 gene and concluded that the gene is made up of 17 exons found on two different chromosomes.[17] Exon 1, which makes up 90% of the 5' untranslated region (UTR), is found on chromosome 7, while the rest of the gene is found on chromosome 1, band q25. They concluded that the mRNAs produced from the two chromosomes then combine to form the full-length mRNA by a novel, as yet undefined trans-splicing event. This full-length mRNA consists of a 1396 bp 5' UTR, a 1.65 kb coding region and a 963 bp 3' UTR that codes for a protein consisting of 550 amino acids. Upon Northern analysis, a heterogeneous banding pattern for ACAT1 mRNA is typically found in almost all tissues.[13] The four-band pattern is similar in most tissues, with bands at approximately 2.0, 2.6, 3.0 and 3.6 kb. The significance of the presence of the first exon on a different chromosome from the rest of the gene remains unknown.

The sequence of the human ACAT2 gene has been determined by two different groups.[18,19] Both groups suggest a more traditional gene map for ACAT2 made up of 15 exons spanning over 18–21 kb of genomic DNA on chromosome 12. The full-length 2040 bp hACAT2 mRNA is made of a 51 bp 5' UTR, a 1.569 kb coding region and a 420 bp 3' UTR that encodes a protein of 522 amino acids. The position of the ACAT2 gene on chromosome 12 places it only about 1300 nucleotide residues downstream of the insulin-like growth factor binding protein-6 structural gene, so that the 5' non-coding region is relatively truncated.[19] In this region, the presence of Cdx-2 binding regions has been identified[20] which could confer the intestine-specific expression that has been noted for ACAT2. Also present in the promoter region HNF-1α and C/EBP-β transcriptional elements and at least the former is likely to be responsible for expression of this enzyme in hepatocytes (Pramfalk et al, manuscript in revision). In a limited epidemiological study of the hACAT2 gene, 91 dyslipidaemic patients were screened for mutations in the ACAT2 gene.[18] Two mutations were found (E14G, T254I) in the coding region. The only phenotypic change observed in the patients possessing the T254I mutation was an increase in apoC-III levels, which has been shown to be an inhibitor of lipoprotein lipase.[21] Even though these elevated apoC-III levels did not result in significant changes in plasma triglyceride levels, further investigation using larger cohorts is required to determine whether mutations in the ACAT2 gene alter plasma lipid and lipoprotein parameters.

The chromosomal location of ACAT1, ACAT2 and DGAT1 in the genome of three non-human primate species has recently been described by in situ hybridization.[22] In the African green monkey, the cynomolgus monkey and the squirrel monkey, each enzyme was found to be in chromosomal regions homologous to those in humans.

STRUCTURAL STUDIES OF ACAT1 AND ACAT2

The comparison of the primary amino acid sequences of primate ACAT1 and ACAT2 proteins has yielded several important insights into the enzyme's structure and function. Comparison of the full-length proteins revealed that the N-terminal 100 amino acids had no sequence similarity, while the remaining C-terminal amino acids had 63% sequence similarity. It has been hypothesized that the unique N-terminal amino acids could be important in the distinct properties of the two isoforms.[15] In an effort to elucidate some of these unique properties, the N-terminal 34 amino acids were deleted from the ARE-2 enzyme, the yeast analogue of ACAT.[23] Significantly decreased activity levels resulted for the truncated protein compared to the wild-type enzyme and this finding led the investigators to speculate that this portion of the protein may play a regulatory role, although further investigation is necessary. In an effort to learn more about the location of the active sites of ACAT1 and ACAT2, Sturley and colleagues[23] compared the amino acid sequences of acyltransferases from several different species that esterify oleoyl-CoA to either sterol (ACAT-like reaction) or diacylglycerol (DGAT-like reaction). All of the acyltransferases had one highly conserved motif consisting of a FY × DWWN heptapeptide that was hypothesized to function in the binding of the oleoyl-CoA molecule. All of the sterol acyltransferases had

another highly conserved motif consisting of an H(Y)SF tripeptide that could function in the binding of the sterol acceptor molecule. Mutation of either of the two conserved motifs in ACAT1 or ACAT2 led to ablation of activity, with no change in protein expression, supporting the hypothesized role of these sites in enzyme activity.

When ACAT1 and ACAT2 were originally cloned, their amino acid sequences were analysed by computer software to determine the probable membrane topology of the two enzymes based on the grouping of hydrophobic amino acids.[8,13] Based on computer predictions that both enzymes had seven to eight transmembrane domains, two different groups have experimentally determined the topology of the two enzymes. Using truncation mutants containing reporter glycosylation sequences inserted after predicted transmembrane domains, Joyce et al[24] found that both enzymes had five transmembrane domains, with the N-terminus of both enzymes in the cytosol of the cell and the C-terminus in the lumen. The DWWN sites were found on the cytoplasmic side for both enzyme models and the H(Y)SF motif was found on the cytoplasmic side of the ACAT1 topology model and on the luminal side of the ACAT2 topology model. The functional significance of this putative active site being on opposite sides of the ER membrane for the two isoforms has yet to be addressed experimentally. Lin et al[25,26] used epitopes inserted after the putative transmembrane domains to construct an entirely different topology model with ACAT1 possessing seven transmembrane domains and ACAT2 possessing only two transmembrane domains. In the Lin topology models, the DWWN and H(Y)SF regions were on the cytoplasmic side of the ER membrane for both enzymes. The experimental methods used by both groups have been used effectively by others,[27–30] making it difficult to determine whether either group's topology model is correct. Any discrepancy in the number and/or locations of utilized transmembrane domains between ACAT1 vs ACAT2 is curious given such high sequence homology (60%) in the predicted transmembrane regions of the two proteins. However, in at least one of the studies[24] the topology for either enzyme was analysed simultaneously with several methods and differences in the utilization of some of the transmembrane domains by ACAT1 and ACAT2 were still predicted.

In the early 1990s, two groups developed data to suggest that the minimum molecular mass of ACAT in rat liver microsomes was between 170 and 224 kDa.[31,32] These data contrast to the apparent molecular weights based on a primary sequence of about 66 000 kDa for ACAT1 and 63 000 kDa for ACAT2, and the apparent molecular weights as seen upon SDS gel electrophoresis of about 50 000 kDa for ACAT1 and 47 000 kDa for ACAT2.[33] The enzymes are not apparently glycosylated,[13] so the reason for the smaller estimate from SDS electrophoresis is unknown. Despite the fact that the experiments did not discern between ACAT1 and ACAT2, it did point to the possibility that one or both of the enzymes existed in an oligomeric state. To investigate the oligomerization of ACAT1, Chang and colleagues performed sedimentation and cross-linking studies on detergent-solubilized enzyme and concluded that ACAT1 existed as a tetramer.[34] Although no studies have examined the oligomeric state of ACAT2, immunoprecipitation studies showed that ACAT1 and ACAT2 did not co-immunoprecipitate, suggesting that the two enzymes do not associate in a hetero-oligomeric state.[35] Experiments in which mutation of prolines in the N-terminal amino acids of the hACAT1 protein led to changes in the oligmerization state brought out the possibility that the isoform-specific oligomerization is due to the involvement of the unique N-terminal amino acids in the self-association of the two isoforms, and that the self-association may be involved in regulation of enzyme activity.[36]

STUDIES SUGGESTING FUNCTIONAL DIFFERENCES OF ACAT1 AND ACAT2

The localization of ACAT1 and ACAT2 mRNA in non-human primate tissues suggested that the two isoforms perform unique physiological functions. To further our knowledge of the location and associated function of the isoforms, antibodies specific for the N-terminal region of ACAT1 and ACAT2 were used to immunohistologically examine the adrenal, kidney, liver and small intestine of African green monkeys.[33] ACAT1 was found in the adrenal cortex, a finding supported by the observation that the adrenals of ACAT1 knock-out mice are depleted of cholesteryl ester (CE).[37] In the kidney, ACAT1 was localized to the distal tubules and podocytes of the kidney, and even though its function in this tissue is not well understood, studies have shown CE enrichment of the tubules during renal injury.[38] ACAT1 was localized within the Kupffer cells of the liver, and goblet cells, interstitial macrophages and Paneth cells of the small intestine, but was not found in the parenchymal cells. ACAT2 localization was limited to the hepatocytes in the liver and the apical portion of the enterocytes in the small intestine, which are both sites of assembly and secretion of apoB-containing lipoprotein particles.[39,40]

In spite of the lack of evidence that both enzymes exist in the same cell types in non-human primates, determination of the location of the isoforms in human liver has met with conflicting results. Immunolocalization experiments in human tissue taken 2 to 24 hours post-mortem found that ACAT1 was localized to the hepatocytes and Kupffer cells of the liver, while ACAT2 was found in fetal, but not adult, hepatocytes.[35,41] In these experiments it was difficult to ascertain the intracellular location of ACAT1 in liver due to low magnification and staining intensity of the images. When similar experiments were carried out in liver biopsies removed surgically from Swedish gallstone patients, the localization of ACAT1 and ACAT2 was identical to that found in non-human primate liver, i.e. ACAT2 was localized to the ER of the hepatocytes and ACAT1 to the ER of the Kupffer cells.[42] Assays with human liver microsomes were used to determine the portion of total ACAT activity that was due either to ACAT1 or to ACAT2. Incubation with the ACAT2–specific inhibitor, pyripyropene

A,[43] showed a 20–70% decrease in ACAT activity in human liver versus >90% inhibition in African green monkey liver microsomes. The data suggested that ACAT2 was responsible for the majority of ACAT activity in almost all liver samples, although relative amounts of ACAT2 activity were lower in human liver microsomes than in those of monkeys. The relative amounts of ACAT1 activity were the same for livers from humans and monkeys. ACAT1 and ACAT2 mRNA levels were quantified in the human livers by real-time PCR. The ratio of ACAT1 mRNA to ACAT2 mRNA was high in liver of both humans and monkeys, although monkeys had relatively higher ACAT2 mRNA levels. Recent studies in which ACAT mRNA was quantified in various human tissues by real-time PCR demonstrated that hepatic ACAT mRNA was 90% ACAT1 mRNA and 10% ACAT2 mRNA.[44] The data seem consistent in showing a relatively higher mRNA abundance for ACAT1 than ACAT2 and this difference is larger than the differences in activity and estimated protein mass for the two enzymes. In transfection studies using AC29 cells (R Temel and L Rudel, unpublished), the ACAT1 protein was found to be 5- to 7-fold more rapidly degraded than the ACAT2 protein. If a similar difference exists in the liver in vivo, then perhaps the relatively higher level of ACAT1 mRNA is related.

REGULATION OF ACAT1 AND ACAT2

Until recently, it was thought that neither ACAT gene was under transcriptional regulation. Despite the absence of detectable SRE[45,46] and LXR elements[47–49] in the 5' flanking regions there were several potential *cis* acting elements that may play a role in sterol dependent transcriptional regulation of the genes. Nevertheless, the only evidence for transcriptional regulation of the ACAT1 mRNA has been upregulation by interferon-γ in macrophages that might provide a partial explanation for some of the pro-atherogenic effects attributed to this cytokine.[50,51] Evidence

of transcriptional regulation of ACAT2 was first observed in vitro where HepG2 cells administered citrus flavonoids showed decreases in cholesterol esterification activity.[52] While the flavonoids inhibited both ACAT isoforms to the same degree, mRNA quantitation showed significant decreases of ACAT2 mRNA with no changes in ACAT1 mRNA. Further evidence for transcriptional regulation of ACAT2 was observed in recent and as yet unpublished studies (Parini, Angelin and Rudel, manuscript in preparation) in which, for 30 days, Swedish patients were administered either atorvastatin, a HMG CoA reductase inhibitor that lowered plasma cholesterol, or placebo. A liver biopsy was then surgically collected and RT-PCR measurements showed a 50% lower level of ACAT2 mRNA in patients receiving the atorvastatin when compared to controls, while ACAT1 mRNA levels were not different.

Additional evidence for transcriptional regulation of ACAT2 was generated when cultured rat hepatocytes were incubated with chylomicron remnants enriched in n-3 polyunsaturated fatty acids. Expression of ACAT2 mRNA dropped when compared to that in hepatocytes incubated with corn-oil-enriched chylomicron remnants.[53] Finally, it was shown that cynomolgus monkeys, a primate species highly responsive to dietary cholesterol challenge, had increased hepatic ACAT2 mRNA when fed a cholesterol-enriched vs low-cholesterol diet.[54] This evidence taken together suggests that ACAT2 may undergo some degree of transcriptional regulation. However, further investigation is required to define the mechanism and extent of this regulation.

Despite the recent evidence supporting a measure of transcriptional regulation of ACAT2, post-transcriptional regulation at both the protein and activity levels appears to be the predominant mechanism of sterol-dependent regulation for both ACAT isoforms. Evidence for post-transcriptional regulation at the activity level derives from studies of the kinetics showing that the cholesterol substrate saturation curves of both enzymes were found to be sigmoidal, raising the strong possibility that cholesterol is an allosteric activator of the

ACAT enzymes,[55] where binding of cholesterol causes a conformational/structural change that converts the enzyme from an inactive form to an active form. Studies by Cheng et al[56] supported this conclusion when they expressed human ACAT1 in Sf9 insect cells and showed that both cholesterol and 25-hydroxycholesterol acted as an ACAT activator in intact cells as well as in vitro.

Post-transcriptional regulation of ACAT1 and ACAT2 at the protein level was recently suggested by Rudel et al[54] when the livers from two species of non-human primate were analysed for total ACAT activity, mRNA abundance for ACAT1 and ACAT2, and ACAT1 and ACAT2 protein mass by quantitative western blotting. Highly dietary-cholesterol-sensitive cynomolgus monkeys and the less responsive African green monkeys were compared when fed either a cholesterol-enriched or low-cholesterol diet. ACAT activity was 75% higher when cholesterol was fed to cynos, but no difference occurred in greens. Given that over 90% of ACAT activity in monkey liver has been found to be due to ACAT2,[43] the increase in total ACAT activity induced by dietary cholesterol in cynomolgus monkeys was probably due to an increase in ACAT2 activity, and a high correlation was found when ACAT activity was correlated to ACAT2 protein mass.[54] No increase in hepatic ACAT2 message or protein in livers of the green monkeys occurred upon challenge with the cholesterol-enriched diet. In contrast, the livers of the cynomolgus monkeys showed an approximate 20% increase in ACAT2 mRNA and a 3-fold increase in ACAT2 protein when the cholesterol-enriched diet was fed. The disparity showing greater increases in protein than in mRNA led to the suggestion that much of the cholesterol-dependent regulation of the protein was post-transcriptional. The observation was made that the relative level of hepatic ACAT2 expression in humans and non-human primates (cynomolgus>African green>human) mirrors the degree of dietary cholesterol responsiveness. This finding has led to speculation that ACAT2 is potentially an important factor in the genetic sensitivity to diet-induced hypercholesterolaemia.

ACAT AND CHOLESTEROL ABSORPTION IN THE SMALL INTESTINE

For many years, it has been recognized that the majority of newly absorbed cholesterol transported in chylomicrons is esterified.[57] ACAT has long been hypothesized to participate in the esterification of cholesterol associated with intestinal cholesterol absorption and enzymatic activity was first demonstrated in rat intestinal mucosa in 1976 by Haugen and Norum.[58] The interest in cholesterol absorption and any role for ACAT is further supported by the correlation that exists between plasma cholesterol concentrations and percentage absorption.[59–62] Development of ACAT inhibitors has been attempted in the pharmaceutical industry for over 20 years.[63] Data suggesting a role for ACAT in cholesterol absorption have been generated by the administration of various ACAT inhibitors to different animal models. Many ACAT inhibitors have decreased intestinal cholesterol absorption, although such an effect has not always been seen in humans and in non-human primates (see review by Sliskovic et al[63,64]).

Most of this work was done before it was known that there are two isoforms of ACAT that must be considered. Linkage analysis of crosses between low and high cholesterol-absorbing mouse strains revealed seven trait loci that influence cholesterol absorption.[65] One locus mapped to the identical region of chromosome 15 where the ACAT2 gene is found, suggesting that regulation of ACAT2 may be involved in the cholesterol absorption pathway. Cholesterol absorption in ACAT1 knockout mice fed either chow or a high-cholesterol diet was not different from wild-type mice, arguing against a role for ACAT1 in cholesterol absorption.[9] However, when ACAT2 knockout mice were challenged with a high-fat, high-cholesterol diet, absorption of cholesterol decreased by 85% when compared to wild-type animals, although cholesterol absorption in chow-fed ACAT2 knockout mice did not show a decrease in cholesterol absorption.[66] This led to the conclusion that mice possess compensatory mechanisms that maintain basal levels of cholesterol absorption in the absence of ACAT2, but are unable to compensate when the animal is challenged with elevated levels of dietary cholesterol. In sum, the strength of the evidence for a role of ACAT2 in regulating intestinal cholesterol absorption is suggestive but not definitive.

Although potentially attractive, intestinal ACAT inhibition as a pharmacological target for plasma cholesterol lowering in humans has yet to be fully exploited. While the mechanism of intestinal cholesterol absorption is not fully understood at this time, a current model is that unesterified plant and animal sterols are transported in bile micelles across the unstirred water layer where they interact with the enterocytes of the duodenum and jejunum. Absorption occurs via a saturable process that is inhibited by ezetimibe (Zetia™), presumably through its effects to limit uptake into the enterocyte via the Niemann-Pick C1 Like 1 (NPC1L1) protein.[67] In the apical portion of the enterocyte, ACAT2 can readily esterify absorbed cholesterol for incorporation into the core of chylomicron particles during MTP-facilitated particle assembly. These lipoproteins are subsequently secreted into the lymph and travel through the blood until the cholesteryl esters are taken up by the liver.[68] Significant plasma LDL lowering with ezetimibe has been found which is additive to that seen with statin administration.[69] Efficacy for ezetimibe is not through any effect on ACAT, but the findings establish the attractiveness of cholesterol absorption inhibition as a target for plasma LDL cholesterol lowering, and ACAT2 represents such a target.

Recent in vitro studies done in AC29 cells stably expressing either ACAT1 or ACAT2 provided evidence of another important role of ACAT2 that may occur during the intestinal absorption of sterols.[70] In these experiments, microsomes isolated from either ACAT1- or ACAT2-expressing cells were loaded with either sitosterol or cholesterol using β-hydroxypropyl cyclodextrin. The mass ratio of esterified cholesterol to esterified sitosterol synthesized by ACAT1 was 1.6 in microsomes from ACAT1 cells and 7.2 in microsomes from

ACAT2 cells, indicating that ACAT2 exhibits significantly more selectivity than ACAT1 and favours the esterification of cholesterol. The authors suggested that ACAT2 could act as a 'gatekeeper' in the intestine that allows cholesterol to enter the circulation in the core of chylomicron particles, while the plant sterols that are not efficiently esterified by ACAT2 are effluxed back into the intestinal lumen via the ABCG5/G8 transporter.[71,72] The hypothesized role of the ABCG5/G8 transporter arises from the finding that mutations in the transporters lead to sitosterolaemia, a disease in which patients have elevated plasma concentrations of plant sterols.[73]

ACAT AND HEPATIC LIPOPROTEIN SECRETION

Over the last 10 years, several groups have investigated the role of ACAT in both CE enrichment and secretion of apoB-containing lipoprotein particles. Both cell culture and in vivo evidence suggest that CE availability may play a regulatory role in the secretion of apoB from cells. Several studies in HepG2 cells, a human hepatoma cell line, as well as in primary hepatocytes, show that chemical inhibition of ACAT decreases the secretion of apoB from the cells.[52,74–78] In vivo administration of ACAT inhibitors to pigs fed a high-cholesterol diet led to a 40% decrease in hepatic VLDL secretion, resulting in a 30% decrease in plasma VLDL cholesterol.[79] Selected ACAT inhibitors administered during perfusion of monkey livers led to significant decreases in both CE and apoB accumulation rates, with some decrease in triglyceride accumulation rates as well, although the patterns of effects on perfusate accumulation rates were specific to individual ACAT inhibitors.[80] Interestingly, none of the three different ACAT inhibitors was limited to specific effects only on CE secretion. A strong association across all three inhibitors was identified when the per cent decrease in apoB secretion was correlated to the per cent decrease in CE secretion. This finding supported a hypothesized role for ACAT2 in coupling CE enrichment with whole-particle secretion of apoB-containing lipoproteins.

Identification of pro-atherogenic properties of hepatic ACAT occurred when lipoprotein CE secretion was monitored for isolated, perfused livers of monkeys that had been fed various fatty-acid-enriched atherogenic diets for a period of 5 years.[81] Liver perfusate CE accumulation rates had highly significant positive correlations ($r \geq 0.8$) to coronary artery atherosclerosis extent. This suggested that the enzyme responsible for hepatic CE synthesis, now known to be ACAT2, was important in facilitating the progression of atherosclerosis. The association between hepatic CE secretion was equally strong in monkeys fed saturated and mono-unsaturated fatty acids, and this occurred in spite of the LDL-cholesterol lowering and higher HDL/LDL-cholesterol ratio in the mono-unsaturated fat group. The secretion of cholesteryl oleate as the primary CE was promoted by dietary mono-unsaturated fat and enrichment of plasma lipoproteins with cholesteryl oleate appeared to be a factor in the atherosclerosis outcome.[82] Studies in coronary heart disease (CHD) patients and controls have been published where the degree of cholesteryl linoleate enrichment in plasma has been found to be higher in controls than in patients.[83–87] The percentage of cholesteryl oleate was inversely associated with the percentage of cholesteryl linoleate, and this may signify that similar effects occur in humans and monkeys, i.e. when hepatic ACAT-derived cholesteryl oleate secretion is higher, more coronary heart disease is found.

ATHEROSCLEROSIS AND ACAT IN MACROPHAGES

A role for the cholesterol esterification reaction in the developing atherosclerotic lesion has long been known. In fact, the most prominent component of the atheromatous gruel from which atherosclerosis derives its name is cholesteryl ester. The original isolation of a cDNA for ACAT1 was from DNA derived from human macrophages.[8] In almost all studies where it has

been examined, ACAT1 has been found to be the enzyme present in macrophages including those associated with the artery wall.[13–15] The process of cholesterol accumulation in the arterial intima appears to follow from the infiltration of plasma LDL, with higher concentrations of plasma LDL promoting more arterial accumulation.[88] The data indicate that the cholesteryl linoleate of LDL is hydrolysed and resynthesized and cholesteryl oleate becomes the predominant CE in lesions. In this hydrolysis, resynthesis appears to involve ACAT1 in macrophages, with the esterification possibly representing conversion of excess amounts of cholesterol into cholesteryl ester, the physical form less damaging to cell membranes. The accumulation of higher melting cholesteryl esters (e.g. enrichment with cholesteryl oleate) in lesions would appear to result in greater accumulation through decreased mobilization.[82,89,90] The isoform of ACAT that participates in CE accumulation in atherogenesis has not been carefully documented in most studies, but since ACAT1 is found in almost all cell types in the artery wall, the evidence favours this enzyme isoform as the predominant player. In most cell types studied in tissue culture, ACAT1 is the isoform expressed. One report describing the appearance of ACAT2 in some cells of atherosclerotic lesions has appeared,[91] but the extent to which this was quantitatively significant was undefined. The factors in the promoters of the ACAT genes that determine tissue and cell type expression remain largely unstudied. It is of interest that, in vivo in most tissues, any one cell type appears to express only ACAT1 or ACAT2, and in some tissues such as the liver, for example, hepatocytes express ACAT2 while the adjacent Kupffer cells express ACAT1.[33] However, when hepatoma cells, such as HepG2 cells, are studied in tissue culture, both ACAT1 and ACAT2 are expressed.[77] Clearly, the factors regulating expression of the ACAT isoforms need to be identified to help us understand the physiological roles of these enzymes.

While it has long been accepted that the intracellular location of the majority of the ACAT enzymes is the membranes of the endoplasmic reticulum, Khelef et al[92] have shown that a small amount of ACAT1 is found in a paranuclear region of macrophages that does not co-localize with resident ER protein. Further characterization of the paranuclear ACAT showed that it was located in a region proximal to the *trans*-Golgi and the endocytic recycling compartment.[93] Because these two organelles are important in the trafficking of internalized cholesterol, it is conceivable that paranuclear ACAT1 may play an important role in the esterification of internalized cholesterol and therefore the development of foam cells. More information is needed to define this relationship.

ATHEROSCLEROSIS IN ACAT1 AND ACAT2 KNOCKOUT MICE

The pathophysiological significance of ACAT1 and ACAT2 in atherogenesis has been most convincingly demonstrated in the gene deletion studies done in mouse models of atherosclerosis where the relative contributions of the two enzymes to the progression of the disease have been studied. After the ACAT1 knockout mouse had been characterized,[9,10] the ACAT1 gene deletion was bred into mice with LDL receptor or apoE gene deletions by Accad et al[94] and by Yagyu et al[95] to examine the effect of the loss of ACAT1 on the development of atherosclerosis. One group fed a 0.15% cholesterol diet to the ACAT1$^{-/-}$, apoE$^{-/-}$ mice and a 1.25% cholesterol diet to the ACAT1$^{-/-}$, LDLr$^{-/-}$ mice for 90 days.[95] At the end of the study, total plasma cholesterol did not change significantly in the ACAT1$^{-/-}$, LDLr$^{-/-}$ mice when compared to ACAT1$^{+/+}$, LDLr$^{-/-}$ controls, but plasma cholesterol in the ACAT1$^{-/-}$ apoE$^{-/-}$ dropped by ~40% when compared to chow-fed animals. When atherosclerosis was measured as aortic CE content the ACAT1$^{-/-}$, LDLr$^{-/-}$ and ACAT1$^{-/-}$, apoE$^{-/-}$ showed decreases of 2-fold and 3-fold, respectively, when compared to controls.

However, the beneficial effects on atherosclerosis were counterbalanced by the dry eye syndrome and cutaneous xanthomatosis observed in the mice lacking ACAT1.

Histological examination of the eye revealed that atrophy of the meibomian glands, a modified sebaceous gland, caused the dry eye in the mice. That fact that ACAT1 is highly expressed in the sebaceous gland suggests that loss of the enzyme led to the inability of the meibomian gland to promote tearing. The cutaneous xanthomatosis was also a serious problem for the mice, causing loss of hair and lesions on the skin. Biochemical and histological examination of the skin revealed that 6- to 7-fold higher skin cholesterol levels had resulted in cholesterol crystal deposition and acute inflammation in the skin.[94] These investigators described the truncal skin as being essentially one massive cholesterol xanthoma.

In an effort to avoid the severe skin pathology observed in the ACAT1 knockout mice, Fazio et al[96] transplanted ACAT1$^{-/-}$ bone marrow into LDLr$^{-/-}$ mice. This procedure generated a mouse with ACAT1-deficient macrophages, but normal ACAT1 expression in other cells. These animals were then placed on a 0.15% cholesterol diet for 12 weeks, and atherosclerosis was measured as the percent of the aorta covered in lesion. Even though the mice with the ACAT1$^{-/-}$ macrophages did not exhibit the skin pathology or dry eye observed in the ACAT1$^{-/-}$ mice, they had 2- to 3-fold more plaque involvement than control mice. Staining of the aortas for macrophages showed that the mice with ACAT1$^{-/-}$ macrophages had fewer macrophages in their lesions than the control mice. It had been shown in tissue culture that inhibition of ACAT1 in macrophages exposed to cholesterol-rich lipoproteins can be cytotoxic due to the cell's inability to store cholesterol in lipid droplets.[4,97,98] To address the possibility that this could occur in vivo, the extent of apoptosis and necrosis in the aorta was examined by TUNEL staining. The mice with ACAT1$^{-/-}$ macrophages had 3-fold more apoptosis than the other mice.[99] Premature death of macrophages was cited by the authors as probably being the principal cause of the increased atherosclerosis in the mice.

Taken together, the results of these studies argue that while modest decreases in atherosclerosis associated with ACAT1 gene deletion were sometimes observed, the noteworthy accompanying negative side-effects in the eye and skin create considerable doubt as to the efficacy of ACAT1 as a pharmaceutical target. The data suggest that even the macrophage-specific ACAT1 deficiency may not lead to desirable decreases in foam cell accumulation and atherosclerosis.

By contrast, the results of studies in the ACAT2$^{-/-}$ mouse indicate that the gene deletion of the ACAT2 isoform is an effective anti-atherosclerotic strategy in mice with minor side-effects. Characterization of the ACAT2$^{-/-}$ mouse showed that ACAT activity in the liver and the small intestine was decreased by greater than 90%.[66] When a chow diet was fed for 3 weeks, plasma cholesterol values for the ACAT2$^{-/-}$ mice were unaffected. However, when these mice were fed the cholesterol, fat and cholate-rich Paigen diet for 3 weeks, plasma cholesterol was 56% less than in ACAT2$^{+/+}$ control mice. The authors speculated that the resistance to dietary cholesterol challenge was related to the >80% decrease in cholesterol absorption observed in the Paigen-diet-fed mice. Adverse side-effects were not observed in ACAT2-deficient mice fed either chow or Paigen diets. The effect of the ACAT2 gene deletion on atherosclerosis was examined by crossing it into the apoE$^{-/-}$ mouse.[100] Absence of ACAT2 in the apoE$^{-/-}$ mice led to a 60% decrease in plasma cholesterol and a 70% decrease in plasma CE when compared to ACAT2$^{+/+}$, apoE$^{-/-}$ controls. After 27 weeks on a chow diet the ACAT2$^{+/+}$, apoE$^{-/-}$ mice had 4.8 ± 2.9% of their aorta surface area covered in lesions compared to 0.1 ± 0.2% in the ACAT2$^{-/-}$, apoE$^{-/-}$ mice. The authors speculated that the loss of ACAT2 was athero-protective due to (1) the replacement of cholesteryl ester with triglyceride in the core of apoB-containing particles and (2) the depletion of pro-atherogenic cholesteryl esters, e.g. cholesteryl oleate, resulting in an enrichment of LCAT-derived CE, e.g. cholesteryl linoleate and cholesteryl arachidonate. Additional studies have recently been completed in LDLr$^{-/-}$, ACAT2$^{-/-}$ mice.[101] In this model, as in the apoE$^{-/-}$, ACAT2$^{-/-}$ mouse, the deficiency of ACAT2 protected the mice against the development of atherosclerosis (aortic lesion surface areas of 1 vs 5% and CE concentrations of 3 vs 25 mg/g protein in ACAT2$^{-/-}$ vs ACAT2$^{+/+}$, LDLr$^{-/-}$ mice, respectively).

CONCLUDING REMARKS

The discovery of the first ACAT gene sequence occurred only about 10 years ago, but the explosion of new knowledge about ACAT1 and ACAT2 in the intervening period of time has been significant. We have tried to discuss many of the discoveries that have contributed to our present understanding of the biochemical and physiological roles of these enzymes in cholesterol homeostasis. In most cases, more information is needed for us to be certain about isoform specificity and associated molecular mechanisms surrounding ACAT-mediated cholesterol esterification as it affects a physiological or pathophysiological process, e.g. intestinal cholesterol absorption and atherosclerosis. Nevertheless, the information that is now available has brought us to a higher level of understanding and has provided a solid database upon which to develop hypotheses for future experimentation.

References

1. Chang TY, Chang CCY, Cheng D. Acyl-coenzyme A: Cholesterol acyltransferase. Annu Rev Biochem 1997; 66:613–38

2. Hamilton JA, Small DM. Solubilization and localization of cholesteryl oleate in egg phosphatidylcholine vesicles. A carbon 13 NMR study. J Biol Chem 1982; 257:7318–21

3. Small DM, Shipley GG. Physical-chemical basis of lipid deposition in atherosclerosis. Science 1974; 185:222–9

4. Warner GJ, Stoudt G, Bamberger M, et al. Cell toxicity induced by inhibition of acyl coenzyme A:cholesterol acyltransferase and accumulation of unesterified cholesterol. J Biol Chem 1995; 270:5772–8

5. Goodman DS, Deykin D, Shiratori T. The formation of cholesterol esters with rat liver enzymes. J Biol Chem 1964; 239:1335–45

6. Doolittle GM, Chang TY. Solubilization, partial purification, and reconstitution in phosphatidylcholine-cholesterol liposomes of acyl-CoA:cholesterol acyltransferase. Biochemistry 1982; 21:674–9

7. Cadigan KM, Heider JG, Chang T-Y. Isolation and characterization of Chinese hamster ovary cell mutants deficient in acyl-coenzyme A:cholesterol acyltransferase activity. J Biol Chem 1988; 263:274–82

8. Chang CCY, Huh HY, Cadigan KM, Chang TY. Molecular cloning and functional expression of human acyl-coenzyme A:cholesterol acyltransferase cDNA in mutant Chinese hamster ovary cells. J Biol Chem 1993; 268:20747–55

9. Meiner V, Tam C, Gunn MD, et al. Tissue expression studies on the mouse acyl-CoA:cholesterol acyltransferase gene (*Acact*): findings supporting the existence of multiple cholesterol esterification enzymes in mice. J Lipid Res 1997; 38:1928–33

10. Meiner VL, Cases S, Myers HM, et al. Disruption of the acyl-CoA:cholesterol acyltransferase gene in mice: evidence suggesting multiple cholesterol esterification enzymes in mammals. Proc Natl Acad Sci USA 1996; 93:14041–6

11. Yang H, Bard M, Bruner DA, et al. Sterol esterification in yeast: a two-gene process. Science 1996; 272:1353–6

12. Cases S, Smith SJ, Zheng YW, et al. Identification of a gene encoding an acyl CoA:diacylglycerol acyltransferase, a key enzyme in triacylglycerol synthesis. Proc Natl Acad Sci USA 1998; 95:13018–23

13. Anderson RA, Joyce C, Davis M, et al. Identification of a form of acyl-CoA:cholesterol acyltransferase specific to liver and intestine in nonhuman primates. J Biol Chem 1998; 273:26747–54

14. Cases S, Novak S, Zheng Y-W, et al. ACAT-2, a second mammalian acyl-CoA:cholesterol acyltransferase. Its cloning, expression, and characterization. J Biol Chem 1998; 273:26755–64

15. Oelkers P, Behari A, Cromley D, et al. Characterization of two human genes encoding acyl coenzyme A:cholesterol acyltransferase-related enzymes. J Biol Chem 1998; 273:26765–71

16. Buhman KF, Accad M, Farese RV Jr. Mammalian acyl-CoA: cholesterol acyltransferases. Biochim Biophys Acta Mol Cell Biol Lipids 2000; 1529:142–54

17. Li BL, Li XL, Duan ZJ, Lee O, et al. Human acyl-CoA:cholesterol acyltransferase-1 (ACAT-1) gene organization and evidence that the 4.3-kilobase ACAT-1 mRNA is produced from two different chromosomes. J Biol Chem 1999; 274:11060–71

18. Katsuren K, Tamura T, Arashiro R, et al. Structure of the human acyl-CoA:cholesterol acyltransferase-2 (ACAT-2) gene and its relation to dyslipidemia. Biochim Biophys Acta Mol Cell Biol Lipids 2001; 1531:230–40

19. Song BL, Qi W, Yang XY, et al. Organization of human ACAT-2 gene and its cell-type-specific promoter activity. Biochem Biophys Res Commun 2001; 282:580–8

20. Song BL, Qi W, Wang CH, et al. Preparation of an anti-Cdx-2 antibody for analysis of different species Cdx-2 binding to *acat*2 promoter. Biochim Biophys Acta Sinica 2003; 35:6–12

21. Wang CS, McConathy WJ, Kloer HU, et al. Modulation of lipoprotein lipase activity by apolipoproteins: effect of apolipoprotein C-III. J Clin Invest 1984; 75:384–90

22. von Kap-herr C, Cockman T, Rudel L, et al. Assignment of acyl-CoA:cholesterol acyltransferase 1 and 2 ((S)AT1, SOAT2)) and diacylglycerol O-acyltransferase 1 (DGAT1) to *M. fascicularis* chromosome band 1p32, 12q13, 8qter; *C. aethiops sabaeus* 13q22, 3q12, 1qter; *S. sciureus* 19q22, 15q21, 16qter by in situ hybridization. Cytogenet Genome Res 2003; 103:203

23. Guo ZM, Cromley D, Billheimer JT, et al. Identification of potential substrate-binding sites in yeast and human acyl-CoA sterol acyltransferases by mutagenesis of conserved sequences. J Lipid Res 2001; 42:1282–91

24. Joyce CW, Shelness GS, Davis MA, et al. ACAT1 and ACAT 2 membrane topology segregates a serine residue essential for activity to opposite sides of the endoplasmic reticulum membrane. Mol Biol Cell 2000; 11:3675–87

25. Lin S, Lu X, Chang CCY, et al. Human acyl-coenzyme A:cholesterol acyltransferase expressed in Chinese hamster ovary cells: membrane topology and active site location. Mol Biol Cell 2003; 14:2447–60

26. Lin S, Cheng D, Liu MS, et al. Human acyl-CoA:cholesterol acyltransferase-1 in the endoplasmic reticulum contains seven transmembrane domains. J Biol Chem 1999; 274:23276–85

27. Galvan DL, Borrego-Diaz E, Perez PJ, et al. Subunit oligomerization, and topology of the inositol 1,4, 5–trisphosphate receptor. J Biol Chem 1999; 274:29483–92

28. Mo C, Holland TC. Determination of the transmembrane topology of herpes simplex virus type 1 glycoprotein K. J Biol Chem 1997; 272:33305–11

29. Heymann JA, Subramaniam S. Integration of deletion mutants of bovine rhodopsin into the membrane of the endoplasmic reticulum. Mol Membr Biol 2000; 17:165–74

30. Manoil C, Traxler B. Insertion of in-frame sequence tags into proteins using transposons. Methods 2000; 20:55–61

31. Billheimer JT, Cromley DA, Kempner ES. The functional size of acyl-coenzyme A (CoA):cholesterol acyltransferase and acyl-CoA hydrolase as determined by radiation inactivation. J Biol Chem 1990; 265:8632–5

32. Erickson SK, Lear SR, McCreery MJ. Functional sizes of hepatic enzymes of cholesteryl ester metabolism determined by radiation inactivation. J Lipid Res 1994; 35:763–9

33. Lee RG, Willingham MC, Davis MA, et al. Differential expression of ACAT1 and ACAT2 among cells within liver, intestine, kidney, and adrenal of nonhuman primates. J Lipid Res 2000; 41:1991–2001

34. Yu CJ, Chen J, Lin S, et al. Human acyl-CoA:cholesterol acyltransferase-1 is a homotetrameric enzyme in intact cells and in vitro. J Biol Chem 1999; 274:36139–45

35. Chang CCY, Sakashita N, Ornvold K, et al. Immunological quantitation and localization of ACAT-1 and ACAT-2 in human liver and small intestine. J Biol Chem 2000; 275:28083–92

36. Yu CJ, Zhang Y, Lu XH, et al. Role of the N-terminal hydrophilic domain of acyl-coenzyme A:cholesterol acyltransferase I on the enzyme's quaternary structure and catalytic efficiency. Biochemistry 2002; 41:3762–9

37. Meiner VL, Welch CL, Cases S, et al. Adrenocortical lipid depletion gene (ald) in AKR mice is associated with an acyl-CoA:cholesterol acyltransferase (ACAT) mutation. J Biol Chem 1998; 273:1064–9

38. Zager RA, Kalhorn TF. Changes in free and esterified cholesterol. Am J Pathol 2000; 157:1007–16

39. Alexander CA, Hamilton RL, Havel RJ. Subcellular localization of B apoprotein of plasma lipoproteins in rat liver. J Cell Biol 1983; 69:241–63

40. Cardell RR, Jr, Badenhausen S, Porter KR. Intestinal triglyceride absorption in the rat. An electron microscopical study. J Cell Biol 1967; 34:123–55

41. Sakashita N, Miyazaki A, Takeya M, et al. Localization of human acyl-coenzyme A:cholesterol acyltransferase-1 (ACAT-1) in macrophages and in various tissues. Am J Pathol 2000; 156:227–36

42. Parini P, Davis M, Lada AT, et al. ACAT2 is localized to hepatocytes and is the major cholesterol-esterifying enzyme in human liver. Circulation 2004; 110:2017–23

43. Lada AT, Davis M, Kent C, et al. Identification of ACAT1– and ACAT2-specific inhibitors using a novel, cell-based fluorescent assay: individual ACAT uniqueness. J Lipid Res 2004; 45:378–86

44. Smith JL, Rangaraj K, Simpson R, et al. Quantitative analysis of expression of ACAT genes in human tissues by real-time PCR. J Lipid Res 2004; 45:686–96

45. Brown MS, Goldstein JL. The SREBP pathway: regulation of cholesterol metabolism by proteolysis of a membrane-bound transcription factor. Cell 1997; 89:331–40

46. Horton JD, Goldstein JL, Brown MS. SREBPs: activators of the complete program of cholesterol and fatty acid synthesis in the liver. J Clin Invest 2002; 109:1125–31

47. Edwards PA, Kast HR, Anisfeld AM. BAREing it all: the adoption of LXR and FXR and their roles in lipid homeostasis. J Lipid Res 2002; 43:2–12

48. Lehmann JM, Kliewer SA, Moore LB, et al. Activation of the nuclear receptor LXR by oxysterols defines a new hormone response pathway. J Biol Chem 1997; 272:3137–40

49. Janowski BA, Willy PJ, Devi TR, et al. An oxysterol signaling pathway mediated by the nuclear receptor LXRα. Nature 1996; 383:728–31

50. Yang JB, Duan ZJ, Yao W, et al. Synergistic transcriptional activation of human acyl-coenzyme A:cholesterol acyltransferase-1 gene by interferon-gamma and all-trans-retinoic acid THP-1 cells. J Biol Chem 2001; 276:20989–98

51. Panousis CG, Zuckerman SH. Regulation of cholesterol distribution in macrophage-derived foam cells by interferon-gamma. J Lipid Res 2000; 41:75–83

52. Wilcox LJ, Borradaile NM, de Dreu LE, et al. The secretion of hepatocyte apoB is inhibited by the flavonoids, naringenin and hesperetin, via reduced activity and expression of ACAT2 and MTP. J Lipid Res 2001; 42:725–34

53. Botham KM, Zheng XZ, Napolitano M, et al. The effects of dietary n-3 polyunsaturated fatty acids delivered in chylomicron remnants on the transcription of genes regulating synthesis and secretion of very-low-density lipoprotein by the liver: modulation by cellular oxidative state. Exp Biol Med. 2003; 228:143–51

54. Rudel LL, Davis M, Sawyer J, et al. Primates highly responsive to dietary cholesterol upregulate hepatic ACAT2 while less responsive primates do not. J Biol Chem 2002; 277:31401–6

55. Chang CCY, Lee C-YC, Chang ET, et al. Recombinant acyl-CoA:cholesterol acyltransferase-1 (ACAT-1) purified to essential homogeneity utilizes cholesterol in mixed micelles or in vesicles in a highly cooperative manner. J Biol Chem 1998; 273:35132–41

56. Cheng D, Chang CCY, Qu X, et al. Activation of acyl-coenzyme A:cholesterol acyltransferase by cholesterol or by oxysterol in a cell-free system. J Biol Chem 1995; 270:685–95

57. Rudel LL, Morris MD, Felts JM. The transport of exogenous cholesterol in the rabbit. I. Role of cholesterol ester of lymph chylomicron and lymph very low density lipoproteins in absorption. J Clin Invest 1972; 51:2686–92

58. Haugen R, Norum KR. Coenzyme-A-dependent esterification of cholesterol in rat intestinal mucosa. Scand J Gastroenterol 1976; 11:615–21

59. Miettinen TA, Kesaniemi A. Cholesterol absorption: regulation of cholesterol synthesis and elimination and within-population variations of serum cholesterol levels. Am J Clin Nutr 1989; 49:629–35

60. Kesaniemi YA, Miettinen TA. Cholesterol absorption efficiency regulates plasma cholesterol level in the Finnish population. Eur J Clin Invest 1987; 17:391–5

61. Miettinen TA, Gylling H. Cholesterol absorption efficiency and sterol metabolism in obesity. Atherosclerosis 2000; 153:241–8

62. Rudel L, Deckelman C, Wilson M, et al. Dietary cholesterol and downregulation of cholesterol 7α-hydroxylase and cholesterol absorption in African green monkeys. J Clin Invest 1994; 93:2463–72

63. Sliskovic DR, Picard JA, Krause BR. ACAT inhibitors: the search for a novel and effective treatment of hypercholesterolemia and atherosclerosis. Prog Medicinal Chem 2002; 39:121–71

64. Wrenn SM Jr, Parks JS, Immermann FW, et al. ACAT

inhibitors CL 283,546 and CL 283,796 reduce LDL cholesterol without affecting cholesterol absorption in African green monkeys. J Lipid Res 1995; 36:1199–210

65. Schwarz M, Davis DLVBR, Russell DW. Genetic analysis of intestinal cholesterol absorption in inbred mice. J Lipid Res 2001; 42:1801–11

66. Buhman KK, Accad M, Novak S, et al. Resistance to diet-induced hypercholesterolemia and gallstone formation in ACAT2–deficient mice. Nature Med 2000; 6:1341–7

67. Altmann SW, Davis HR Jr, Zhu L, et al. Niemann-Pick C1 like 1 protein is critical for intestinal cholesterol absorption. Science 2004; 303:1201–4

68. Goodman DS. The metabolism of chylomicron cholesteryl ester in the rat. J Clin Invest 1962; 41:1886–96

69. Bruckert E, Giral P, Tellier P. Perspectives in cholesterol-lowering therapy – The role of ezetimibe, a new selective inhibitor of intestinal cholesterol absorption. Circulation 2003; 107:3124–8

70. Temel RE, Gebre AK, Parks JS, et al. Compared with acyl-CoA:cholesterol O-acyltransferase (ACAT)1 and lecithin:cholesterol acyltransferase, ACAT2 displays the greatest capacity to differentiate cholesterol from sitosterol. J Biol Chem 2003; 278:47594–601

71. Yu LQ, Hammer RE, Li-Hawkins J, et al. Disruption of Abcg5 and Abcg8 in mice reveals their crucial role in biliary cholesterol secretion. Proc Natl Acad Sci USA 2002; 99:16237–42

72. Yu L, Li-Hawkins J, Hammer RE, et al. Overexpression of ABCG5 and ABCG8 promotes biliary cholesterol secretion and reduces fractional absorption of dietary cholesterol. J Clin Invest 2002; 110:671–80

73. Lee MH, Lu K, Patel SB. Genetic basis of sitosterolemia. Curr Opin Lipidol 2001; 12:141–9

74. Avramoglu RK, Cianflone K, Sniderman AD. Role of the neutral lipid accessible pool in the regulation of secretion of apoB-100 lipoprotein particles by HepG2 cells. J Lipid Res 1995; 36:2513–28

75. Cianflone KM, Yasruel Z, Rodriquez MA, et al. Regulation of apoB secretion from HepG2 cells: evidence for a critical role for cholesteryl ester synthesis in the response to a fatty acid challenge. J Lipid Res 1990; 31:2045–55

76. Sniderman AD, Zhang Z, Genest J, et al. Effects on apoB-100 secretion and bile acid synthesis by redirecting cholesterol efflux from HepG2 cells. J Lipid Res 2003; 44:527–32

77. Wilcox LJ, Barrett PHR, Newton RS, et al. ApoB100 secretion from HepG2 cells is decreased by the ACAT inhibitor CI-1011 – an effect associated with enhanced intracellular degradation of ApoB. Arterioscler Thromb Vasc Biol 1999; 19:939–49

78. Zhang ZJ, Cianflone K, Sniderman AD. Role of cholesterol ester mass in regulation of secretion of ApoB100 lipoprotein particles by hamster hepatocytes and effects of statins on that relationship. Arterioscler Thromb Vasc Biol 1999; 19:743–52

79. Huff MW, Telford DE, Barrett PHR, et al. Inhibition of hepatic ACAT decreases apoB secretion in miniature pigs fed a cholesterol-free diet. Arterioscler Thromb 1994; 14:1498–508

80. Carr TP, Hamilton RL Jr, Rudel LL. ACAT inhibitors decrease secretion of cholesteryl esters and apolipoprotein B by perfused livers of African green monkeys. J Lipid Res 1995; 36:25–36

81. Rudel LL, Haines J, Sawyer JK, et al. Hepatic origin of cholesteryl oleate in coronary artery atherosclerosis in African green monkeys. Enrichment by dietary monounsaturated fat. J Clin Invest 1997; 100:74–83

82. Lada AT, Rudel LL, St Clair RW. Effects of LDL enriched with different dietary fatty acids on cholesteryl ester accumulation and turnover in THP-1 macrophages. J Lipid Res 2003; 44:770–9

83. Logan RL, Thomson M, Riemersma RA, et al. Risk factors for ischaemic heart-disease in normal men aged 40. Lancet 1978; i:949–51

84. Lewis B. Composition of plasma cholesterol ester in relation to coronary-artery disease and dietary fat. Lancet 1958; ii:71–3

85. Kingsbury KJ, Brett C, Stovold R, et al. Abnormal fatty acid composition and human atherosclerosis. Postgrad Med J 1974; 50:425–40

86. Kingsbury KJ, Morgan DM, Stovold R, et al. Polyunsaturated fatty acids and myocardial infarction. Follow-up of patients with aortoiliac and femoropopliteal atherosclerosis. Lancet 1969; ii:1325–9

87. Lawrie TDV, McAlpine SG, Rifkind BM, et al. Serum fatty-acid patterns in coronary-artery disease. Lancet 1961; 14:421–4

88. Smith EB. The relationship between plasma and tissue lipids in human atherosclerosis. Adv Lipid Res 1974; 12:1–49

89. Mahlberg FH, Glick JM, Jerome WG, et al. Metabolism of cholesteryl ester lipid droplets in a J774 macrophage foam cell model. Biochim Biophys Acta 1990; 1045:291–8

90. Glick JM, Adelman SJ, Phillips MC, et al. Cellular cholesteryl ester clearance. Relationship to the physical state of cholesteryl ester inclusions. J Biol Chem 1983; 258:13425–30

91. Sakashita N, Miyazaki A, Chang CCY, et al. Acyl-coenzyme A:cholesterol acyltransferase 2 (ACAT2) is induced in monocyte-derived macrophages: in vivo and in vitro studies. Lab Invest 2003; 83:1569–81

92. Khelef N, Buton X, Beatini N, et al. Immunolocalization of acyl-coenzyme A:cholesterol O-acyltransferase in macrophages. J Biol Chem 1998; 273:11218–24

93. Khelef N, Soe TT, Quehenberger O, et al. Enrichment of acyl coenzyme A:cholesterol o-acyltransferase near trans-Golgi network and endocytic recycling compartment. Arterioscler Thromb Vasc Biol 2000; 20:1769–76

94. Accad M, Smith SJ, Newland DL, et al. Massive xanthomatosis and altered composition of atherosclerotic lesions in hyperlipidemic mice lacking acyl

CoA:cholesterol acyltransferase 1. J Clin Invest 2000; 105:711–19

95. Yagyu H, Kitamine T, Osuga J, et al. Absence of ACAT-1 attenuates atherosclerosis but causes dry eye and cutaneous xanthomatosis in mice with congenital hyperlipidemia. J Biol Chem 2000; 275:21324–30

96. Fazio S, Liu L, Major AS, et al. Accelerated atherosclerosis in LDL receptor null mice reconstituted with ACAT negative macrophage. Circulation 1999; 100:1-613

97. Kellner-Weibel G, Jerome WG, Small DM, et al. Effects of intracellular free cholesterol accumulation on macrophage viability: a model for foam cell death. Arterioscler Thromb Vasc Biol 1998; 18:423–31

98. Maccarrone M, Bellincampi L, Melino G, et al. Cholesterol, but not its esters, triggers programmed cell death in human erythroleukemia K562 cells. Eur J Biochem 1998; 253:107–13

99. Fazio S, Major AS, Swift LL, et al. Increased atherosclerosis in LDL receptor-null mice lacking ACAT1 in macrophages. J Clin Invest 2001; 107:163–71

100. Willner EL, Tow B, Buhman KK, et al. Deficiency of acyl CoA:cholesterol acyltransferase 2 prevents atherosclerosis in apolipoprotein E-deficient mice. Proc Natl Acad Sci USA 2003; 100:1262–7

101. Lee RG, Kelley KL, Sawyer JK, et al. Plasma cholesteryl esters provided by lecithin:cholesterol acyltransferase and acyl-Coenzyme A:cholesterol acyltransferase 2 have opposite atherogenic potential. Circ Res 2004; 95:998–1004

Overview of intestinal lipid metabolism 5

T.A. Miettinen and H. Gylling

INTRODUCTION

One of the most important problems in modern Western society is increasing body weight and obesity. This is due to increased absolute amount of calorie consumption in relation to decreased energy utilization by limited physical activity. Even though the excess calorie intake is not solely due to enhanced consumption of fat-containing food, weight reduction of obese subjects has renewed the idea of using low-carbohydrate diet, not only for acute weight control but also for long-term maintenance of body weight.[1] The resulting relative increase in fat intake involves mainly less-saturated vegetable oil products and also fish oil products.

Vegetable oils are the major sources of dietary phytosterols (plant sterols: mainly campesterol and sitosterol and their 5α-saturated stanols). Plant sterols from the natural plant products and especially from artificial functional food preparations inhibit cholesterol absorption and lower serum cholesterol levels. For that purpose, poorly soluble plant stanols were converted to fat-soluble esters and used as a plant stanol ester margarine[2] and later a plant sterol ester spread[3] was developed for serum cholesterol lowering. Dramatic reduction of cardiovascular risk with long-term statin treatment, even in subjects with a relatively low baseline cholesterol level,[4] has increased interest in lowering serum cholesterol concentration through the long-term consumption of diets enriched with phyto-sterols.[5] Fat-soluble plant stanol or sterol esters are the major products used for that purpose.[6] Their increased use has raised several interesting scientific and also practical questions concerning the role of the matrix of the fat in the diet, mechanism of cholesterol absorption and inhibition, regulation of plant sterol absorption and interference of saturated plant stanols in sterol absorption. Recent findings on the role of the enterocyte ATP-binding cassette half-transporters ABC G5 and G8 gene expressions in sterol absorption,[7] and the introduction of a specific inhibitor of cholesterol absorption, ezetimibe,[8] have widened the understanding of intestinal sterol metabolism. Recently the Niemann-Pick C1 like 1 protein has been introduced as a putative cholesterol.[9] However, the exact mechanisms of intestinal sterol metabolism at the molecular level are still poorly understood. This chapter will review the principles of fat, acidic and, especially, neutral sterol metabolism primarily in the small intestine of man, not dealing specifically with chylomicron formation in enterocytes or bacterial metabolic phenomena in the large bowel. Several review articles on different aspects of the intestinal lipid metabolism have recently been published.[6,10–13]

PRINCIPLES OF DIETARY FAT METABOLISM

The largest component of dietary lipids consists of triglycerides (about 60–80 g/day), the actual fats, followed by phospholipids (about 5 g/day) and cholesterol (about 200–500 mg/day). In addition to dietary intake, lipids enter the gastrointestinal tract from desquamated epithelial cells, and cholesterol and phospholipids are also delivered to the intestine by bile. Even though the molecular structures of lipids differ markedly from each other, they have one feature in common: they are all hydrophobic compounds, which makes their digestion, absorption and transport in aqueous medium complicated. Phospholipids, derived from both diet and bile, have both hydrophilic and hydrophobic groups in their structure, which enables them to act as bridges between hydrophobic and hydrophilic milieu. The following section deals mainly with fats, even though cholesterol and phospholipids are also mentioned.

Emulsification and lipolysis of fats in the stomach

Digestion of dietary fats consists of emulsification of fats in the stomach, lipolysis by lipases in the stomach and especially in the duodenum, solubilization with bile salts in the duodenum and absorption in the small intestine. Digestion starts in the oral cavity, where salivation and mastication start to separate fats from food and disperse the large fat droplets into smaller ones. The stomach contributes to fat digestion by both emulsification and hydrolysis of triglycerides by gastric lipase. The fats are warmed to body temperature and then enter a liquid phase. The grinding action of the antrum contributes to the emulsification, yielding smaller and smaller fat droplets and a greater surface area, which enhances lipolysis.

Gastric lipase is the main enzyme performing intragastric lipolysis, whereas the importance of lingual lipase is minimal in humans.[14] Gastric lipase is secreted by principal cells of the stomach, and it acts in an acidic milieu. It is substrate-specific and hydrolyses only triglycerides and only the fatty acids in the sn-3 position. Accordingly, the major products of gastric lipase action are short-, medium- or long-chain free fatty acids and diglycerides.

However, intragastric hydrolysis is important for triglyceride cleavage, because it is assumed that about one-third of fat lipolysis takes place in the stomach.[14] This is the reason why patients lacking pancreatic lipase can escape massive steatorrhoea. Mastication, antral grinding and lipolysis lead to an unstable gastric emulsion called chyme, which is released into the duodenum in a volume of 3 ml twice a minute.

The release of long-chain fatty acids in the stomach stimulates the release of cholecystokinin, which in turn stimulates the secretion of pancreatic lipase. Accordingly, gastric lipolysis prepares the intraduodenal circumstances for fat digestion. In addition, a complicated interplay regulates the motility of the gastrointestinal tract in order to secure as complete fat digestion as possible. For example, dietary fats regulate the emptying rate of the stomach. In the duodenal mucosa there are lipid-sensitive receptors, which, in connection with neural pathways, are capable of slowing gastric emptying in order to potentiate gastric emulsification and lipolysis. A similar 'brake' system operates in the terminal ileum and proximal colon. Intraluminal fats, bile salts and complex carbohydrates arriving to these parts of the gastrointestinal tract activate an endocrine–neurohumoral cascade, which decreases gastric emptying and small bowel transit.

Lipolysis in the small intestine

The entry of chyme into the duodenum stimulates the marked release of cholecystokinin, which inhibits gut mobility and enhances secretion of bile acids from the gall bladder and pancreatic juice with several lipases. Of these lipolytic enzymes, the most important ones for fat digestion are colipase and pancreatic lipase. The pancreatic lipase is an interfacial enzyme, which works best in a heterogeneous milieu of water–oil interface. To optimize the lipolytic effect, emulsified fats are solubilized by bile salts and phospholipids to form aggregates called mixed micelles. The mixed micelles also contain free fatty acids, cholesterol and other sterols and fat-soluble vitamins. In bile, when the concentration of conjugated bile acids exceeds 2 mmol/l, they aggregate and form micelles with cholesterol and phospholipids. The concentration of bile salts needed for micelle formation is called the critical micellar concentration. However, if the concentration of bile salts exceeds the critical micellar concentration, they inhibit the lipase activity by a physical competition for the lipid interface.

Pancreatic lipase hydrolyses fatty acids from the glyceride backbone at the sn-1 and sn-3 positions, releasing free fatty acids and monoglycerides. Pancreatic lipase is activated after colipase anchors it to the substrate interface, after which lipolysis can be started. In addition, colipase can overcome the competition between surplus bile salts and lipase activity. Two other lipases secreted from the pancreas are phospholipase A2, which releases fatty acid from phospholipid, and cholesterol esterase (also called bile-salt-stimulated lipase), which hydrolyses cholesterol esters and fat-soluble vitamin esters.

Fat absorption

The products of fat hydrolysis, i.e. fatty acids and mono- or diglycerides together with free cholesterol, phospholipids and fat-soluble vitamins, are carried in mixed micelles through the unstirred water layer to the apical membrane of enterocytes. The absorption of long-chain fatty acids and monoglycerides across the cell membrane to the enterocyte is completed by receptor uptake and also by a diffusion gradient. The receptor is called fatty acid binding protein, and it is located in the cell membrane. In the enterocyte, the long-chain fatty acids are transported protein-bound to the endoplasmic reticulum, where, following re-esterification, they are incorporated into chylomicrons by microsomal transfer protein (MTP). Short- and medium-chain fatty acids can be absorbed readily into enterocytes even without micellar transport, and they can be transported to the portal system without assembly to chylomicrons. The absorption of triglycerides (and probably also that of phospholipids) is very effective so that over 90% of triglycerides are absorbed.

PRINCIPLES OF CHOLESTEROL ABSORPTION

Hydrolysis of dietary cholesterol

Of dietary cholesterol roughly 20% is esterified. As described above, dietary lipids, including cholesterol and plant sterols, are already mixed in the mouth to a crude emulsion and further processed in the stomach which contains lingual and especially gastric lipases. Cell-membrane cholesterol from food, e.g. from animal or fish meat, should be released from the membranes before emulsification. Pancreatic juice contains several enzymes including cholesterol esterase (E.C. 3.1.1.13), which hydrolyses the small amount of dietary cholesterol esters. However, hydrolysis does not seem to be complete in the small intestine, because in colectomy patients, small amounts of ester cholesterol are found in ileal excreta.[15] Hydrolysis of esterified cholesterol seems to be necessary for cholesterol absorption in experimental animals.[16] Preliminary studies in man have shown that a cholesterol esterase inhibitor did not change the percentage of cholesterol absorption or serum cholesterol level;[17] thus, cholesterol esterase does not appear to be a cholesterol transporter into enterocytes in man.

Micelle formation with biliary lipids

Bile transports from 800 mg to 1200 mg of cholesterol per day mainly in micellar form into the intestinal lumen, indicating that the daily cholesterol load for intestinal absorption can be up to 1700 mg.[18] During intestinal digestion, bile acids, free fatty acids, monoglycerides, phospholipids and lysophospholipids form with cholesterol mixed micelles which can easily dissolve dietary water-insoluble compounds, including fat-soluble vitamins and sterols. Dietary cholesterol is incorporated into these micelles and absorbed, apparently in increasing proportion to bile cholesterol, when moved more distally in the intestine. The absorption rate of cholesterol ester may be slower, depending on its hydrolysis. Interestingly, the amount of cholesterol ester may actually increase in the duodenum, suggesting that under some conditions, e.g. in the presence of other sterol esters and fat, hydrolysis of dietary cholesterol esters may be inhibited, and cholesterol esterase could even form cholesterol esters retarding cholesterol absorption.[15,19] Bile cholesterol may be absorbed preferentially in the upper part of the small intestine owing to its micelle form in bile, and its absorption decreases when it moves to a more caudal direction, while absorption of dietary cholesterol could increase progressively when passing through the upper small intestinal lumen. Transfer of cholesterol to the micellar phase depends on many factors, including the amount of bile acids (critical micellar concentration), the amount and type of phospholipids and hydrolysis of triglycerides. A large oil phase tends to trap cholesterol and competes in general for micellar solubility of sterols. Thus, pancreatic insufficiency, use of a lipase inhibitor or olestra[20] and the presence of other sterols, mainly plant sterols and stanol esters in large amounts,[21] can retard transfer of cholesterol to micelles. The role of plant sterols/stanols will be dealt with later. Also, increased secretion of bile cholesterol, as in obesity or in type 2 diabetes, could supersaturate bile and prevent the transfer of dietary cholesterol to the micellar phase. In this case, the fractional absorption of dietary cholesterol is lowered despite normal or even increased total cholesterol absorption. In fact, in obesity the percentage absorption of dietary cholesterol is negatively, but not significantly, related to intestinal cholesterol flux, whereas it is significantly negatively related to biliary cholesterol concentration.[22] Accordingly, supersaturated bile cannot dissolve dietary cholesterol until 'extra' cholesterol is absorbed in the upper small intestine from the micellar phase. In general, cholesterol not entering the micellar phase is not absorbed and is finally excreted in the colon. Colonic bacterial action saturates the $\Delta 5$ double bond of cholesterol to the 5β position, causing formation of coprostanol and 3-ketocoprostanone, in which form up to 85% of cholesterol is eliminated from the body.

Cholesterol transfer to enterocytes

Micellar solubilization of cholesterol in the upper duodenum is considered to be essential for its transfer to the enterocyte through the unstirred water layer to the intestinal brush-border of the enterocyte membrane.[13] Apparently micellar structure is disaggregated in the membrane and cholesterol is taken up by the enterocyte through mechanism(s) not currently understood. The extracellular vs intracellular concentration gradient of free cholesterol may partly facilitate its enterocyte entry, even though current opinions consider that several membrane-located proteins, cholesterol transporters, are responsible for this transfer. Adenosine-triphosphate-binding cassette (ABC) transporters, ABCA1 and ABC G5/G8, appear to regulate the intracellular vs extracellular transport of cholesterol, and the scavenger receptor class B1 type (SR-B1) and another scavenger receptor, CD36, may enhance cholesterol uptake. A new candidate receptor protein has recently been introduced.[9] Experiments with gene-modified animals have raised questions about the possible role of ABCA1, SR-B1 and CD36 as specific cholesterol transporters in enterocytes.[23,24] Mutation of ABC G5/G8 genes, half transporters of sterols (sterol pumps) in enterocytes and hepatocytes, results in sitosterolaemia because of enhanced sterol uptake by enterocytes and decreased secretion by hepatocytes.[7]

Ezetimibe, a specific inhibitor of cholesterol absorption, seems to inhibit cholesterol and plant sterol absorption[25] in sitosterolaemic patients, also lowering their serum LDL cholesterol and plant sterol levels.[26] In mice with high cholesterol absorption, an ezetimibe derivative reduces ABC G5/G8 expression in enterocytes for animals on both low- and high-cholesterol diets. The findings have been interpreted to indicate that cholesterol and plant sterols are taken up by the enterocyte through a common permease blocked by ezetimibe independently of the ABC-transporter family.[13] The amount of intracellular sterols would then regulate expression of the ABC G5/G8 proteins.

After absorption, cholesterol is partially esterified by acyl CoA:cholesterol acyltransferase-2 (ACAT 2) in the enterocyte. Esterification reduces free cholesterol and changes the intracellular vs extracellular gradient to one more favourable for additional absorption. Esterified cholesterol is incorporated into chylomicron particles, formation of which is facilitated by MTP, apoprotein B48 and triglycerides. The role of ACAT-2 and MTP in cholesterol absorption in man seems to be limited, and inhibition of the latter may result in side-effects.[27]

Chylomicrons, or remnants thereof, are finally taken up by the liver. It has been calculated that about 1.2–1.6 g of cholesterol (200–500 mg from diet and 900–1100 mg from bile and intestinal mucosa) enters the intestinal lumen daily. Since the mean absorption of dietary cholesterol, and probably also of bile cholesterol, is about 50% in a random male population,[28] and in other populations,[25,29] up to 1 g of intestinal cholesterol can enter the liver daily. Thus, inhibition of cholesterol absorption, e.g. by plant stanols/sterols or ezetimibe, can easily affect the hepatic cholesterol balance, also changing lipoprotein and cholesterol synthesis, with a final lowering of LDL-cholesterol.

INTESTINAL METABOLISM OF PLANT STEROLS/STANOLS AND THEIR CONTRIBUTION TO CHOLESTEROL ABSORPTION

Dietary plant sterols and stanols

Our daily food contains about 250–350 mg/day of plant sterols, consisting of a large number of phytosterols (over 200), mainly sitostosterol, campesterol, stigmasterol and avenasterol (for example, see references 10–12). Their chemical structure differs from that of cholesterol mainly by the presence of either a methyl or ethyl group, with or without an additional double bond in the side chain. In vegetarian food the amounts can be higher, because any dietary plant material also contains plant sterols. Since small amounts of plant sterols are also present in meat and fish, it is actually difficult to have a diet free from plant sterols. In fact, like cholesterol

in the mammalian organism, plant sterols are necessary for normal cellular function, being structural components of plant cell membranes. The highest amounts of plant sterols are obtained from vegetable oils and oil products, especially from corn and rapeseed oils, however cereal grains, cereal products and nuts are also rich in these sterols. The Δ5 double bond of plant sterols can be saturated in nature to form the respective plant stanols, of which sitostanol and campestanol are the most important. About 10% of dietary plant sterols are plant stanols originating from, e.g., cereals, especially rye and wheat, corn and some corn products. Dietary plant sterols can be free, esterified at 3β-OH to a fatty acid or hydroxycinnamic acid or the hydroxyl group can be glycosylated with a hexose or a fatty acid–hexose. Thus, the conjugated forms of plant sterols are more complicated than that of mammalian cholesterol, which is only esterified with different fatty acids.

Hydrolysis of dietary sterols

Dietary phytosterols lower serum cholesterol by inhibiting intestinal cholesterol absorption. It is generally considered that they compete with cholesterol for incorporation into mixed micelles, resulting in reduced transfer of cholesterol into enterocytes.[30] However, micelle solubility requires free sterols, indicating that dietary natural phytosterol conjugates or phytosterol esters of functional foods should first be hydrolysed. Free plant sterols are apparently poorly incorporated into micelles, indicating that they should be presented in fat-soluble form or esterified, but even then the food matrix should contain some fat.[31–35] As noted above, dietary plant sterols, together with food fat and cholesterol, form a crude emulsion in the mouth and stomach, and a finer emulsion in the upper intestine. However, owing to rough plant material, sterols incorporated into cells in constrained plant tissues may not be released as easily as mammalian cholesterol to emulsion droplets, retarding hydrolysis of several types of conjugated plant sterols. On the other hand, most of these conjugates, especially plant sterol esters, appear to be already hydrolysed within a short segment of the upper small intestine, even though hydrolysis of glycosylated sterols is less known. Hydrolysis of plant sterols from fine emulsions favours transfer of free sterols to micelles. Intubation studies have shown[15,19] that, at low plant sterol and stanol concentrations, with high respective ester percentages of infused sterols, the amounts of ester cholesterol, cholestanol and their esterification percentages increased and those of plant sterols and stanols decreased in the upper small intestine when the infusate had passed 60 cm more distally in the duodenum. Hydrolysis of plant sterols was 60–80% and that of plant stanols about 55%. After a large amount of plant stanol esters had been added to the infusate, including a small amount of plant sterol esters (ester percentage of non-cholesterol sterols 56–96%), the amount of jejunal ester cholesterol was further increased, but hydrolysis of the respective plant sterols and stanols, including cholestanol, was about 40%. This finding suggests that, at low ester percentages, large amounts of free sterols in the intestinal contents might even increase ester formation, while markedly increased sterol esters, shown in fact after plant stanol ester infusion, could overload the hydrolysis process and even increase the amount of esters of the sterols with a low baseline ester percentage like cholesterol. The increase in cholesterol esters may explain why plant stanol esters, perhaps also plant sterol esters, retard cholesterol absorption. The increase in cholesterol esters may be temporary, indicating that, in the more distal intestine, hydrolysis may proceed after further absorption of free cholesterol. In fact, virtually no increase was seen in cholesterol esters, and only a small increase in sitostanol esters of ileal excreta of colectomy patients after consumption of large amounts of plant stanol esters.

Role of plant sterols in micelle formation

Infusion of a vegetable oil/egg yolk/glycerol/mono-oleate/water mixture (experiments shown above[15]) in the upper duodenum showed that campesterol, sitosterol and the respective stanols after hydrolysis were incorporated up to 70% into mixed micelles with free cholesterol and cholestanol (70–80%). Addition of a large amount of stanol esters (about 150-fold) with slightly increased plant sterol esters to the infusion mixture revealed, as shown above, a rapid hydrolysis. Subsequently, free intestinal plant stanols were transferred into the mixed micellar phase, such that the absolute concentration of campestanol and sitostanol were increased 100–200 times. Respective infusate increased unsaturated plant sterols only by up to 45%, while that of cholesterol decreased by one-third and also that of cholestanol tended to decrease in the micellar phase. No precipitation of sterols was found when the intestinal contents moved 60 cm more distally in the upper small intestine. The small quantities of plant sterols in the infusion material indicated that larger amounts might have similar effects on their micellar solubility with plant stanols, but no data in man are available.

Plant sterol/stanol absorption

Micelle transfer through the enterocyte membrane by permease would allow further metabolism of sterols. However, recent developments in the understanding of plant sterol absorption in sitosterolaemia have indicated that the sterol pump proteins, expression of which is regulated by the ABC G5/G8 genes, enhance the output of absorbed plant sterols and cholesterol from the enterocyte back to the intestinal lumen (see reference 7). Accordingly, specificity of this pumping out may limit plant sterol absorption to less than one-fifth of that for cholesterol, to less than 10% vs about 50% for cholesterol. However, even with the markedly high micelle concentration of plant stanols, as in the perfusion study[15] cited above, their absorption is low, <1%, suggesting that their transfer to enterocytes and further to blood and tissues is limited. Thus, consumption of plant stanol esters increases serum plant stanol concentrations only slightly.[36,37] A high dietary plant sterol intake, on the other hand, most likely increases plant sterols in micelles and subsequently enhances their bypass of the sterol pump in the enterocytes, resulting ultimately in increased serum plant sterol levels. The fact that serum levels of both cholestanol and plant stanols are also increased in sitosterolaemia, and that some of the dietary plant stanols are even absorbed normally, indicate that their absorption is also regulated by the sterol pump system. Competition of plant stanols with cholesterol, cholestanol and plant sterols for intestinal absorption includes enhanced ester formation and reduced micellar solubility of cholesterol, some reduction of cholestanol concentration but only a relative reduction of micellar plant sterols in the total intestinal sterols. The specificity of sterol output from enterocytes back to the intestinal lumen may effectively regulate sterol absorption according to the size of sterol molecules and their saturation.

Experiments with caco-2 cells in vitro have shown that mixed micelles with sitostanol or cholesterol plus sitostanol induced expression of ABCA1. Thus, increased enterocyte plant stanols, and possibly also plant sterols, might increase the ABCA1-mediated sterol efflux back into the intestinal lumen and the LXR pathway may regulate intestinal lipid metabolism.[38] Stimulation of ABCA1 gene expression by plant sterols may explain the finding that one daily dose of plant stanols or sterols in man lowers serum cholesterol by a similar extent as three doses.[34,39]

References

1. Foster GD, Wyatt HR, Hill JO, et al. A randomized trial of a low-carbohydrate diet for obesity. New Engl J Med 2003; 348:2082–90
2. Miettinen TA, Puska P, Gylling H, et al. Reduction of serum cholesterol with sitostanol-ester margarine in a mildly hypercholesterolemic population. N Engl J Med 1995; 333:1308–12
3. Weststrate JA, Meijer GW. Plant sterol-enriched margarines and reduction of plasma total- and LDL-cholesterol concentrations in normocholesterolaemic and mildly hypercholesterolaemic subjects. Eur J Clin Nutr 1998; 52:334–43
4. Heart Protection Study Collaborative Group. MRC/BHF Heart Protection Study of cholesterol lowering with simvastatin in 20536 high-risk individuals: a randomised placebo-controlled trial. Lancet 2002; 361:2005–16
5. Miettinen TA, Gylling H. Plant stanol and sterol esters in prevention of cardiovascular disease. Ann Med 2004; 36(2):126–34
6. Katan MB, Grundy SM, Jones P, et al. for the Stresa Workshop Participants. Efficacy and safety of plant stanols and sterols in the management of blood cholesterol levels. Mayo Clin Proc 2003; 78:965–78
7. Berge KE. Sitosterolemia: a gateway to new knowledge about cholesterol metabolism. Ann Med 2003; 35: 502–11
8. Darkes MJM, Poole RM, Goa KL. Ezetimibe. Am J Cardiovasc Drugs 2003; 3:67–76
9. Altmann SW, Davis Jr HR, Zhu L-j, et al. Niemann-Pick C1 like 1 protein is critical for intestinal cholesterol absorption. Science 2004; 303:1201–4
10. Piironen V, Lindsay DG, Miettinen TA, et al. Plant sterols: biosynthesis, biological function and their importance to human nutrition. J Sci Food Agric 2000; 80:939–66
11. Moreau RA, Whitaker BD, Hicks KB. Phytosterols, phytostanols, and their conjugates in foods: structural diversity, quantitative analysis, and health-promoting uses. Progr Lipid Res 2002; 41:457–500
12. Ostlund RE Jr. Phytosterols in human nutrition. Annu Rev Nutr 2002; 22:533–49
13. Turley SD, Dietschy JM. Sterol absorption by the small intestine. Curr Opin Lipidol 2003; 14:233–40
14. Hamosh M. Preduodenal fat digestion. In Christophe AB, de Vriese S, eds. Fat Digestion and Absorption. Champaign, Ill: AOCS Press, 2000:1–12
15. Nissinen M, Gylling H, Vuoristo M, et al. Micellar distribution of cholesterol and phytosterols after duodenal plant sterol ester infusion. Am J Physiol 2002; 282:G1009–15
16. Howles PN, Carter CP, Hui DY. Dietary free and esterified cholesterol absorption in cholesterol esterase (bile salt-stimulated lipase) gene-targeted mice. J Biol Chem 1996; 271:7196–202
17. Bosner MS, Wolff AA, Ostlund RE Jr. Lack of effect of cholesterol esterase inhibitor CVT-1 on cholesterol absorption and LDL cholesterol in humans. Cardiovasc Drugs Ther 1999; 13:449–54
18. Mitchell JC, Stone BG, Logan GM, et al. Role of

cholesterol synthesis in regulation of bile acid synthesis and biliary cholesterol secretion in humans. J Lipid Res 1991; 32:1143–9

19. Miettinen TA, Siurala M. Bile salts, sterols, sterol esters, glycerides and fatty acids in micellar and oil phases of intestinal contents during fat digestion in man. Z Klin Chem Klin Biochem 1971; 9:47–52

20. Mittendorfer B, Ostlund RE Jr, Patterson BW, et al. Orlistat inhibits dietary cholesterol absorption. Obes Res 2001; 9:599–604

21. Miettinen TA. Cholesterol absorption inhibition: a strategy for cholesterol lowering therapy. Int J Clin Pract 2001; 55:599–604

22. Miettinen TA, Gylling H. Cholesterol absorption efficiency and sterol metabolism in obesity. Atherosclerosis 2000; 153:241–8

23. Dropnik W, Lindenthal B, Lieser B, et al. ATP-binding cassette transporter A 1 (ABCA1) affects total body cholesterol. Gastroenterology 2001; 120:1203–11

24. Mardones P, Quinones V, Amigo L, et al. Hepatic cholesterol and bile acid metabolism and intestinal cholesterol absorption in scavenger receptor class B type I-deficient mice. J Lipid Res 2001; 42:170–80

25. Sudhop T, Lütjohann D, Kodal A, et al. Inhibition of intestinal cholesterol absorption by ezetimibe in humans. Circulation 2002; 106:1943–8

26. Salen G, von Bergmann K, Kwiterovich P, et al. Ezetimibe is an effective treatment for homozygous sitosterolemia. Circulation 2002; 106 (Suppl): 929

27. Sudhop T, von Bergmann K. Cholesterol absorption inhibitors for the treatment of hyperlipidemia. Drugs 2002; 62:2333–47

28. Miettinen TA, Kesäniemi YA. Cholesterol absorption: regulation of cholesterol synthesis and elimination and within-population variations of serum cholesterol levels. Am J Clin Nutr 1989; 49:629–35

29. Bosner MS, Lange LG, Stenson WE, et al. Percent cholesterol absorption in normal women and men quantified with dual stable isotopic tracers and negative ion mass spectrometry. J Lipid Res 1999; 40:302–8

30. Ikeda I, Tanabe Y, Sugano M. Effects of sitosterol and sitostanol on micellar solubility of cholesterol. J Nutr Sci Vitaminol 1989; 35:361–9

31. Denke MA. Lack of efficacy with low-dose sitostanol therapy as an adjunct to a cholesterol-lowering diet in men with moderate hypercholesterolemia. Am J Clin Nutr 1995; 61:392–6

32. Plat J, van Onselen ENM, van Heugten MMA, et al. Effects on serum lipids, lipoproteins and fat-soluble antioxidant concentrations of consumption frequency of margarines and shortenings enriched with plant stanol esters. Eur J Clin Nutr 2000; 54: 671–7

33. Nestel P, Cehun M, Pomeroy S, et al. Cholesterol-lowering effects of plant sterol esters and non-esterified plant stanols in margarine, butter and low-fat foods. Eur J Clin Nutr 2001; 55:1084–90

34. Mensink RP, Ebbing S, Lindhout M, et al. Effects of plant stanol ester supplied in low-fat yoghurt on serum lipids and lipoproteins, non-cholesterol sterols and fat soluble antioxidant concentrations. Atherosclerosis 2002; 160:205–13

35. Jones PJH, Vanstone CA, Raeini-Sarjaz M, et al. Phytosterols in low- and nonfat beverages as part of a controlled diet fail to lower lipid levels. J Lipid Res 2003; 44:1713–9

36. Miettinen TA, Vuoristo M, Nissinen M, et al. Serum, biliary and fecal cholesterol and plant sterols in colectomized patients before and during consumption of stanol ester margarine. Am J Clin Nutr 2000; 71:1095–102

37. Ostlund RE Jr, McGill JB, Zeng C-M, et al. Gastrointestinal absorption and plasma kinetics of soy delta(5)-phytosterols and phytostanols in humans. Am J Physiol Endocrinol Metab 2002; 282:E911–6

38. Plat J, Mensink RP. Increased intestinal ABCA1 expression contributes to the decrease in cholesterol absorption after plant stanol consumption. FASEB J 2002; 16:1248–53

39. Matvienco OA, Lewish DE, Swanson M, et al. A single daily dose of soybean phytosterols in ground beef decreases serum total cholesterol and LDL cholesterol in young, mildly hypercholesterolemic men. Am J Clin Nutr 2002; 76:57–64

The role of non-cholesterol sterols in the pathogenesis of atherosclerosis and their modulation by the sitosterolaemia locus

E.L. Klett and S.B. Patel

INTRODUCTION

Elevated blood cholesterol levels have been shown to be one of the major risk factors for the development of cardiovascular disease. While a great deal is known about how cholesterol is transported in the body via lipoproteins, very little is known about the molecular mechanisms by which cholesterol exerts its potential metabolic effects. Additionally, it remains to be shown that cholesterol itself functions as a bioactive molecule resulting directly in atherosclerosis. Despite these reservations, one cannot overlook the important link between cholesterol and cardiovascular disease. This review will focus on the pathways of dietary cholesterol and non-cholesterol entry and excretion by the body. In particular, the role of the newly described transporters, ABCG5 and ABCG8, in these processes will be highlighted. Further, we draw attention to the difference between bioactive molecules, versus biomarkers of disease. Cholesterol is clearly an important biomarker, but how good is it as a bioactive molecule and if it is not a bioactive molecule with respect to the pathogenesis of atherosclerosis, which sterol molecules are? This chapter will focus only on the sterol molecules and other chapters in this book highlight the roles of other potent molecules.

Sterol homeostasis is a tightly regulated process; mechanisms of dietary sterol absorption, endogenous *de novo* synthesis and excretion and/or breakdown of sterols ensure balance is maintained. For mammals, cholesterol is the major sterol; it is synthesized endogenously, is not a dietary necessity and excess cholesterol is metabolized by the body and excreted as biliary cholesterol or bile acids. The use of inhibitors of *de novo* cholesterol synthesis, namely 3-hydroxy-3-methyl glutaryl coenzyme A reductase inhibitors or statins, has had a significant impact on reducing the risk of cardiovascular events as shown by multiple trials (4S, CARE, LIPID, HPS, etc.).[1-4] Based upon present knowledge, statin efficacy on cardiovascular disease is based upon the reduction in serum cholesterol levels as well as potential 'pleiotropic' effects. Irrespective of these mechanisms and despite the availability of very potent statins, the risk reduction with appropriate use of statins is only ~20–30% in many clinical studies.[1-4] The major mechanism whereby statins are likely to exert their effects is the increased clearance of blood lipoprotein particles by the liver (upregulation of the LDL receptors) that results in a reduction of cholesterol as well as any bioactive sterols (oxysterol as well as non-cholesterol sterols) carried in these particles. Note that, on statin therapy, whole-body sterol balance does not change and, at the cellular level, the free cholesterol content is also unlikely to be reduced, but stored pools of cholesterol (as cholesterol esters) are reduced, especially atheromatous plaques as they regress. The thesis of this treatise is to explore the hypothesis that the bioactive molecule(s) track with cholesterol, use pathways that cholesterol may use and that the proteins ABCG5 and ABCG8 may play a key role in keeping these molecules from accumulating.

A typical Western diet contains ~400 mg of cholesterol per day, derived from animal sources, and about 200–400 mg of non-cholesterol sterols, derived mostly from plants.[5,6] On average, about 55% of the dietary cholesterol is absorbed and retained on a daily basis, but almost none of the non-cholesterol sterols (such as the plant sterols – sitosterol, campesterol, brassicasterol, etc.) are retained.[7] Additionally, cooked foods contribute oxidized sterols to the dietary intake pool of which the metabolic fate is relatively unknown. While most of the total body pool of cholesterol is derived from *de novo* cholesterol synthesis, it is now clear that dietary sources play a crucial role in maintaining total body sterol balance. Influx of cholesterol from the diet regulates the amount of *de novo* synthesis. The liver is the central organ in maintaining this balance. Excess body cholesterol, derived from endogenous synthesis or from dietary absorption, is excreted exclusively by the liver, either by direct excretion as free cholesterol into bile, or by breakdown to bile acids and excretion as bile acid conjugates into bile. A small amount of dietary non-cholesterol also enters the body. However, the liver rapidly excretes these sterols into bile, thus resulting in a very low net daily absorption.[8] Why have mechanism(s) evolved that regulate dietary non-cholesterol (or dietary cholesterol), if these non-cholesterol sterols are thought not to be biologically active in our bodies? Our group and others have hypothesized that the body has evolved very efficient mechanisms that allow for the separation and/or exclusion of potentially deleterious dietary compounds since within the bulk of these dietary sterols there are potent and bioactive sterols or sterol derivatives that have potentially deleterious effects in our bodies. It is only when these mechanisms are perturbed that atherosclerosis develops. This review will focus on the potential role of two ABC half-transporters, ABCG5 and ABCG8, in this process of abrogating dietary-induced atherosclerosis.

CLUES FROM A RARE GENETIC DISORDER, SITOSTEROLAEMIA

The identification of a rare autosomal recessive disorder of sterol absorption/excretion termed sitosterolaemia (also known as phytosterolaemia, MIM 210250), has helped to shed light on the molecular mechanisms by which the intestinal cells traffic sterols and has led to the identification of the elusive hepatobiliary cholesterol exporter(s).[9,10] Patients with this disease can present with tendon xanthomas (usually involving the Achilles tendon), haemolytic episodes, arthritis/arthralgias and, most strikingly, accelerated atherosclerosis. The key feature of this disease is the disruption of the normal pathways that prevent the accumulation of non-cholesterol sterols, such as plant sterols.[9,11,12] The gene(s) causing sitosterolaemia was mapped to the *STSL* locus on human chromosome 2p21.[13–15] Elucidation of the molecular defects of sitosterolaemia showed that the *STSL* locus comprises two genes, *ABCG5* and *ABCG8*, encoding sterolin-1 and sterolin-2, respectively, and mutation in either one of these genes is sufficient to cause sitosterolaemia.[13] In the absence of functioning sterolin-1 (ABCG5) or sterolin-2 (ABCG8), patients hyper-absorb all non-cholesterol sterols (and cholesterol), retain these in the body and fail to excrete sterols into bile.[8,16–19] Based on this it would be expected that these patients would have tremendously high serum cholesterols, but paradoxically they have normal to only slightly elevated serum cholesterol.[11] Since patients with sitosterolaemia have accelerated atherosclerosis and since the defective genes alter non-cholesterol sterol levels (all of which are of dietary origin), this raises the possibility that ABCG5/ABCG8 evolved to keep bioactive non-cholesterol sterols out of the body. The *STSL* locus is highly conserved and these genes are found in animals as disparate as fish and mammals, and since one important role for these proteins is the biliary excretion of sterols, the possibility that these proteins may also be responsible for clearance of bioactive sterols from the body has also been raised.

Genetics of ABCG5 and ABCG8

Genetic analyses of sitosterolaemia pedigrees allowed the mapping of the *STSL* locus to human chromosome 2p21, between D2S2294 and D2S2298.[20,21] By using positional cloning procedures or by screening for genes induced by exposure to LXR agonists, two groups identified not one but two genes, *ABCG5* and *ABCG8*, that encode the proteins sterolin-1 and sterolin-2, mutations of which cause sitosterolaemia.[14,15] To date, no patient with sitosterolaemia has been identified with mutations in both genes. *ABCG5* and *ABCG8* are organized in a head-to-head configuration with the two initiator ATGs of the two genes separated by only 340 bp.[13] The bi-directional promoter for the two genes has not been definitively defined, but ~140 bp of DNA separates the two transcription start sites. Each gene is made up of 13 exons and 13 introns. Although LXR agonists have been used to stimulate the mRNA expression from the *STSL* locus, no motifs suggestive of LXR recognition sequences in the intergenic region have been identified.[22] Recently, regulation of this locus through LRH has been reported and suggests that LXR modulation of this locus may be indirect.[23]

The *STSL* locus is polymorphic but, unusually, while *ABCG8* is highly polymorphic, *ABCG5* seems almost invariant in humans.[13] Despite the closeness of *ABCG5* and *ABCG8*, the increased polymorphic frequency of *ABCG8* or the relative 'conservation' of *ABCG5* suggests that there may be a biological pressure for these genetic changes. Many of the polymorphic changes detected at the *STSL* locus are in linkage disequilibrium, suggesting many of these changes are relatively new.

Since *STSL* locus defects cause sitosterolaemia, the heritability of plasma plant sterol levels has been examined as a prelude to whether natural variation at this locus is a strong determinant of these levels. In both nuclear families, as well as twin studies, plant sterols are highly heritable.[24] Preliminary evidence suggests an association with certain polymorphic variations and plant sterol levels,

but a study to formally examine this has not been performed.

ARE NON-CHOLESTEROL STEROLS INVOLVED IN ATHEROGENESIS?

Although Bhattacharyya and Connor were the first to propose that sitosterol may be a factor in causing atherosclerosis,[9] Glueck and colleagues were the first to show that plasma plant sterols are present in atheromatous plaques and subsequently showed that these are elevated in patients with proven heart disease and may be genetically determined.[25,26] Miettinen and colleagues,[27] as well as von Bergmann and colleagues,[28] have also reported case-controlled studies showing the association of plant sterols with proven coronary heart disease. Data from the PROCAM study, presented at the American Heart Association Scientific Sessions 2003, also suggests plasma sitosterol levels as independent predictors of future CVD.[29] More recently, association studies between the responsiveness to statin drugs and genetic variations at the *STSL* locus have been reported, although it should be pointed out that this locus shows significant linkage disequilibrium amongst the multiple polymorphisms thus-far identified.[30–32]

Oxysterols are products of cholesterol oxidation and have been implicated in the initiation and/or development of atherosclerosis.[33,34] However, there is no direct evidence in humans that oxysterols contribute to the development of atherosclerosis, despite observational reports such as detection of non-enzymatically derived oxysterols in atherosclerotic plaques (such as 7-ketocholesterol) or limited epidemiological studies.[35–39] A possible connection between cardiovascular disease and diet may be the dietary-derived oxidatively modified sterols. The identification of nuclear receptors LXRα and LXRβ, which bind with high affinity to oxidized sterols, as regulators of cholesterol homeostasis has implicated oxysterols as important modulators of these pathways. To date, the endogenous physiological ligand for LXR has not been identified, although a number of potential candidates have been proposed, a major one being 27-OH cholesterol. LXRα strongly modulates the transcription of several genes involved in the metabolism and transport of sterols including *Cyp7a1, SREBP-1c, CETP, ApoE, ABCA1, ABCG1* and *ABCG5/ABCG8*.[40,41] Two pools of oxysterols exist, those derived endogenously and those that arise from the diet. Dietary oxysterols are produced as a result of heating in air (cooking) or prolonged storage of foods.[33] Absorption of dietary oxysterols, as determined by lymphatic cannulation, has been shown in rats to range from 6 to 30%.[42,43] Once dietary-derived oxysterols enter the circulation their fate is not known. Given their capacity to alter gene expression and their direct toxic effects on the vasculature,[34] it is likely that oxysterols may utilize the same cholesterol transport and clearance mechanisms for rapid removal, and it remains to be seen whether ABCG5/ABCG8 play a major role. Current dogma suggests that most oxysterols are rapidly taken up by the liver and metabolized via the bile acid synthesis pathways, and some may be excreted directly into bile. Given the high biological activity and relatively low levels, it is apparent from a teleological perspective that organisms have evolved certain protective mechanisms to specifically exclude and/or excrete these potentially deleterious compounds.

DO ABCG5/ABCG8 PLAY A CRUCIAL ROLE IN CARDIOVASCULAR RISK AND ARE THESE PROTEINS OR THEIR ACTIVITIES 'TARGETABLE' FOR THERAPEUTIC INTERVENTION?

At present, there are no data that directly link the *STSL* locus and a predisposition to atheromatous cardiovascular disease. Interestingly, statin responsiveness in humans has been linked in some preliminary analyses, but the best study to date has not reproduced these findings. There are lines of investigation that are indirect. For example, sitosterolaemic rats prone to hypertension (SHRSP) show increased morbidity and mortality when fed

diets rich in plant sterols (although dietary studies are known for not controlling for the dietary constituents).[44] Feeding high quantities of plant sterols to such hypertensive rats also raised their blood pressure even higher. And, as stated above, plant sterol levels in the plasma seem to act as a biomarker of predisposition to cardiovascular disease. We have proposed a model whereby the dietary entry of sterols (cholesterol and non-cholesterol sterols) may be initially regulated by the activity of NPC1L1 and subsequently by activity of ABCG5/ABCG8 in the intestine.[45–47] On the other hand, the rates of sterol excretion via the hepatobiliary system may be primarily determined by ABCG5/ABCG8 activity. Currently, we have no further biochemical characterization of how ABCG5/ABCG8 act to 'pump' sterols out. It is not clear whether their activity is increased by any allosteric interactions and thus direct modulation by small molecules seems unlikely. In contrast, transcriptional activation by therapeutic ligands seems feasible. To date, only two transcriptional factors are known, LXR and LRH, and both of these have a multitude of effects and a specific targeted ABCG5/ABCG8 activation does not seem to be possible at this time.

CONCLUSIONS

The identification of the molecular defects underlying sitosterolaemia has afforded considerable insight into the molecular mechanisms by which dietary cholesterol is absorbed, how non-cholesterol sterols may be prevented from entry and how sterols are excreted into the biliary system. The renewed interest in non-cholesterol sterols has also led to a renewed interest in defining the bioactive sterol or sterol metabolite that is likely to play a key role in atherogenic cardiovascular disease and may finally lead to a molecular basis for the connection between diet and heart disease. Currently, the lack of biochemical characterization of how ABCG5/ABCG8 may act to pump sterols out, the lack of clear understanding of how the *STSL* locus is regulated and the fact that any therapeutic intervention will need to activate, rather than inactivate, this pathway suggests that these proteins are unlikely to be 'targetable'. However, the continued investigation of these pathways has shed considerable light onto the role of sterol trafficking and this, in itself, has already led to significant advancement in our understanding of these physiological processes. Perhaps this insight may allow us to better identify the bioactive sterols and move away from the biomarkers, with newer therapies targeted at these molecules.

References

1. Randomised trial of cholesterol lowering in 4444 patients with coronary heart disease: the Scandinavian Simvastatin Survival Study (4S). Lancet 1994; 344:1383–9

2. Prevention of cardiovascular events and death with pravastatin in patients with coronary heart disease and a broad range of initial cholesterol levels. The Long-Term Intervention with Pravastatin in Ischaemic Disease (LIPID) Study Group. N Engl J Med 1998; 339:1349–57

3. Sacks FM, Pfeffer MA, Moye LA, et al. The effect of pravastatin on coronary events after myocardial infarction in patients with average cholesterol levels. Cholesterol and Recurrent Events Trial investigators. N Engl J Med 1996; 335:1001–9

4. Shepherd J, Cobbe SM, Ford I, et al. Prevention of coronary heart disease with pravastatin in men with hypercholesterolemia. West of Scotland Coronary Prevention Study Group. N Engl J Med 1995; 333:1301–7

5. Weihrauch JL, Gardner JM. Sterol content of foods of plant origin. J Am Diet Assoc 1978; 73:39–47

6. Nair PP, Turjman N, Kessie G, et al. Diet, nutrition intake, and metabolism in populations at high and low risk for colon cancer. Dietary cholesterol, beta-sitosterol, and stigmasterol. Am J Clin Nutr 1984; 40(4 Suppl):927–30

7. Wilson MD, Rudel LL. Review of cholesterol absorption with emphasis on dietary and biliary cholesterol. J Lipid Res 1994; 35:943–55

8. Salen G, Tint GS, Shefer S, et al. Increased sitosterol absorption is offset by rapid elimination to prevent accumulation in heterozygotes with sitosterolemia. Arterioscler Thromb 1992; 12:563–8

9. Bhattacharyya AK, Connor WE. Beta-sitosterolemia and xanthomatosis. A newly described lipid storage disease in two sisters. J Clin Invest 1974; 53:1033–43

10. Rao MK, Perkins EG, Connor WE, et al. Identification of beta-sitosterol, campesterol, and stigmasterol in human serum. Lipids 1975; 10:566–8

11. Salen G, Shefer S, Nguyen L, et al. Sitosterolemia. J Lipid Res 1992; 33:945–55

12. Salen G, Patel SB, Batta AK. Sitosterolemia. Cardiovasc Drug Rev 2002; 20:255–70

13. Lu K, Lee M-H, Hazard S, et al. Two genes that map to the *STSL* locus cause sitosterolemia: genomic structure and spectrum of mutations involving sterolin-1 and sterolin-2, encoded by *ABCG5* and *ABCG8* respectively. Am J Hum Genet 2001; 69: 278–90

14. Berge KE, Tian H, Graf GA, et al. Accumulation of dietary cholesterol in sitosterolemia caused by mutations in adjacent ABC transporters. Science 2000; 290:1771–5

15. Lee M-H, Lu K, Hazard S, et al. Identification of a gene, ABCG5, important in the regulation of dietary cholesterol absorption. Nat Genet 2001; 27:79–83

16. Miettinen TA. Phytosterolaemia, xanthomatosis and premature atherosclerotic arterial disease: a case with high plant sterol absorption, impaired sterol elimination and low cholesterol synthesis. Eur J Clin Invest 1980; 10:27–35

17. Bhattacharyya AK, Connor WE, Lin DS, et al. Sluggish sitosterol turnover and hepatic failure to excrete sitosterol into bile cause expansion of body pool of sitosterol in patients with sitosterolemia and xanthomatosis. Arterioscler Thromb 1991; 11:1287–94

18. Gregg RE, Connor WE, Lin DS, et al. Abnormal metabolism of shellfish sterols in a patient with sitosterolemia and xanthomatosis. J Clin Invest 1986; 77:1864–72

19. Salen G, Shore V, Tint GS, et al. Increased sitosterol absorption, decreased removal, and expanded body pools compensate for reduced cholesterol synthesis in sitosterolemia with xanthomatosis. J Lipid Res 1989; 30:1319–30

20. Lee M-H, Gordon D, Ott J, et al. Fine mapping of a gene responsible for regulating dietary cholesterol absorption; founder effects underlie cases of phytosterolemia in multiple communities. Eur J Hum Genet 2001; 9:375–84

21. Lu K, Lee M-H, Carpten JD, et al. High-resolution physical and transcript map of human chromosome 2p21 containing the sitosterolemia locus. Eur J Hum Genet 2001; 9:364–74

22. Remaley AT, Bark S, Walts AD, et al. Comparative genome analysis of potential regulatory elements in the ABCG5–ABCG8 gene cluster. Biochem Biophys Res Commun 2002; 295:276–82

23. Freeman LA, Kennedy A, Wu J, et al. The orphan nuclear receptor LRH-1 activates the ABCG5/ABCG8 intergenic promoter. J Lipid Res 2004; 45:1197–206

24. Berge KE, von Bergmann K, Lutjohann D, et al. Heritability of plasma noncholesterol sterols and relationship to DNA sequence polymorphism in ABCG5 and ABCG8. J Lipid Res 2002; 43:486–94

25. Mellies MJ, Ishikawa TT, Glueck CJ, et al. Phytosterols in aortic tissue in adults and infants. J Lab Clin Med 1976; 88:914–21

26. Glueck CJ, Speirs J, Tracy T, et al. Relationships of serum plant sterols (phytosterols) and cholesterol in 595 hypercholesterolemic subjects, and familial aggregation of phytosterols, cholesterol, and premature coronary heart disease in hyperphytosterolemic probands and their first-degree relatives. Metabolism 1991; 40:842–8

27. Rajaratnam RA, Gylling H, Miettinen TA. Independent association of serum squalene and noncholesterol sterols with coronary artery disease in postmenopausal women. J Am Coll Cardiol 2000; 35:1185–91

28. Sudhop T, Gottwald BM, von Bergmann K. Serum plant sterols as a potential risk factor for coronary heart disease. Metabolism 2002; 51:1519–21

29. Assman G, Cullen P, Erbey JR, et al. Elevation in plasma sitosterol concentration is associated with an increased risk for coronary events in the PROCAM study. American Heart Association Scientific Sessions 2003, Abstract 3300. Circulation 2003; 108(Suppl 4):730

30. Miettinen TA, Gylling H, Lindbohm N, et al. Serum noncholesterol sterols during inhibition of cholesterol synthesis by statins. J Lab Clin Med 2003; 141:131–7

31. Kajinami K, Brousseau ME, Nartsupha C, et al. ATP binding cassette transporter G5 and G8 genotypes and plasma lipoprotein levels before and after treatment with atorvastatin. J Lipid Res 2004; 45:653–6

32. Gylling H, Hallikainen M, Pihlajamaki J, et al. Polymorphisms in the ABCG5 and ABCG8 genes associate with cholesterol absorption and insulin sensitivity. J Lipid Res 2004; 45:1660–5

33. Brown AJ, Jessup W. Oxysterols and atherosclerosis. Atherosclerosis 1999; 142:1–28

34. Garcia-Cruset S, Carpenter K, Codony R, et al. Cholesterol oxidation products and atherosclerosis. In: Guardiola F, Dutta P, Codony R, Savage G, eds. Cholesterol and Phytosterol Oxidation Products: Analysis, Occurrence, and Biological Effects. Champaign, Illinois: AOCS Press, 2002: 241–77

35. Jacobson MS. Cholesterol oxides in Indian ghee: possible cause of unexplained high risk of atherosclerosis in Indian immigrant populations. Lancet 1987; 2:656–8

36. Brown AJ, Leong SL, Dean RT, et al. 7-Hydroperoxycholesterol and its products in oxidized low density lipoprotein and human atherosclerotic plaque. J Lipid Res 1997; 38:1730–45

37. Bjorkhem I, Andersson O, Diczfalusy U, et al. Atherosclerosis and sterol 27–hydroxylase: evidence for a role of this enzyme in elimination of cholesterol from human macrophages. Proc Natl Acad Sci USA 1994; 91:8592–6

38. Crisby M, Nilsson J, Kostulas V, et al. Localization of sterol 27-hydroxylase immuno-reactivity in human atherosclerotic plaques. Biochim Biophys Acta 1997; 1344:278–85

39. Suarna C, Dean RT, May J, et al. Human atherosclerotic plaque contains both oxidized lipids and relatively large amounts of alpha-tocopherol and ascorbate. Arterioscler Thromb Vasc Biol 1995; 15:1616–24

40. Lu TT, Repa JJ, Mangelsdorf DJ. Orphan nuclear receptors as eLiXiRs and FiXeRs of sterol metabolism. J Biol Chem 2001; 276:37735–8

41. Repa JJ, Berge KE, Pomajzl C, et al. Regulation of ATP-binding cassette sterol transporters ABCG5 and ABCG8 by the liver X receptors alpha and beta. J Biol Chem 2002; 277:18793–800

42. Osada K, Sasaki E, Sugano M. Lymphatic absorption of oxidized cholesterol in rats. Lipids 1994; 29:555–9

43. Vine DF, Croft KD, Beilin LJ, et al. Absorption of dietary cholesterol oxidation products and incorporation into rat lymph chylomicrons. Lipids 1997; 32:887–93

44. Ratnayake WM, Plouffe L, Hollywood R, et al. Influence of sources of dietary oils on the life span of stroke-prone spontaneously hypertensive rats. Lipids 2000; 35:409–20

45. Klett EL, Patel SB. Biomedicine. Will the real cholesterol transporter please stand up. Science 2004; 303:1149–50

46. Altmann SW, Davis HR Jr, Zhu LJ, et al. Niemann-Pick C1 Like 1 protein is critical for intestinal cholesterol absorption. Science 2004; 303:1201–4

47. Davis HR Jr, Zhu LJ, Hoos LM, et al. Niemann-Pick C1 Like 1 (NPC1L1) is the intestinal phytosterol and cholesterol transporter and a key modulator of whole-body cholesterol homeostasis. J Biol Chem 2004; 279:33586–92

FXR: the molecular link between bile acid and lipid metabolism 7

T. Claudel, E. Sturm, B. Staels and F. Kuipers

INTRODUCTION

Bile acids (BAs) are synthesized from cholesterol exclusively by the liver. The biosynthetic steps that collectively accomplish the conversion of hydrophobic, water-insoluble cholesterol molecules into more water-soluble compounds also confer detergent properties to the BA that are crucial for their physiological functions in bile formation and intestinal fat absorption. Bile acids are actively secreted by the hepatocytes into the bile canaliculi that drain into intrahepatic bile ducts, stored in the gallbladder and expelled into the intestinal lumen in response to a fatty meal. In the small intestine, BAs act as detergents to emulsify and facilitate the absorption of dietary fats and lipid-soluble vitamins. Subsequently, BAs are reabsorbed from the terminal ileum by the actions of specific transporter proteins: about 95% returns to the liver to be secreted again into the bile, completing the so-called entero-hepatic circulation, whereas 5% escapes reabsorption and is lost via the faeces. The fraction of BAs that are lost per cycle is compensated for by hepatic synthesis from cholesterol, which maintains BA pool size. Although the fractional loss of BAs per cycle is relatively small, daily BA synthesis in adult humans amounts up to ~500 mg, which accounts for about 90% of the cholesterol that is actively metabolized in the body.

The detergent properties of BAs, determined in part by the number of hydroxyl groups present at the steroid moiety, are crucial for most of their biological functions, i.e. in generating bile flow, promoting biliary excretion of hydrophobic compounds and facilitating intestinal fat absorption. The physical characteristics of BAs, which allow them to form micelles, also impose a certain risk to cells that are exposed to high concentrations of these natural detergents. When present at high concentrations, BAs may become cytotoxic. Hepatocytes and bile duct cells, in particular, are at risk, for instance in conditions of disturbed bile formation or stasis of bile in the ductular system (cholestasis), and protective mechanisms appear to become active when intracellular BA concentrations are elevated. Obviously, both the maintenance of physiological control of the enterohepatic circulation and the initiation of cell-protective reactions require a mode of 'bile acid sensing' in particular cells. Recently, it became clear that BAs themselves are directly involved in regulation of gene expression in liver and intestine via interaction with a nuclear receptor called farnesoid X receptor (FXR), which provides such a sensor function. Nuclear receptors are ligand-activated transcription factors that, in general, bind small molecules of endogenous or dietary origin, such as oxysterols, fatty acids, vitamins or certain drugs. FXR is involved in the regulation of several steps of BA biology, including synthesis, detoxification and transport. Moreover, a direct link has recently been established between BA–FXR activation and various aspects of lipid metabolism. Therefore, FXR modulation may constitute a new pharmaceutical target with potential application in the treatment of lipid disorders.

THE BIOLOGY OF FXR

FXR (or NR1H4) was cloned independently by two groups using different strategies in 1995. In a quest for new retinoid X receptor (RXR) partners, the RXR interacting protein (RIP14) was isolated by Seol et al. Two isoforms were subsequently cloned in mouse, that were expressed in the liver and in the intestine.[1] Simultaneously, Forman et al cloned a new sequence of a nuclear receptor by liver cDNA bank screening.[2] Since it was originally shown to be activated by the isoprenoid farnesol, this receptor was designated farnesoid X receptor.[2] FXR expression was detected in the liver, the intestine, the kidney and in the adrenals of adult rats and similar expression patterns have been reported in mice.[3] Being closely related to the insect ecdysone receptor (EcR), it was shown that FXR, after heterodimerization with its partner RXR, also binds to the EcR response element inverted repeat-1 (IR-1).

Analysis of the FXR locus demonstrated the expression of four splice variants with different N-terminal domains (FXRα or FXRβ) and a four-amino-acid insertion between the DNA- and the ligand-binding domains (FXRα1, FXRα2, FXRβ1, FXRβ2). Two promoters drive the expression of the two FXR isoforms that are expressed in a developmental and tissue-specific manner with distinct transcriptional activities.[4,5]

Relatively little is known about the regulation of FXR expression. Very recently, we were able to show that the expression of the FXR gene is suppressed in rat models of diabetes. Using rat hepatocytes in culture, it was demonstrated that glucose positively regulates FXR gene expression in a dose- and time-dependent manner, probably by acting at the transcriptional level through the actions of metabolites of the pentose-phosphate shunt.[6]

In 1999, three groups identified BAs as natural FXR ligands.[7–9] Interestingly, FXR can be activated by several primary and secondary BA species conjugated to either taurine or glycine (Figure 1) with an affinity in the micromolar range.

To evaluate the potential beneficial effects of pharmacological FXR activation, several groups

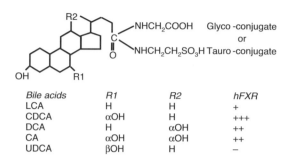

Bile acids	R1	R2	hFXR
LCA	H	H	+
CDCA	αOH	H	+++
DCA	H	αOH	++
CA	αOH	αOH	++
UDCA	βOH	H	−

Figure 1 FXR is a bile acid receptor. LCA, lithocholic acid; CDCA, chenodeoxycholic acid; DCA, deoxycholic acid; CA, cholic acid; UDCA, ursodeoxycholic acid. The +/– indicate the relative potencies of the bile acids to activate the human FXR receptor

started the search for synthetic, non-steroidal FXR agonists. The first compound isolated was the potent FXR agonist GW4064, an isoxazole derivative, which is often used as a 'chemical tool' to show that BA-target genes are regulated in an FXR-specific manner[10] since BAs are also able to activate FXR-independent pathways.[11] Soon thereafter, several new synthetic compounds were described. By modification of the BA backbone to increase its affinity for FXR, Pellicciari et al produced 6-ethyl CDCA, a more potent FXR agonist than the natural BA chenodeoxycholic acid (CDCA, see further) in in vitro experiments that conferred protection against cholestasis induced by the toxic BA species lithocholic acid in rats.[12] Analysis by Downes et al of the properties of another agonist, FeXaRamine, in comparison to the synthetic agonist GW4064 and the natural agonist CDCA, showed that these compounds do not regulate the same genes.[13] In addition, Dussault et al characterized the mixed properties of AGN34, a molecule structurally derived from a relatively weak and non-specific FXR agonist, which was shown to act either as an agonist, an antagonist or neutral on different FXR target genes.[14] In analogy with the oestrogen receptor (ER), for which different ligands called selective oestrogen receptor modulators, or SERMs, were shown to induce distinct biological responses depending on the response element structure in the promoter of the target gene, the co-factor recruitment and

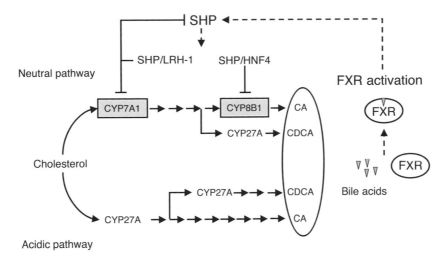

Figure 2 FXR controls the bile acid biosynthetic pathways. CYP7A1 is the key enzyme of the neutral pathway, whereas CYP27A is the key enzyme of the acidic pathway. CYP7A1 and CYP8B1 are negatively regulated by FXR (grey boxes) after induction of SHP. The inactive SHP/LRH-1 complex will subsequently impair CYP7A1, whereas SHP/HNF4 will impair CYP8B1 promoter *trans*-activation. Moreover, SHP/LRH-1 will also turn off SHP induction and thus the repression mechanism. The normal arrows show activation, the block arrows inhibition

the target tissue, these observations led to the new concept of selective Bile Acid Receptor Modulator or BARM. The BARM concept will be of crucial importance for the development of potential therapeutic applications of FXR modulators.

THE ROLE OF FXR IN THE CONTROL OF BILE ACID METABOLISM

Bile acids are amphipathic molecules with detergent-like properties that are essential for their physiological functions. As a BA receptor, FXR controls several of the adaptive changes that are required to maintain optimal BA concentrations at the sites of their physiological actions, i.e. in the biliary tree to generate bile flow and in the intestinal lumen to facilitate fat absorption. At the same time, FXR is crucial for the protection of cells contributing to the enterohepatic circulation from BA-induced toxicity, for instance when the capacity of liver cells to secrete BAs into the bile is perturbed in cholestatic liver disease. During the past few

years, it has become clear that FXR has a crucial role in control of BA synthesis and transport as well as in their 'detoxification' when intracellular concentrations exceed a certain threshold.

Bile acid synthesis

Bile acids are endproducts of a series of cholesterol-converting enzymatic reactions. Chenodeoxycholic acid (CDCA) and cholic acid (CA) are the major primary BAs in humans that can be synthesized by two different pathways: the neutral pathway produces both CDCA and CA, whereas the acidic pathway gives rise to CDCA only (Figure 2).

Microsomal CYP7A1 is the rate-controlling enzyme of the neutral pathway. It has been known for decades that BAs exert a negative feedback regulation on their own synthesis. Recently, FXR was identified as a key player in BA-induced downregulation of CYP7A1 expression, through an indirect mechanism.[15] The original observation that SHP (small heterodimer partner or NR0B2) expression was reduced in FXR-deficient mice whereas CYP7A1 expression was increased, combined with the fact that the atypical nuclear receptor SHP was devoid of a DNA-binding domain and closely related to another orphan nuclear Dax-1 (dosage-sensitive sex reversal – congenital adrenal hypoplasia or NR0B1), led to a new hypothesis based on the model of the Dax-1/SF-1 (steroidogenic factor 1 or NR5A2) interaction. FXR activation was found to increase gene expression of SHP. Subsequently, the interaction between SHP and LRH-1 (liver receptor homologue-1 or NR5A2) inhibits LRH-1 trans-activation of CYP7A1[16,17] (Figure 2). Moreover, the basal gene expression of SHP is also activated by LRH-1, therefore the inactive SHP/LRH-1 complex reduces SHP expression and turns off the negative feedback signal (Figure 2). FXR also induces the expression of a secreted growth factor that activates the FGF4 receptor isotype in hepatocytes: fibroblast growth factor-19 (FGF-19).[18] FGF-19 represses CYP7A1 expression in human and mouse hepatocytes via a signalling cascade involving the c-Jun N-terminal kinase pathway. Interestingly, FGFR4-deficient mice display an increased BA pool size and higher hepatobiliary BA excretion rate[19] and CYP7A1 expression is unresponsive to dietary cholesterol, but can be repressed by BA in these mice.

However, CYP7A1 regulation is extremely complex and several other, FXR-independent mechanisms have been invoked in the negative feedback regulation exerted by circulating BA.[11,20] Discussion of these mechanisms is beyond the scope of this chapter, but can be found in excellent recent reviews.[21,22]

The CYP8B1 enzyme controls the hydrophobicity of the BA pool by modulating the relative amount of CA synthesized. Einarrsson et al demonstrated that CYP8B1 expression is upregulated after ileal resection, suggesting alleviation of negative feedback control by BA.[23] Underlying mechanisms may involve a decreased expression of HNF4α and/or a decreased trans-activation of the CYP8B1 promoter by HNF4α due to SHP induction[24] (Figure 2).

Finally, it is important to know that the acidic pathway is not under the control of BA, since the key enzyme CYP27 is not regulated by BA nor changed in FXR-deficient mice.[25]

Bile acid transport within the enterohepatic circulation

After conjugation with either taurine or glycine on their side chain, a process also regulated at the transcriptional level by FXR,[26] BAs become more hydrophilic and require a transporter network to cycle between liver and intestine.

During their enterohepatic cycle, BAs are taken up by the liver via the Na⁺ taurocholate co-transporting polypeptide (NTCP),[27–29] expressed exclusively at the basolateral plasma membrane of hepatocytes,[30,31] which represents almost 75% of BA uptake (Figure 3). NTCP expression is downregulated by FXR since it is reduced in wild-type but not in FXR-deficient mice upon CA treatment,[25] but its basal expression is not different between wild-type and FXR-deficient mice.[25,32] FXR acts, via SHP induction, to inhibit RXR/RAR trans-activation of the NTCP promoter, at least in rats.[33] Given the fact that the RXR/RAR site is lacking in human and mouse NTCP promoters, it is unlikely that a negative transcriptional regulation by BA will occur in these species.[34]

A Na⁺-independent BA uptake is mediated by the organic anion transporter polypeptides (OATPs). In humans, OATP-C is the most abundant Na⁺-independent BA transporter localized at the basolateral membrane[35–37] (Figure 3). In mice, OATP1 expression is either repressed or not affected by BA treatment.[25,38] Importantly, FXR deficiency did not change OATP1 gene expression at the basal level in mice.[25,32]

Within the hepatocytes, BAs traffic from the basolateral membrane across the cells to the canalicular pole prior to their secretion into bile. The mechanism(s) of trans-cellular BA transport remain poorly understood and it is unclear whether FXR is functionally involved in the regulation of this process. Several proteins were identified as potential intracellular BA carriers, like the liver fatty-acid-binding protein (L-FABP), which is induced by CA treatment in wild-type but not in FXR-deficient mice.[25]

BA secretion at the canalicular membrane is an ATP-dependent process mediated by the bile salt export pump (BSEP or ABCB11).[39–43] BSEP mutations underlie the bile secretion

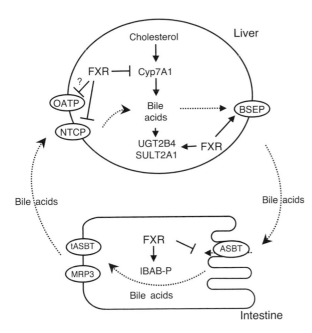

Figure 3 FXR controls the bile acid enterohepatic cycle. At the hepatic level, FXR represses the expression of NTCP and CYP7A1. Simultaneously, FXR induces the expression of the detoxification enzymes SULT2A1 and UGT2B4 and promotes BA clearance by the induction of BSEP. At the intestinal level, FXR represses ileal Apical Sodium-dependent Bile acid Transporter (ASBT) expression and induces the expression of the putative intracellular transporter IBABP. BAs will subsequently go to the portal circulation after excretion by MRP3 or tASBT. The normal arrows show activation, the block arrows inhibition

the overabundant expression of BSEP under normal conditions provides the hepatocytes with a safety valve to deal with situations in which the liver is exposed to a high BA influx, e.g. in the post-prandial period.

Bile acid absorption at the intestinal level occurs with an extremely high efficiency (~95%). BAs cross the enterocyte membranes via the action of the apical sodium-dependent bile acid transporter (ASBT) protein.[48–52] BA does not regulate rat ASBT gene expression,[53] but FXR influences the transcription factor network involved in the BA response[54,55] (Figure 3). In the enterocytes, FXR induces the expression of IBABP (ileal bile acid binding protein), a small cytosolic protein.[56] Until recently, it was believed that IBABP acts as a shuttle delivering BA from the apical to the basolateral membrane.[57] Yet, the observation that IBABP expression is strongly decreased in FXR-deficient mice while BA absorption is enhanced indicates that the exact physiological role of IBABP remains to be defined.[32] It is plausible to suggest that IBABP may act as a 'BA sink' to protect enterocytes from BA toxicity when exposed to high concentrations. Bile acids may cross the basolateral membrane of enterocytes to enter the portal blood stream using the MRP3 transporter[58] or the tABST protein[59] (Figure 3).

Bile acid detoxification

As mentioned previously, relatively hydrophobic BA species, as exemplified by CDCA and its bacterial metabolite lithocholic acid, are potentially toxic agents and readily induce cholestasis when administered to rodents. Sulphation and glucuronidation are common phase II detoxification reactions to facilitate removal of poorly water-soluble endo- and xenobiotics from the body. It has been known for more than 30 years that these reactions also occur with BA, especially in conditions associated with cholestatic liver disease. Dehydroepiandrosterone– sulphotransferase SULT2A1 is a cytosolic enzyme that promotes 3α-OH sulphation of BAs.[60] SULT2A1 gene expression is induced by FXR.[61] The human uridine glucuronosyltransferase 2B4, that converts BAs

failure in patients with progressive familial intrahepatic cholestasis type II (PFIC 2).[44] Inactivation of BSEP in mice results in a less severe phenotype than in humans,[45] which may be due to differences in BA metabolism between the species. BA–FXR activation increases BSEP expression in rodents as well as in human liver cells[46,47] (Figure 3).

Taken together, FXR activation decreases BA uptake by NTCP downregulation and increases BA excretion via BSEP induction, a mechanism that will protect the hepatocytes from a potentially toxic BA overload. Since FXR-deficient mice display low BSEP expression but have normal biliary BA excretion,[32] BSEP expression is not limiting for biliary BA secretion at the basal level. This suggests that into more hydrophilic glucuronide deriva-tives,[62,63] is positively regulated by FXR binding to a monomeric FXRE localized in its pro-moter.[64] Since glucuronidated and sulphated BAs are usually more water-soluble, FXR may reduce BA toxicity as well by enhancing their clearance via bile and/or urine. Thus, a major physiological role of the BA receptor FXR is to protect cells from the deleterious effects of BA overload by decreasing endogenous BA production and promoting BA biotransforma-tion and clearance.

AN EMERGING ROLE FOR FXR IN THE CONTROL OF LIPID METABOLISM

In the past few years, several studies have demonstrated that BAs, via FXR, are potent modulators of lipid and lipoprotein metabo-lism in a way that goes far beyond their estab-lished functions as 'catabolites' of cholesterol and as 'soaps' that facilitate the absorption of fat and cholesterol from the intestine. This newly established physiological function of BA is of potentially great interest for the develop-ment of alternative strategies for the treatment of hyperlipidaemias.

FXR and HDL

The resins cholestyramine, colestipol and colesevelam are non-absorbable drugs with high affinity for BAs in the intestine. After binding to the BAs, the resin/BA complex is eliminated via the faeces. As a consequence of the interruption of the enterohepatic circula-tion, CY7A1 expression in the liver will be induced which, in turn, will increase the conversion of cholesterol into BA. The ensuing hepatic cholesterol depletion will then lead to an increase in surface-active LDL receptors and therefore to a fall in low density lipoprotein (LDL)-cholesterol levels due to increased clearance of apoB-100- and apoE-containing lipoproteins. A side-effect of this modification in hepatic cholesterol homeostasis is a rise in hepatic HMG-CoA reductase activity in

conjunction with an increased very low density lipoprotein (VLDL) triglyceride production (see below).

Interestingly, treatment with BA-binding resins also leads to an increase in high density lipoprotein (HDL)-cholesterol levels,[65,66] thereby promoting the reverse cholesterol transport pathway (Figure 4). Intriguingly, patients with gallstones and cerebrotendinous xanthomatosis (CTX) treated with BAs display lower levels of HDL-cholesterol.[67,68] Moreover, patients with progressive familial intrahepatic cholestasis (PFIC), a disease characterized by intrahepatic accumulation of BA, have low serum levels of apoA-I, the major HDL apolipoprotein.[69] The molecular basis for this interaction between BA and HDL metabolism has remained enigmatic for many years. Recently, we were able to demonstrate that both the human and mouse *apo A-I* genes are negatively regulated by FXR, that binds as a monomer to a negative response element in the *apo A-I* promoter.[69] In line with this, chow-fed FXR-deficient mice displayed higher HDL-cholesterol levels than wild-type mice.[25] In addition, FXR was also shown to induce the expression of the phospholipid transfer protein (PLTP),[70] an enzyme involved in HDL remodelling (Figure 4).

FXR and triglyceride metabolism

As already described previously, disruption of the enterohepatic cycle of BAs in humans using either sequestrants[71] or ileal bypass surgery[72] results in an increase in serum triglyc-eride levels.[73] Furthermore, hypertriglyceri-daemia in type IV hyperlipoproteinaemia patients is associated with impaired absorption of BA[74] due to diminished ASBT expression.[73] Conversely, triglyceride levels decrease in gallstone patients as well as in hyperlipaemic patients treated with BA.[75–78] Finally, FXR-deficient mice have higher triglyceride levels than wild-type mice, mainly confined to the VLDL-sized lipoprotein fractions.[25] Taken together, these results suggest that FXR activation by BA also modulates triglyceride metabolism.

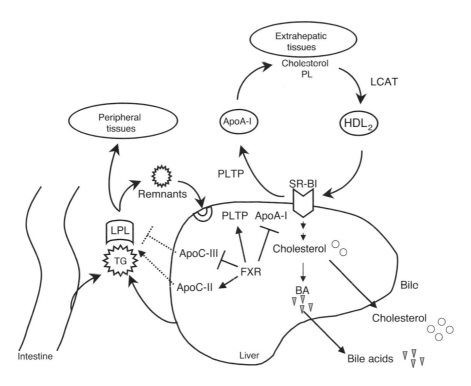

Figure 4 FXR controls plasma HDL and triglyceride metabolism. HDL-cholesterol promotes cholesterol excretion from the peripheral tissues to the liver. FXR represses apoA-I and induces PLTP gene expression, respectively. Simultaneously, FXR induces apoC-II (LPL co-factor) and represses apoC-III (LPL inhibitor) gene expression, respectively, and therefore increases LPL activity and triglyceride clearance. The normal arrows show activation, the block arrows inhibition. PL, phospholipid; LCAT, lecithin:cholesterol acyltransferase; PLTP, phospholipid transfer protein; LPL, lipoprotein lipase; TG, triglycerides

A key player in the control of plasma triglyceride metabolism is the lipoprotein lipase (LPL), an enzyme that mediates lipolysis of triglyceride-rich lipoproteins. ApoC-II and apoA-V are activators, whereas apoC-III is an inhibitor of LPL activity. Since FXR activation increases apoC-II expression[79] and simultaneously inhibits apoC-III gene expression in the liver[80] and since, although not confirmed by in vivo data, FXR *trans*-activated the promoter of the human apoA-V gene,[81] the overall effect of FXR activation will be to increase the LPL activity and therefore to accelerate triglyceride clearance.

The peroxisome proliferator-activated receptor α (PPAR-α) is a nuclear receptor activated by fatty acids[82] and the synthetic drugs fibrates[83] that also regulates BA synthesis and pool composition.[84,85] Moreover, PPAR-α activation increases LPL activity and subsequently lowers triglyceride levels. PPAR-α is a species-specific FXR-target gene, i.e. in humans, but not in mice, FXR increases PPAR-α gene expression.[86] The existence of such a cross-talk between these nuclear receptors suggests the existence of a delicate co-ordination between fatty acid and BA metabolism.

The peroxisome proliferator activated receptor gamma coactivator 1α (PGC-1α) is a nuclear receptor co-factor involved in the control of adaptive thermogenesis and glucose metabolism as well as CYP7A1 expression.[87] Under fasting conditions the expression of the FXRβ isoform is induced via a mechanism implicating PGC-1α and PGC-1α was also identified as a potential FXR cofactor involved in the increase in triglyceride clearance and the lowering of triglyceride synthesis mediated by FXR.[88]

Finally, the trans-membrane heparan sulphate proteoglycan syndecan 1 is expressed in the liver and binds several lipoproteins and proteins, such as LPL.[89] Remnant lipoprotein particles are believed to bind to syndecan 1 prior to their transfer to receptors, such as the LDL-receptor, which increases lipoprotein catabolism. FXR increases syndecan 1 gene expression in an isoform-dependent manner, i.e. FXR-α2 and FXR-β2 are involved in the trans-activation promoter.[90]

Taken together, it is evident that BA activated-FXR modulates several aspects of triglyceride metabolism. Therefore, it is attractive to speculate that stimulation of the entero-hepatic BA flux upon ingestion of a (fatty) meal provides a signal that prepares the body to adequately handle the 'upcoming' fat load and that blunts the post-prandial hyperlipidaemia.

NATURAL NON-BILE ACID FXR MODULATORS: THE GUGGULSTERONE STORY

Guggulipid, a resin extract of the tree *Commiphora mukul*, is a traditional medicinal herb used in India to treat obesity and lipid disorders.[91,92] Given the therapeutic interest in FXR modulators, several recent studies have focused on the action mechanism of E- and Z-guggulsterone, which are believed to be the active components of guggulipid.[93] Urizar et al demonstrated that guggulsterone acted as FXR antagonist and pregnane X receptor (PXR) partial agonist.[94] Moreover, in vivo experiments using mice on a high-cholesterol diet showed that guggulsterone treatment decreased the

hepatic cholesterol content in an FXR-dependent manner.[94] Nevertheless, guggulsterone seems to act both as FXR and PXR modulator.[95] It was subsequently proposed that the FXR modulation properties of the drug explained its hypolipidaemic effect. Until recently, appropriately well-designed human studies on the effects of the guggulsterones were lacking, especially with patients from Western countries. In 2003, Szapary et al demonstrated a complete failure of guggulsterone to decrease the cholesterol levels in hypercholesterolaemic patients.[96] Therefore, despite a plausible mechanism of action via FXR, guggulsterone seems not to be 'the' appropriate FXR modulator suitable for the treatment of obesity or hyperlipidaemia. The quest for such a compound is still open.

CONCLUSION

FXR is a nuclear receptor that acts at the cross-road of BA and lipid metabolism. It is evident that FXR constitutes a potential attractive target for treatment of cholestatic liver diseases as well as of (specific forms of) hyperlipidaemia. From its multitude of actions, it is clear that selective FXR modulators are required to limit potential undesirable side-effects. Since such selective modulators have already been generated, exciting results from this area of research can be expected in the coming years.

ACKNOWLEDGEMENTS

Thierry Claudel was supported by Grant number 2002B017 from the Nederlandse Hartstichting.

References

1. Seol W, Choi HS, Moore DD. Isolation of proteins that interact specifically with the retinoid X receptor: two novel orphan receptors. Mol Endocrinol 1995; 9:72–85

2. Forman BM, Goode E, Chen J, et al. Identification of a nuclear receptor that is activated by farnesol metabolites. Cell 1995; 81:687–93

3. Repa JJ, Mangelsdorf DJ. Nuclear receptor regulation

of cholesterol and bile acid metabolism. Curr Opin Biotechnol 1999; 10:557–63

4. Huber RM, Murphy K, Miao B, et al. Generation of multiple farnesoid-X-receptor isoforms through the use of alternative promoters. Gene 2002; 290:35–43

5. Zhang Y, Kast-Woelbern HR, Edwards PA. Natural structural variants of the nuclear receptor farnesoid X receptor affect transcriptional activation. J Biol Chem 2003; 278:104–10

6. Duran-Sandoval D, Mautino G, Martin G, et al. Glucose regulates the expression of the farnesoid X receptor in liver. Diabetes 2004; 53:890–8

7. Wang H, Chen J, Hollister K, et al. Endogenous bile acids are ligands for the nuclear receptor FXR/BAR. Mol Cell 1999; 3:543–53

8. Makishima M, Okamoto AY, Repa JJ, et al. Identification of a nuclear receptor for bile acids. Science 1999; 284:1362–5

9. Parks DJ, Blanchard SG, Bledsoe RK , et al. Bile acids: natural ligands for an orphan nuclear receptor. Science 1999; 284:1365–8

10. Maloney PR, Parks DJ, Haffner CD, et al. Identification of a chemical tool for the orphan nuclear receptor FXR. J Med Chem 2000; 43:2971–4

11. Gupta S, Stravitz RT, Dent P, et al. Down-regulation of cholesterol 7alpha-hydroxylase (CYP7A1) gene expression by bile acids in primary rat hepatocytes is mediated by the c-Jun N-terminal kinase pathway. J Biol Chem 2001; 276:15816–22

12. Pellicciari R, Fiorucci S, Camaioni E, et al. 6alpha-ethyl-chenodeoxycholic acid (6α-ECDCA), a potent and selective FXR agonist endowed with anticholestatic activity. J Med Chem 2002; 45:3569–72

13. Downes M, Verdecia MA, Roecker AJ, et al. A chemical, genetic, and structural analysis of the nuclear bile acid receptor FXR. Mol Cell 2003; 11:1079–92

14. Dussault I, Beard R, Lin M, et al. Identification of gene-selective modulators of the bile acid receptor FXR. J Biol Chem 2003; 278:7027–33

15. Chiang JY, Kimmel R, Weinberger C, et al. Farnesoid X receptor responds to bile acids and represses cholesterol 7alpha-hydroxylase gene (CYP7A1) transcription. J Biol Chem 2000; 275:10918–24

16. Goodwin B, Jones SA, Price RR, et al. A regulatory cascade of the nuclear receptors FXR, SHP-1, and LRH-1 represses bile acid biosynthesis. Mol Cell 2000; 6:517–26

17. Lu TT, Makishima M, Repa JJ, et al. Molecular basis for feedback regulation of bile acid synthesis by nuclear receptors. Mol Cell 2000; 6:507–15

18. Holt JA, Luo G, Billin AN, et al. Definition of a novel growth factor-dependent signal cascade for the suppression of bile acid biosynthesis. Genes Dev 2003; 17:1581–91

19. Yu C, Wang F, Kan M, et al. Elevated cholesterol metabolism and bile acid synthesis in mice lacking membrane tyrosine kinase receptor FGFR4. J Biol Chem 2000; 275:15482–9

20. Miyake JH, Wang SL, Davis RA. Bile acid induction of cytokine expression by macrophages correlates with repression of hepatic cholesterol 7alpha-hydroxylase. J Biol Chem 2000; 275:21805–8

21. Russell DW. The enzymes, regulation, and genetics of bile acid synthesis. Annu Rev Biochem 2003; 72:137–74

22. Chiang JY. Regulation of bile acid synthesis: pathways, nuclear receptors, and mechanisms. J Hepatol 2004; 40:539–51

23. Einarsson K, Akerlund JE, Reihner E, et al. 12 alpha-hydroxylase activity in human liver and its relation to cholesterol 7 alpha-hydroxylase activity. J Lipid Res 1992; 33:1591–5

24. Zhang M, Chiang JY. Transcriptional regulation of the human sterol 12alpha-hydroxylase gene (CYP8B1). Roles of hepatocyte nuclear factor 4alpha in mediating bile acid repression. J Biol Chem 2001; 276:41690–9

25. Sinal CJ, Tohkin M, Miyata M, et al. Targeted disruption of the nuclear receptor FXR/BAR impairs bile acid and lipid homeostasis. Cell 2000; 102:731–44

26. Pircher PC, Kitto JL, Petrowski ML, et al. Farnesoid X receptor regulates bile acid-amino acid conjugation. J Biol Chem 2003; 278:27703–11

27. Hagenbuch B, Stieger B, Foguet M, et al. Functional expression cloning and characterization of the hepatocyte Na+/bile acid cotransport system. Proc Natl Acad Sci USA 1991; 88:10629–33

28. Hagenbuch B, Meier PJ. Molecular cloning, chromosomal localization, and functional characterization of a human liver Na+/bile acid cotransporter. J Clin Invest 1994; 93:1326–31

29. Cattori V, Eckhardt U, Hagenbuch B. Molecular cloning and functional characterization of two alternatively spliced Ntcp isoforms from mouse liver1. Biochim Biophys Acta 1999; 1445:154–9

30. Stieger B, Hagenbuch B, Landmann L, et al. In situ localization of the hepatocytic Na+/taurocholate cotransporting polypeptide in rat liver. Gastroenterology 1994; 107:1781–7

31. Ananthanarayanan M, Ng OC, Boyer JL, et al. Characterization of cloned rat liver Na(+)-bile acid cotransporter using peptide and fusion protein antibodies. Am J Physiol 1994; 267:G637–43

32. Kok T, Hulzebos CV, Wolters H, et al. Enterohepatic circulation of bile salts in farnesoid X receptor-deficient mice: efficient intestinal bile salt absorption in the absence of ileal bile acid-binding protein. J Biol Chem 2003; 278:41930–7

33. Denson LA, Sturm E, Echevarria W, et al. The orphan nuclear receptor, shp, mediates bile acid-induced inhibition of the rat bile acid transporter, ntcp. Gastroenterology 2001; 121:140–7

34. Jung D, Hagenbuch B, Fried M, et al. Role of liver-enriched transcription factors and nuclear receptors in regulating the human, mouse, and rat NTCP gene. Am J Physiol Gastrointest Liver Physiol 2004; 286:G752–61

35. Abe T, Kakyo M, Tokui T, et al. Identification of a

novel gene family encoding human liver-specific organic anion transporter LST-1. J Biol Chem 1999; 274:17159–63

36. Hsiang B, Zhu Y, Wang Z, et al. A novel human hepatic organic anion transporting polypeptide (OATP2). Identification of a liver-specific human organic anion transporting polypeptide and identification of rat and human hydroxymethylglutaryl-CoA reductase inhibitor transporters. J Biol Chem 1999; 274:37161–8

37. Konig J, Cui Y, Nies AT, et al. A novel human organic anion transporting polypeptide localized to the basolateral hepatocyte membrane. Am J Physiol Gastrointest Liver Physiol 2000; 278:G156–64

38. Fickert P, Zollner G, Fuchsbichler A, et al. Effects of ursodeoxycholic and cholic acid feeding on hepatocellular transporter expression in mouse liver. Gastroenterology 2001; 121:170–83

39. Adachi Y, Kamisako T, Yamamoto T. The effects of temporary occlusion of the superior mesenteric vein or splenic vein on biliary bilirubin and bile acid excretion in rats. J Lab Clin Med 1991; 118:261–8

40. Muller M, Ishikawa T, Berger U, et al. ATP-dependent transport of taurocholate across the hepatocyte canalicular membrane mediated by a 110-kDa glycoprotein binding ATP and bile salt. J Biol Chem 1991; 266:18920–6

41. Nishida T, Gatmaitan Z, Che M, et al. Rat liver canalicular membrane vesicles contain an ATP-dependent bile acid transport system. Proc Natl Acad Sci USA 1991; 88:6590–4

42. Gerloff T, Stieger B, Hagenbuch B, et al. The sister of P-glycoprotein represents the canalicular bile salt export pump of mammalian liver. J Biol Chem 1998; 273:10046–50

43. Green RM, Hoda F, Ward KL. Molecular cloning and characterization of the murine bile salt export pump. Gene 2000; 241:117–23

44. Jansen PL, Strautnieks SS, Jacquemin E, et al. Hepatocanalicular bile salt export pump deficiency in patients with progressive familial intrahepatic cholestasis. Gastroenterology 1999; 117:1370–9

45. Wang R, Salem M, Yousef IM, et al. Targeted inactivation of sister of P-glycoprotein gene (spgp) in mice results in nonprogressive but persistent intrahepatic cholestasis. Proc Natl Acad Sci USA 2001; 98:2011–16

46. Ananthanarayanan M, Balasubramanian N, Makishima M, et al. Human bile salt export pump promoter is transactivated by the farnesoid X receptor/bile acid receptor. J Biol Chem 2001; 276:28857–65

47. Plass JR, Mol O, Heegsma J, et al. Farnesoid X receptor and bile salts are involved in transcriptional regulation of the gene encoding the human bile salt export pump. Hepatology 2002; 35:589–96

48. Wong MH, Oelkers P, Craddock AL, Dawson PA. Expression cloning and characterization of the hamster ileal sodium-dependent bile acid transporter. J Biol Chem 1994; 269:1340–7

49. Wong MH, Oelkers P, Dawson PA. Identification of a mutation in the ileal sodium-dependent bile acid transporter gene that abolishes transport activity. J Biol Chem 1995; 270:27228–34

50. Shneider BL, Dawson PA, Christie DM, et al. Cloning and molecular characterization of the ontogeny of a rat ileal sodium-dependent bile acid transporter. J Clin Invest 1995; 95:745–54

51. Saeki T, Matoba K, Furukawa H, et al. Characterization, cDNA cloning, and functional expression of mouse ileal sodium-dependent bile acid transporter. J Biochem (Tokyo) 1999; 125:846–51

52. Dawson PA, Haywood J, Craddock AL, et al. Targeted deletion of the ileal bile acid transporter eliminates enterohepatic cycling of bile acids in mice. J Biol Chem 2003; 278:33920–7

53. Arrese M, Trauner M, Sacchiero RJ, et al. Neither intestinal sequestration of bile acids nor common bile duct ligation modulate the expression and function of the rat ileal bile acid transporter. Hepatology 1998; 28:1081–7

54. Chen F, Ma L, Dawson PA, et al. Liver receptor homologue-1 mediates species- and cell line-specific bile acid-dependent negative feedback regulation of the apical sodium-dependent bile acid transporter. J Biol Chem 2003; 278:19909–16

55. Neimark E, Chen F, Li X, et al. Bile acid-induced negative feedback regulation of the human ileal bile acid transporter. Hepatology 2004; 40:149–56

56. Grober J, Zaghini I, Fujii H, et al. Identification of a bile acid-responsive element in the human ileal bile acid-binding protein gene. Involvement of the farnesoid X receptor/9–cis-retinoic acid receptor heterodimer. J Biol Chem 1999; 274:29749–54

57. Kramer W, Corsiero D, Friedrich M, et al. Intestinal absorption of bile acids: paradoxical behaviour of the 14 kDa ileal lipid-binding protein in differential photoaffinity labelling. Biochem J 1998; 333 (Pt 2):335–41

58. Inokuchi A, Hinoshita E, Iwamoto Y, et al. Enhanced expression of the human multidrug resistance protein 3 by bile salt in human enterocytes. A transcriptional control of a plausible bile acid transporter. J Biol Chem 2001; 276:46822–9

59. Lazaridis KN, Tietz P, Wu T, et al. Alternative splicing of the rat sodium/bile acid transporter changes its cellular localization and transport properties. Proc Natl Acad Sci USA 2000; 97:11092–7

60. Barnes S, Buchina ES, King RJ, et al. Bile acid sulfotransferase I from rat liver sulfates bile acids and 3–hydroxy steroids: purification, N-terminal amino acid sequence, and kinetic properties. J Lipid Res 1989; 30:529–40

61. Song CS, Echchgadda I, Baek BS, et al. Dehydroepiandrosterone sulfotransferase gene induction by bile acid activated farnesoid x receptor. J Biol Chem 2001; 276:42549–56

62. Pillot T, Ouzzine M, Fournel-Gigleux S, et al. Glucuronidation of hyodeoxycholic acid in human

liver. Evidence for a selective role of UDP-glucuronosyltransferase 2B4. J Biol Chem 1993; 268:25636–42

63. Monaghan G, Burchell B, Boxer M. Structure of the human UGT2B4 gene encoding a bile acid UDP-glucuronosyltransferase. Mamm Genome 1997; 8:692–4

64. Barbier O, Torra IP, Sirvent A, et al. FXR induces the UGT2B4 enzyme in hepatocytes: a potential mechanism of negative feedback control of FXR activity. Gastroenterology 2003; 124:1926–40

65. Bard JM, Parra HJ, Douste-Blazy P, et al. Effect of pravastatin, an HMG CoA reductase inhibitor, and cholestyramine, a bile acid sequestrant, on lipoprotein particles defined by their apolipoprotein composition. Metabolism 1990; 39:269–73

66. Hagen E, Istad H, Ose L, et al. Fluvastatin efficacy and tolerability in comparison and in combination with cholestyramine. Eur J Clin Pharmacol 1994; 46:445–9

67. Leiss O, von Bergmann K. Different effects of chenodeoxycholic acid and ursodeoxycholic acid on serum lipoprotein concentrations in patients with radiolucent gallstones. Scand J Gastroenterol 1982; 17:587–92

68. Kuriyama M, Tokimura Y, Fujiyama J, et al. Treatment of cerebrotendinous xanthomatosis: effects of chenodeoxycholic acid, pravastatin, and combined use. J Neurol Sci 1994; 125:22–8

69. Claudel T, Sturm E, Duez H, et al. Bile acid-activated nuclear receptor FXR suppresses apolipoprotein A-I transcription via a negative FXR response element. J Clin Invest 2002; 109:961–71

70. Urizar NL, Dowhan DH, Moore DD. The farnesoid X-activated receptor mediates bile acid activation of phospholipid transfer protein gene expression. J Biol Chem 2000; 275:39313–17

71. Molgaard J, von Schenck H, Olsson AG. Comparative effects of simvastatin and cholestyramine in treatment of patients with hypercholesterolemia. Eur J Clin Pharmacol 1989; 36:455–60

72. Buchwald H, Varco RL, Matts JP, et al. Effect of partial ileal bypass surgery on mortality and morbidity from coronary heart disease in patients with hypercholesterolemia. Report of the Program on the Surgical Control of the Hyperlipidemias (POSCH). N Engl J Med 1990; 323:946–55

73. Duane WC, Hartich LA, Bartman AE, et al. Diminished gene expression of ileal apical sodium bile acid transporter explains impaired absorption of bile acid in patients with hypertriglyceridemia. J Lipid Res 2000; 41:1384–9

74. Angelin B, Hershon KS, Brunzell JD. Bile acid metabolism in hereditary forms of hypertriglyceridemia: evidence for an increased synthesis rate in monogenic familial hypertriglyceridemia. Proc Natl Acad Sci USA 1987; 84:5434–8

75. Miller NE, Nestel PJ. Triglyceride-lowering effect of chenodeoxycholic acid in patients with endogenous hypertriglyceridaemia. Lancet 1974; 2:929–31

76. Begemann F. Influence of chenodeoxycholic acid on the kinetics of endogenous triglyceride transport in man. Eur J Clin Invest 1978; 8:283–8

77. Angelin B, Einarsson K, Hellstrom K, et al. Effects of cholestyramine and chenodeoxycholic acid on the metabolism of endogenous triglyceride in hyperlipoproteinemia. J Lipid Res 1978; 19:1017–24

78. Bateson MC, Maclean D, Evans JR, et al. Chenodeoxycholic acid therapy for hypertriglyceridaemia in men. Br J Clin Pharmacol 1978; 5:249–54

79. Kast HR, Nguyen CM, Sinal CJ, et al. Farnesoid X-activated receptor induces apolipoprotein C-II transcription: a molecular mechanism linking plasma triglyceride levels to bile acids. Mol Endocrinol 2001; 15:1720–8

80. Claudel T, Inoue Y, Barbier O, et al. Farnesoid X receptor agonists suppress hepatic apolipoprotein CIII expression. Gastroenterology 2003; 125:544–55

81. Prieur X, Coste H, Rodriguez JC. The human apolipoprotein AV gene is regulated by peroxisome proliferator-activated receptor-alpha and contains a novel farnesoid X-activated receptor response element. J Biol Chem 2003; 278:25468–80

82. Willson TM, Brown PJ, Sternbach DD, et al. The PPARs: from orphan receptors to drug discovery. J Med Chem 2000; 43:527–50

83. Staels B, Dallongeville J, Auwerx J, et al. Mechanism of action of fibrates on lipid and lipoprotein metabolism. Circulation 1998; 98:2088–93

84. Patel DD, Knight BL, Soutar AK, et al. The effect of peroxisome-proliferator-activated receptor-alpha on the activity of the cholesterol 7 alpha-hydroxylase gene. Biochem J 2000; 351 (Pt 3):747–53

85. Post SM, Duez H, Gervois PP, et al. Fibrates suppress bile acid synthesis via peroxisome proliferator-activated receptor-alpha-mediated downregulation of cholesterol 7alpha-hydroxylase and sterol 27-hydroxylase expression. Arterioscler Thromb Vasc Biol 2001; 21:1840–5

86. Pineda Torra I, Claudel T, Duval C, et al. Bile acids induce the expression of the human peroxisome proliferator-activated receptor alpha gene via activation of the farnesoid X receptor. Mol Endocrinol 2003; 17:259–72

87. De Fabiani E, Mitro N, Gilardi F, et al. Coordinated control of cholesterol catabolism to bile acids and of gluconeogenesis via a novel mechanism of transcription regulation linked to the fasted-to-fed cycle. J Biol Chem 2003; 278:39124–32

88. Zhang Y, Castellani LW, Sinal CJ, et al. Peroxisome proliferator-activated receptor-gamma coactivator 1alpha (PGC-1alpha) regulates triglyceride metabolism by activation of the nuclear receptor FXR. Genes Dev 2004; 18:157–69

89. Williams KJ, Fless GM, Petrie KA, et al. Mechanisms by which lipoprotein lipase alters cellular metabolism of lipoprotein(a), low density lipoprotein, and nascent lipoproteins. Roles for low density lipoprotein receptors and heparan sulfate proteoglycans. J Biol Chem 1992; 267:13284–92

90. Anisfeld AM, Kast-Woelbern HR, Meyer ME, et al. Syndecan-1 expression is regulated in an isoform specific manner by the farnesoid-X receptor. J Biol Chem 2003; 26:26

91. Dev S. Ethnotherapeutics and modern drug development the potential of Ayurveda. Curr Sci 1997; 73:909–28

92. Satyavati GV, Dwarakanath C, Tripathi SN. Experimental studies on the hypocholesterolemic effect of *Commiphora mukul. Engl.* (Guggul). Indian J Med Res 1969; 57:1950–62

93. Nityanand S, Kapoor NK. Cholesterol lowering activity of the various fractions of guggul. Indian J Exp Biol 1973; 11:395–8

94. Urizar NL, Liverman AB, Dodds DT, et al. A natural product that lowers cholesterol as an antagonist ligand for FXR. Science 2002; 296:1703–6

95. Cui J, Huang L, Zhao A, et al. Guggulsterone is a farnesoid X receptor antagonist in coactivator association assays but acts to enhance transcription of bile salt export pump. J Biol Chem 2003; 278:10214–20

96. Szapary PO, Wolfe ML, Bloedon LT, et al. Guggulipid for the treatment of hypercholesterolemia: a randomized controlled trial. JAMA 2003; 290:765–72

Overview of HDL and reverse cholesterol transport

P. Barter

8

INTRODUCTION

The concentration of cholesterol in high density lipoproteins (HDLs) has long been known to correlate inversely with the risk of developing premature coronary heart disease.[1–8] In animal studies this relationship has been shown to be one of cause and effect. Increasing the concentration of HDLs in several animal models leads to an inhibition of atherosclerosis.[9–11] The mechanism by which HDLs protect is still uncertain, although several of the known functions of these lipoproteins have anti-atherogenic potential. These functions include the ability of HDL particles to act as extracellular acceptors of cholesterol in the first step of the reverse cholesterol transport (RCT) pathway as well as anti-oxidant, anti-inflammatory and anti-thrombotic properties of these lipoproteins. The best-documented function relates to the role of HDLs in RCT.

Reverse cholesterol transport is the term used to describe the transport of cholesterol from extrahepatic tissues to the liver, either for recycling or for elimination from the body through bile.[12,13] Not only is this pathway fundamental to normal cell function, but there is also compelling evidence that it is anti-atherogenic. The RCT pathway is facilitated and regulated by several factors that operate in plasma. Some of these factors are potential targets for therapies designed to prevent atherosclerosis. In order to exploit this potential to its fullest, it is necessary to understand how RCT operates, how it is regulated and which plasma factors should be targeted therapeutically.

This chapter provides an overview of HDLs and the pathway of RCT and identifies possible targets for therapeutic intervention.

COMPOSITION AND STRUCTURE OF HDLS

High density lipoproteins are the smallest and densest of the plasma lipoproteins. As with other plasma lipoproteins, most of the HDLs in plasma consist of a hydrophobic core (mainly cholesteryl esters plus a small amount of triglyceride) surrounded by a surface monolayer consisting of phospholipids, unesterified cholesterol and apolipoproteins. There are two main HDL apolipoproteins, apoA-I and apoA-II, that collectively account for about 90% of total. Human HDLs also contain several other minor apolipoproteins, including apoA-IV, apoA-V, the C apolipoproteins, apoD, apoE, apoJ and apoL. In addition, HDLs act as a transport vehicle for several other proteins that are involved in plasma lipid metabolism and RCT. These include cholesteryl ester transfer protein (CETP), lecithin:cholesterol acyltransferase (LCAT) and phospholipid transfer protein (PLTP).

HDL SUBPOPULATIONS

The HDL fraction in human plasma is heterogeneous, consisting of several distinct subpopulations of particles that differ in shape, size, density, composition and surface charge (Figure 1).

HDL heterogeneity

Shape
Spherical HDLs
Discoidal HDLs

Size and density
HDL_{2b}, HDL_{2a}, HDL_{3a}, HDL_{3b}, HDL_{3c}, lipid-free apoA-I

Apolipoprotein composition
apoA-I containing HDLs
apoA-I/apoA-II containing HDLs
apoE containing HDLs

Electrophoretic mobility
Alpha-migrating HDLs
Pre-beta-migrating HDLs
Gamma-migrating HDLs
Pre-alpha-migrating HDLs

Figure 1 High density lipoproteins (HDLs) in human plasma are heterogeneous in terms of shape, size, density, apolipoprotein composition and electrophoretic mobility

Most of the HDLs circulating in normal human plasma are spherical, with discoidal particles accounting for a very small percentage of the total. When isolated on the basis of density by ultracentrifugation, human HDLs separate into two major subfractions, HDL_2 ($1.063 < d < 1.125$ g/ml) and HDL_3 ($1.125 < d < 1.21$ g/ml), and one minor subfraction, very high density lipoproteins (VHDL) ($1.21 < d < 1.25$ g/ml). Non-denaturing polyacrylamide gradient gel electrophoresis separates HDLs on the basis of particle size into at least five distinct subpopulations of particles with diameters ranging from 7.6 to 10.6 nm.[14]

HDLs can also be divided into two main subpopulations on the basis of their apolipoprotein composition. One subpopulation comprises HDLs containing apoA-I but no apoA-II (A-I HDLs), while another comprises particles containing both apoA-I and apoA-II (A-I/A-II HDLs).[15,16] ApoA-I is distributed approximately equally between A-I HDLs and A-I/A-II HDLs in most subjects, while almost all of the apoA-II is in A-I/A-II HDLs.[16] Most of the

A-I/A-II HDLs are found in the HDL_3 density range, while A-I HDLs are prominent components of both HDL_2 and HDL_3.[16]

The HDL fraction is also heterogeneous in terms of its electrophoretic mobility. When subjected to agarose gel electrophoresis, the human HDLs include subpopulations with alpha, pre-alpha, pre-beta and gamma migration.[17-20] Most human plasma HDLs are spherical particles with an alpha mobility. The minor pool of pre-beta-migrating HDLs consists mainly of discoidal apoA-I-containing particles. Gamma-migrating HDLs are discoidal, apoE-containing particles.

These HDL subpopulations are closely interrelated and are potentially interconvertible by factors acting in the vascular compartment.

The functional implications of HDL heterogeneity are still uncertain. There is evidence that the preferred extracellular acceptor of cell cholesterol in the process mediated by the ATP-binding cassette A1 (ABCA1) is a minor subfraction of lipid-poor (or even lipid-free) apoA-I.[21] There is also evidence that discoidal HDLs are the preferred substrates for LCAT,[22] while larger, spherical HDLs are the preferred acceptors of cell cholesterol in the efflux process mediated by the scavenger receptor type B1 (SR-B1).[23] But, overall, there is poor understanding of either functional or antiatherogenic differences between the various HDL subpopulations.

METABOLISM OF HDLS

Formation of HDLs

apoA-I and apoA-II originate mainly in the liver. Once in plasma they are rapidly lipidated. A proportion of the lipid-free apoA-I and apoA-II interacts with ABCA1 in cell membranes,[24] in a process that generates discoidal HDLs containing apolipoproteins, phospholipids and a small amount of unesterified cholesterol. Discoidal HDLs are also generated from the interaction of lipid-poor apoA-I with redundant surface components that are shed from triglyceride-rich lipoproteins following hydrolysis of their triglyceride by lipoprotein lipase.[25,26]

Once formed, discoidal HDLs acquire additional unesterified cholesterol that is passively transferred either from other plasma lipoproteins or from cell membranes. The unesterified cholesterol in A-I HDL discs is then rapidly esterified by LCAT in a reaction that provides the particle with a core of cholesteryl esters and converts the disc into a small sphere.[22] The rapidity with which LCAT catalyses cholesterol esterification in discoidal HDLs explains why most of the HDLs in plasma are spherical rather than discoidal.

LCAT is also involved in the formation of A-I/A-II HDLs.[27] It is probable that apoA-I and apoA-II are secreted into plasma separately and are assembled into A-I/A-II HDLs only after their entry into the circulation. As with apoA-I, apoA-II is synthesized mainly (or exclusively) in the liver and is most likely secreted in a lipid-free/lipid-poor form. Once in the extracellular space, this hydrophobic protein acquires phospholipids and unesterified cholesterol from cell membranes, probably in an ABCA1-dependent process, to form discoidal complexes containing apoA-II, phospholipids and unesterified cholesterol. However, unlike discoidal A-I HDLs, discoidal A-II HDLs are non-reactive with LCAT and are thus not converted into spherical particles. The presence of apoA-II in spherical A-I/A-II HDLs depends on a process in which discoidal A-II HDLs fuse with A-I HDLs in a reaction catalysed by LCAT.[27]

The initial product of an interaction of LCAT with discoidal A-I HDLs is a small spherical A-I HDL particle that contains the same number of apoA-I molecules (two) as the precursor discoidal particles. Continuing activity of LCAT results in an increase in the cholesteryl ester content of these small, spherical A-I HDLs. To accommodate the expanding particle core, the HDL particle must acquire additional apolipoproteins in the surface monolayer. This may be achieved in two ways. One mechanism involves fusion of the expanding particle with discoidal A-I HDLs to form a larger spherical A-I HDL in which the number of molecules of apoA-I is also increased.[28] A second mechanism involves fusion of the expanding spherical A-I HDLs with discoidal A-II HDLs to form spherical A-I/A-II HDLs.[27]

Catabolism of HDL

Once formed, the subsequent metabolism of spherical HDLs is complex. Most of the HDL constituents are metabolized as discrete entities rather than being removed from the circulation as an uptake of intact HDL particles. For example, HDL-cholesteryl esters are either transferred to very low density lipoproteins (VLDLs) and low density lipoproteins (LDLs) by CETP[29,30] or are selectively taken up by the liver in a process dependent on the binding of HDLs to SR-B1 (also known as CLA-1).[31] HDL triglyceride and phospholipids are removed from the particle by hydrolysis in reactions catalysed by lipases, including hepatic lipase (HL), endothelial lipase (EL) and secretory phospholipase A2 (sPLA2). The apoA-I in HDLs may also be independently metabolized

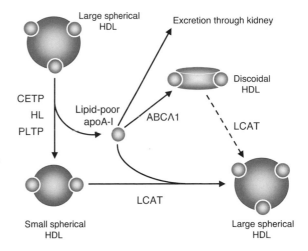

Figure 2 Cycling of apolipoprotein (apo)A-I between lipid-poor and lipid-rich pools. Large, spherical high density lipoproteins (HDLs) are reduced in size by cholesteryl ester transfer protein (CETP), hepatic lipase (HL) and phospholipid transfer protein (PLTP) in a process that results in the dissociation of lipid-poor/lipid-free apoA-I from the particle. The dissociated apoA-I may be excreted in urine, relipidated by the ATP-binding cassette A1 (ABCA1) to form discoidal HDLs or re-incorporated into pre-existing HDLs as they are increased in size by lecithin:cholesterol acyltransferase (LCAT)

following its dissociation from the particle during HDL remodelling.[32,33] The presence of apoA-II in the particle (e.g. in A-I/A-II HDLs) reduces this dissociation of apoA-I.[34] Once dissociated from HDLs, lipid-poor/lipid-free apoA-I may be excreted in urine[35] or it may be recycled into the HDL fraction as part of the continual remodelling of HDLs in plasma (Figure 2).

REMODELLING OF HDLS IN PLASMA

As outlined above, discoidal HDLs are rapidly converted into spherical particles by the action of LCAT. Once formed, spherical HDLs are also subject to continuous remodelling during their circulation in plasma.

Factors that increase the size of spherical HDLs

Small, spherical A-I HDLs retain a degree of reactivity with LCAT and continue to acquire cholesteryl esters in an expanding particle core. Additional surface constituents (including apolipoproteins) are then required to accommodate the expanded lipoprotein core. Additional apoA-I is provided, either in the form of lipid-free apolipoprotein[33] or in a process involving the fusion of the particle with an A-I HDL disc.[28] Additional apolipoprotein may also be provided in the form of apoA-II by fusion of the expanding particle with an A-II HDL disc.[27] Additional phospholipids and unesterified cholesterol are acquired as transfers from other plasma lipoproteins or as diffusion from cell membranes.

The size of spherical, A-I HDLs may also be increased by PLTP in a process of particle fusion that is accompanied by dissociation of lipid-poor apoA-I from the fusion product.[36,37] Remodelling of HDLs by PLTP is enhanced by the presence of triglyceride in the particle.[38]

Factors that decrease the size of spherical HDL

The combined activities of CETP and HL in the presence of triglyceride-rich lipoproteins are especially effective in reducing the particle size of HDLs.[39] CETP promotes a net mass transfer of cholesteryl esters from HDLs to triglyceride-rich lipoproteins in exchange for triglyceride that is transferred into HDLs. This exchange results in formation of HDLs that are depleted of cholesteryl esters and enriched in triglyceride. The triglyceride enrichment not only enhances the interaction of HDLs with PLTP but also provides the particles with the preferred substrate for HL. When HL hydrolyses the newly acquired HDL triglyceride, the consequent reduction in HDL core volume is accompanied by a decrease in HDL particle size and dissociation of lipid-free/lipid-poor apoA-I from the particle[39] (Figure 2).

Metabolism of lipid-free/lipid-poor apoA-I in plasma

As outlined above, one byproduct of the remodelling of spherical HDLs by PLTP, CETP and HL is a pool of lipid-poor (or lipid-free) apoA-I. A small proportion of this newly generated apoA-I may be excreted in urine,[35] although most appears to be re-incorporated into the HDL fraction. There are at least three mechanisms by which lipid-poor apoA-I returns to the HDL fraction. The simplest involves incorporation directly into pre-existing spherical HDLs that are expanding as a consequence of an interaction with LCAT.[33] ApoA-I may also be relipidated by acquiring phospholipids and unesterified cholesterol from cells in the ABCA1-mediated process[21] to form new discoidal HDL particles. Third, apoA-I may form discoidal complexes with phospholipids released as redundant surface constituents from triglyceride-rich lipoproteins following hydrolysis of their triglyceride by lipoprotein lipase.[40] Of all these potential metabolic fates of lipid-poor apoA-I, the most important physiologically is probably the interaction with ABCA1 in the first step of RCT.

HDL AND REVERSE CHOLESTEROL TRANSPORT

Reverse cholesterol transport involves several discrete steps:

(1) Unesterified cholesterol in cell membranes is transferred to acceptors in the extracellular space where it becomes incorporated into HDL particles;

(2) The unesterified cholesterol in HDL is then either delivered directly to the liver (and possibly other tissues) or is converted into cholesteryl esters by LCAT;

(3) The newly formed HDL cholesteryl esters may then either be delivered directly to the liver (and steroidogenic tissues) in a process dependent on SR-B1 (CLA-1) or be transferred by CETP to VLDL/LDL;

(4) The cholesteryl esters in VLDL/LDL are delivered to the liver as a component of the receptor-mediated uptake of LDL.

Efflux of cellular unesterified cholesterol to extracellular acceptors

There are at least three distinct processes that promote the efflux of cholesterol from cell membranes to acceptors in the extracellular space. One involves ABCA1, another ABCG1, a third involves SR-B1 and a fourth involves passive diffusion (Figure 3).

ABCA1 translocates phospholipids and cholesterol from the inner to the outer leaflets of cell membranes where they are picked up by apoA-I (or apoA-II) in the extracellular space.[21,41,42] This interaction is limited to apolipoproteins that contain no or very little lipid. Precisely how lipid-poor apolipoproteins remove cholesterol from cells is not known. According to one view, there is a simultaneous transfer of both cellular phospholipids and cholesterol to the apolipoproteins in a process that results in formation of discoidal complexes containing apolipoproteins, phospholipids and unesterified cholesterol. An alternative view holds that the lipid-poor apolipoproteins first acquire phospholipids from cells in an ABCA1-mediated process that generates discoidal complexes of apolipoprotein and phospholipid. These discoidal particles are then able to accept unesterified cholesterol from cell membranes in a diffusion process that may not require ABCA1.[44] Once formed by either mechanism, the discoidal

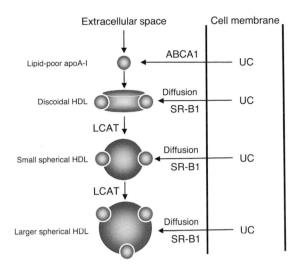

Figure 3   Efflux of unesterified cholesterol (UC) from cells. UC in cell membranes is transferred (with phospholipids) to lipid-free apolipoprotein (apoA)-I in the extracellular space to form discoidal high density lipoproteins (HDLs). The discoidal HDLs are sequentially converted into small and then larger spherical HDLs by lecithin:cholesterol acyltransferase (LCAT). The discoidal and the spherical HDLs acquire additional UC from cells either by passive diffusion or by diffusion facilitated by scavenger receptor type B1 (SR-B1). ABCG1 promotes the active transfer of cell cholesterol to spherical HDLs.

complexes of apolipoprotein, phospholipids and unesterified cholesterol (nascent HDLs) are subsequently transported, via lymphatics, to the plasma compartment where they are further metabolised as outlined above.

ABCG1 promotes the transfer of cholesterol from cells, including macrophages, to preformed, spherical HDL in the extracellular space.[45,46]

SR-BI is an HDL receptor.[47] Its best known function is to promote the selective hepatic uptake of HDL cholesteryl esters.[31] However, it has also been implicated in the efflux of unesterified cholesterol from cells to HDLs.[48,49] In contrast to the efflux promoted by ABCA1, SR-B1 mediates the bidirectional transfer of unesterified cholesterol between cells and HDLs and promotes a net efflux only if there is a concentration gradient of unesterified cholesterol from the donor cell to the acceptor HDL. Larger, spherical HDLs are preferred as acceptors in the efflux promoted by SR-B1.[23] The contribution made by SR-B1 to overall RCT is uncertain.

Mature, spherical HDLs in plasma also accept unesterified cholesterol efflux from cells in a process of passive aqueous diffusion that requires neither ABCA1 nor SR-B1.[50] Unesterified cholesterol in cell membranes is spontaneously released into the aqueous, extracellular space where it collides with and incorporates into any preformed HDL particles that are present. This is a bidirectional process in which unesterified cholesterol exchanges between HDLs and cell membranes. However, a net transfer of cholesterol into HDLs may be achieved by the formation of a concentration gradient generated by LCAT-mediated esterification of cholesterol on the HDL surface. The relative contribution made by these three efflux processes to overall RCT is not known.

Once cell cholesterol has been transferred to extracellular acceptors and ultimately incorporated into HDLs, it may be transported to the liver for elimination from the body by several pathways.

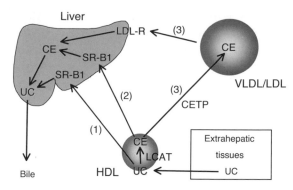

Figure 4 Pathways for delivery of cholesterol from extrahepatic tissues to the liver. Following the incorporation of cellular unesterified cholesterol (UC) into HDL, it may be delivered directly to the liver in a process involving binding of HDLs to hepatic scavenger receptor type B1 (SR-B1) (pathway 1) or it may be esterified by lecithin:cholesterol acyltransferase (LCAT) to form cholesteryl esters (CE). The HDL CE may then be delivered directly to the liver, again in a process involving binding of HDLs to hepatic SR-B1 (pathway 2), or it may first be transferred by cholesteryl ester transfer protein (CETP) to the VLDL/LDL fraction and then delivered to the liver as a component of the LDL receptor-mediated uptake of LDLs (pathway 3)

Delivery of HDL-cholesterol to the liver (Figure 4)

The unesterified cholesterol incorporated into HDLs may be taken up directly by the liver in a process that probably involves binding of HDLs to SR-B1 (pathway 1 in Figure 4). Alternatively, it may be converted by LCAT into cholesteryl esters that are then delivered to the liver by either a direct (pathway 2 in Figure 4) or indirect (pathway 3 in Figure 4) pathway. The direct pathway involves binding of HDL to hepatic SR-B1 (CLA-1).[47] Binding to SR-B1 results in a selective uptake of cholesteryl esters from HDLs,[31] leaving core-lipid-depleted particles to return to the circulation where they are available to participate further in the RCT process. In the indirect pathway, HDL cholesteryl esters are transferred by CETP to the VLDL/LDL fraction and then delivered to the liver as a consequence of the receptor-mediated uptake of LDLs.

The relative contribution made by each of these various pathways is not known. On the basis of mathematical modelling following injections into humans of HDL radiolabelled in the unesterified cholesterol moiety, it has been concluded that an hepatic uptake of HDL unesterified cholesterol represents the major pathway by which peripheral cholesterol is returned to the liver.[50] Another view holds that the predominant fate of unesterified cholesterol in HDL is to be esterified by LCAT, with a subsequent delivery to the liver being achieved as an uptake of cholesteryl esters. In this latter case, it is not known what proportion of the HDL cholesteryl esters is subsequently taken up directly by the liver via the SR-B1 pathway and what proportion is first transferred by CETP to other lipoproteins before being taken up by the liver.

It is important to discover the contribution of each of these pathways to overall RCT. If, for example, the predominant pathway is via CETP-mediated transfers of cholesteryl esters from HDLs to the VLDL/LDL pool, it follows that therapeutic inhibition of CETP may compromise RCT. If, on the other hand, the major pathway involves the direct SR-B1-mediated hepatic uptake of either HDL unesterified cholesterol or HDL cholesteryl esters, inhibition of CETP would be predicted to be anti-atherogenic by virtue of partitioning cholesterol in HDLs at the expense of LDLs without compromising RCT. Further research in this area is clearly required.

POTENTIAL MECHANISMS BY WHICH HDLS PROTECT AGAINST ATHEROSCLEROSIS

HDL-mediated cell cholesterol efflux

There is compelling evidence that HDLs counteract the effects of elevated levels of LDLs by removing cholesterol from cells in the arterial intima. In cultured fibroblasts harvested from humans with mutations of ABCA1, ABCA1-mediated efflux of cholesterol correlates positively and significantly with the concentration of HDL-cholesterol in the plasma of the fibroblast donor.[52] Another study of apoA-I and HDL-mediated efflux in carriers of ABCA1 mutations revealed a positive correlation of efflux with both HDL-cholesterol levels in plasma and carotid intima-media thickness.[53] These observations suggest a direct link between cholesterol efflux, HDL levels and the development of atherosclerosis. Further direct evidence that cholesterol efflux is anti-atherogenic has been provided in mice in studies in which selective expression of ABCA1 in macrophages was found to be anti-atherogenic, in this case without any change in HDL concentration in plasma.[54]

Anti-oxidant properties of HDLs

LDL oxidation within the arterial intima is an early event in atherogenesis.[55] The ability of HDLs to inhibit this oxidation is thus potentially anti-atherogenic. HDLs inhibit the transmigration of monocytes induced by oxidized LDLs,[56] the cytotoxicity induced by oxidized LDLs[57] and the oxidized LDL-induced adhesion of monocytes to endothelial cells.[58] HDLs also inhibit LDL oxidation in vitro[59,60] and in vivo.[61] Paraoxonase may be involved in this effect of HDLs,[62–64] although apoA-I and apoA-II have also been shown to have anti-oxidant properties.[65] The importance of these anti-oxidant properties of HDLs to their anti-atherogenic function in vivo in humans remains to be determined.

HDL-mediated inhibition of adhesion molecule expression

HDLs inhibit the cytokine-induced expression of VCAM-1, ICAM-1 and E-selectin in endothelial cells growing in tissue culture in a concentration-dependent manner[66] in a process that may involve an HDL-mediated inhibition of endothelial cell sphingosine kinase.[67] HDL-mediated inhibition of VCAM-I and E-selectin protein expression is paralleled by significant reductions in the steady-state mRNA levels of these adhesion molecules.[66] The in vivo significance of these findings has been supported by the finding of a significant reduction of plasma sICAM-1 and sE-selectin concentrations in patients whose HDL levels were increased by treatment with fenofibrate.[68] It remains to be determined whether this anti-inflammatory property of HDLs contributes to their ability to protect against atherosclerosis.

Stimulation of endothelial NO production

Another potential mechanism by which HDLs protect relates to their ability to modulate endothelial function.[69] The probable mechanism of this effect is a stimulation of the production of endothelial NO, a known anti-atherogenic mediator.[70] An effect of HDL on endothelial function has also been demonstrated in vivo in human studies in which short-term intravenous infusion of reconstituted HDLs (rHDLs) containing apoA-I complexed with phospholipids normalized endothelial-dependent vasodilatation.[71]

INTERVENTION STUDIES WITH HDLS

Experimental animals

There is clear evidence of a direct anti-atherogenic of HDLs in experimental animals.

Weekly infusions of HDLs into cholesterol-fed rabbits have been shown to reduce aortic lipid deposition and promote regression of aortic atherosclerosis.[72] A similar beneficial effect has been observed in rabbits infused with reconstituted HDL (rHDL) containing apoA-I$_{Milano}$ complexed with phospholipid.[73]

Additional compelling evidence of a direct cardio-protective effect of HDLs has been provided by studies of genetically modified animals. Overexpression of the human apoA-I gene in rabbits[9] and mice[10,11] increases the concentration of HDL-cholesterol and protects against diet-induced atherosclerosis[10] and the spontaneous atherosclerosis that develops in LDL-receptor-deficient,[74] apoE-deficient[11] and LP(a)[75] transgenic animals. This effect is not confined to overexpression of apoA-I. Mice overexpressing the combination of human apoA-I and apoA-II[76] or human apoA-II alone[77] are also protected. In contrast, mice overexpressing murine (as distinct from human) apoA-II have an increased susceptibility to atherosclerosis.[78]

Human studies

Until recently, the evidence that HDL inhibited atherosclerosis in humans was circumstantial, depending on the analysis of results from intervention trials in which an increase in HDL concentration appeared to be a predictor of benefit that was independent of effects on other lipoprotein fractions.[79–81] However, there is now compelling direct evidence that HDL is anti-atherogenic in humans. Human subjects with coronary atherosclerosis received weekly intravenous injections of rHDL (complexes of apoA-I$_{Milano}$ and phospholipid) for 5 weeks. Coronary atherosclerosis was assessed by intravascular ultrasound. In subjects receiving the infusions of rHDL there was a statistically significant reduction in the atherosclerosis burden after only 5 weeks of treatment.[82] There is now a clear need to repeat this study in a larger cohort of subjects. Confirmation of the result will provide the stimulus for a massive research effort directed towards the development of new strategies designed to increase HDL concentration.

POTENTIAL NEW THERAPIES

Current therapies for raising the HDL concentration are, at best, only moderately effective. PPAR-α activists such as fibrates raise HDL-cholesterol levels by 5–25%. This is achieved by at least two mechanisms: directly by stimulating the synthesis of apoA-I and apoA-II and indirectly by increasing lipoprotein lipase.[83,84] Statins also increase HDL-cholesterol, both by increasing apoA-I synthesis[85] and by inhibiting CETP,[86] although the effect is relatively small with increases tending to be less than 10%. Nicotinic acid is the most effective of currently available agents, raising HDL levels by up to 30% by a mechanism that remains to be determined.

The mounting evidence in both animal and human studies that raising HDL levels retards or even reverses the progression of atherosclerosis has stimulated great interest in developing new therapies designed to increase the concentration of HDLs and to enhance the pathway of RCT. Potential approaches to raising HDLs include:

(1) More potent PPAR-α agonists and other agents designed to increase the synthesis of apoA-I;
(2) Therapies with the potential to increase the activities of ABCA1, LCAT and lipoprotein lipase and
(3) Therapies that inhibit CETP.

It should be noted, however, that an elevation of HDL concentration might not automatically translate into an increased protection against atherosclerosis.

It may also be possible to increase RCT by strategies that could be accompanied by a paradoxical decrease in the concentration of HDL. One such approach would be activation of SR-B1 in a process that simultaneously increases the delivery of HDL-cholesterol to the liver and reduces the concentration of HDL-cholesterol in plasma. This latter approach is underpinned by the concept that HDL function is more important than HDL concentration in protecting against atherosclerosis. The problem here is that it is still not known which of the documented functions of HDLs is responsible for their ability to inhibit atherosclerosis.

CONCLUSIONS

With a growing understanding of the metabolism and regulation of HDLs and their involvement in several potential anti-atherogenic processes, there has been a major interest in exploiting the knowledge with a view to developing novel approaches for the prevention of atherosclerosis. The potential of these new approaches is considerable, but only time will tell whether the potential will translate into safe and effective new therapies.

References

1. Gordon DJ, Knoke J, Probstfield JL, et al. High-density lipoprotein cholesterol and coronary heart disease in hypercholesterolemic men: the Lipid Research Clinics Coronary Primary Prevention Trial. Circulation 1986; 74:1217–25

2. Enger SC, Hjermann I, Foss OP, et al. High density lipoprotein cholesterol and myocardial infarction or sudden coronary death: a prospective case-control study in middle-aged men of the Oslo study. Artery 1979; 5:170–81

3. Miller NE, Thelle DS, Forde OH, et al. The Tromso heart-study. High-density lipoprotein and coronary heart-disease: a prospective case-control study. Lancet 1977; 1:965–8

4. Goldbourt U, Medalie JH. High density lipoprotein cholesterol and incidence of coronary heart disease – the Israeli Ischemic Heart Disease Study. Am J Epidemiol 1979; 109:296–308

5. Gordon T, Castelli WP, Hjortland MC, et al. High density lipoprotein as a protective factor against coronary heart disease. The Framingham Study. Am J Med 1977; 62:707–14

6. Jacobs DR Jr, Mebane IL, Bangdiwala SI, et al. High density lipoprotein cholesterol as a predictor of cardiovascular disease mortality in men and women: the follow-up study of the Lipid Research Clinics Prevalence Study. Am J Epidemiol 1990; 131:32–47

7. Miller M, Seidler A, Kwiterovich PO, et al. Long-term predictors of subsequent cardiovascular events with coronary artery disease and 'desirable' levels of plasma total cholesterol. Circulation 1992; 86:1165–70

8. Pekkanen J, Linn S, Heiss G, et al. Ten-year mortality from cardiovascular disease in relation to cholesterol level among men with and without preexisting cardiovascular disease. N Engl J Med 1990; 322:1700–7

9. Duverger N, Kruth H, Emmanuel F, et al. Inhibition of atherosclerosis development in cholesterol-fed human apolipoprotein A-I-transgenic rabbits. Circulation 1996; 94:713–17

10. Rubin EM, Krauss RM, Spangler EA, et al. Inhibition of early atherogenesis in transgenic mice by human apolipoprotein AI. Nature 1991; 353:265–7

11. Plump AS, Scott CJ, Breslow JL. Human apolipoprotein A-I gene expression increases high density lipoprotein and suppresses atherosclerosis in the apolipoprotein E-deficient mouse. Proc Natl Acad Sci USA 1994; 91:9607–11

12. Barter PJ. HDL and reverse cholesterol transport. Curr Opin Lipidol 1993; 4:210–17

13. Fielding CJ, Fielding PE. Molecular physiology of reverse cholesterol transport. J Lipid Res 1995; 36:211–28

14. Blanche PJ, Gong EL, Forte TM, et al. Characterization of human high-density lipoproteins by gradient gel electrophoresis. Biochim Biophys Acta 1981; 665:408–19

15. Cheung MC, Albers JJ. Distribution of high density lipoprotein particles with different apoprotein composition: particles with A-I and A-II and particles with A-I but no A-II. J Lipid Res 1982; 23:747–53

16. Cheung MC, Albers JJ. Characterization of lipoprotein particles isolated by immunoaffinity chromatography. Particles containing A-I and A-II and particles containing A-I but no A-II. J Biol Chem 1984; 259:12201–9

17. Asztalos BF, Sloop CH, Wong L, et al. Two-dimensional electrophoresis of plasma lipoproteins: recognition of new apo A-I-containing subpopulations. Biochim Biophys Acta 1993; 1169:291–300

18. Huang Y, von Eckardstein A, Wu S, et al. Effects of the apolipoprotein E polymorphism on uptake and transfer of cell-derived cholesterol in plasma. J Clin Invest 1995; 96:2693–701

19. Kunitake ST, La Sala KJ, Kane JP. Apolipoprotein A-I-containing lipoproteins with pre-beta electrophoretic mobility. J Lipid Res 1985; 26:549–55

20. Sparks DL, Lund-Katz S, Phillips MC. The charge and structural stability of apolipoprotein A-I in discoidal and spherical recombinant high density lipoprotein particles. J Biol Chem 1992; 267:25839–47

21. Oram JF. HDL Apolipoproteins and ABCA1. Partners

in the removal of excess cellular cholesterol. Arterioscler Thromb Vasc Biol 2003; 23:720–7

22. Jonas A, von Eckardstein A, Kezdy KE, et al. Structural and functional properties of reconstituted high density lipoprotein discs prepared with six apolipoprotein A-I variants. J Lipid Res 1991; 32: 97–106

23. Liadaki KN, Liu T, Xu S, et al. Binding of high density lipoprotein (HDL) and discoidal reconstituted HDL to the HDL receptor scavenger receptor class B type I. Effect of lipid association and APOA-I mutations on receptor binding. J Biol Chem 2000; 275:21262–71

24. Lawn RM, Wade DP, Garvin MR, et al. The Tangier disease gene product ABC1 controls the cellular apolipoprotein-mediated lipid removal pathway. J Clin Invest 1999; 104:R25–R31

25. Redgrave TG, Small DM. Quantitation of the transfer of surface phospholipid of chylomicrons to the high density lipoprotein fraction during the catabolism of chylomicrons in the rat. J Clin Invest 1979; 64:162–71

26. Tall AR, Blum CB, Forester GP, et al. Changes in the distribution and composition of plasma high density lipoproteins after ingestion of fat. J Biol Chem 1982; 257:198–207

27. Clay MA, Pyle DH, Rye K-A, et al. Formation of spherical, reconstituted high density lipoproteins containing both apolipoproteins A-I and A-II is mediated by lecithin:cholesterol acyltransferase. J Biol Chem 2000; 275:9019–25

28. Liang H-Q, Rye K-A, Barter PJ., Remodelling of reconstituted high density lipoproteins by lecithin: cholesterol acyltransferase. J Lipid Res 1996; 37:1962–70

29. Barter PJ, Hopkins GJ, Calvert GD. Pathways for the incorporation of esterified cholesterol into very low density and low density lipoproteins in plasma incubated in vitro. Biochim Biophys Acta 1982; 713:136–48

30. Tall AR. Plasma cholesteryl ester transfer protein. J Lipid Res 1993; 34:1255–74

31. Glass C, Pittman RC, Weinstein DB, et al. Dissociation of tissue uptake of cholesterol ester from that of apoprotein A-I of rat plasma high density lipoprotein: selective delivery of cholesterol ester to liver, adrenal, and gonad. Proc Natl Acad Sci USA 1983; 80:5435–9

32. Liang HQ, Rye KA, Barter PJ. Dissociation of lipid-free apolipoprotein A-I from high density lipoproteins. J Lipid Res 1994; 35:1187–99

33. Liang HQ, Rye KA, Barter PJ. Cycling of apolipoprotein A-I between lipid-associated and lipid-free pools. Biochim Biophys Acta 1995; 1257:31–7

34. Rye K-A, Wee K, Curtiss L, et al. Apolipoproteins A-II inhibits high density lipoprotein remodeling and lipid-poor apolipoproteins A-I formation. J Biol Chem 2003; 278:22530–6

35. Horowitz BS, Goldberg IJ, Merab J, et al. Increased plasma and renal clearance of an exchangeable pool of apolipoprotein A-I in subjects with low levels of high density lipoprotein cholesterol. J Clin Invest 1993; 91:1743–52

36. van Tol A. Phospholipid transfer protein. Curr Opin Lipidol 2002; 13:135–9

37. Lusa S, Jauhiainen M, Metso J, et al. The mechanism of human plasma phospholipid transfer protein-induced enlargement of high-density lipoprotein particles: evidence for particle fusion. Biochem J 1996; 313:275–82

38. Rye KA, Jauhiainen M, Barter PJ, et al. Triglyceride-enrichment of high density lipoproteins enhances their remodelling by phospholipid transfer protein. J Lipid Res 1998; 39:613–22

39. Rye KA, Clay MA, Barter PJ. Remodelling of high density lipoproteins by plasma factors. Atherosclerosis 1999; 145:227–38

40. Clay MA, Barter PJ. Formation of new HDL particles from lipid-free apolipoprotein A-I. J Lipid Res 1996; 7:1722–32

41. Wang N, Tall AR. Regulation and mechanism of ATP-binding cassette transporter A-mediated cellular cholesterol efflux. Arterioscler Thromb Vasc Biol 2003; 23:1178–84

42. Francis GA, Knopp RH, Oram JF. Defective removal of cellular cholesterol and phospholipids by apolipoprotein A-I in Tangier disease. J Clin Invest 1995; 96:78–87

43. Oram JF, Lawn RM. ABCA1: the gatekeeper for eliminating excess tissue cholesterol. J Lipid Res 2001; 42:1173–9

44. Wang N, Lan D, Chen W, et al. ATP-binding cassette transporters G1 and G4 mediate cellular cholesterol efflux to high-density lipoproteins. Proc Natl Acad Sci USA 2004; 101:9774–9.

45. Nakamura K, Kennedy MA, Baldan A, et al. Expression and regulation of multiple murine ATP-binding cassette transporter G1 mRNAs/isoforms that stimulate cellular cholesterol efflux to high density lipoprotein. J Biol Chem 2004; 279:45980–9.

46. Fielding PE, Nagao K, Hakamata H, et al. A two-step mechanism for free cholesterol and phospholipid efflux from human vascular cells to apolipoprotein A-1. Biochemistry 2000; 39:14113–20

47. Acton S, Rigotti A, Landschulz KT, et al. Identification of scavenger receptor SR-BI as a high density lipoprotein receptor. Science 1996; 271:518–20

48. Ji Y, Jian B, Wang N, et al. Scavenger receptor BI promotes high density lipoprotein-mediated cellular cholesterol efflux. J Biol Chem 1997; 272: 20982–5

49. Gu X, Kozarsky K, Krieger M. Scavenger receptor class B, type I-mediated [3H]cholesterol efflux to high and low density lipoproteins is dependent on lipoprotein binding to the receptor. J Biol Chem 2000; 275:29993–30001

50. Yancey PG, Bortnick AE, Kellner-Weibel G, et al. Importance of different pathways of cellular cholesterol efflux. Arterioscler Thromb Vasc Biol 2003; 23:712–19

51. Schwartz CC, Zech LA, VandenBroek JM, et al. Cholesterol kinetics in subjects with bile fistula.

Positive relationship between size of the bile acid precursor pool and bile acid synthetic rate. J Clin Invest 1993; 91:923–38

52. Clee SM, Kastelein JJ, van Dam M, et al. Age and residual cholesterol efflux affect HDL cholesterol levels and coronary artery disease in ABCA1 heterozygotes. J Clin Invest 2000; 106:1263–70

53. Attie AD, Kastelein JP, Hayden MR. Pivotal role of ABCA1 in reverse cholesterol transport influencing HDL levels and susceptibility to atherosclerosis. J Lipid Res 2001; 42:1717–26

54. Aiello RJ, Brees, D, Bourassa P-A, et al. Increased atherosclerosis in hyperlipidemic mice with inactivation of ABCA1 in macrophages. Arterioscler Thromb Vasc Biol 2002; 22:630–7

55. Steinberg D, Parthasarathy S, Carew TE, et al. Beyond cholesterol. Modifications of low-density lipoprotein that increase its atherogenicity. N Engl J Med 1989; 320:915–24

56. Navab M, Imes SS, Hama SY, et al. Monocyte transmigration induced by modification of low density lipoprotein in cocultures of human aortic wall cells is due to induction of monocyte chemotactic protein 1 synthesis and is abolished by high density lipoprotein. J Clin Invest 1991; 88:2039–46

57. Hessler JR, Robertson AL Jr, Chisolm GM III. LDL-induced cytotoxicity and its inhibition by HDL in human vascular smooth muscle and endothelial cells in culture. Atherosclerosis 1979; 32:213–29

58. Maier JA, Barenghi L, Bradamante S, et al. Modulators of oxidized LDL-induced hyperadhesiveness in human endothelial cells. Biochem Biophys Res Commun 1994; 204:673–7

59. Decossin C, Tailleux A, Fruchart JC, et al. Prevention of in vitro low-density lipoprotein oxidation by an albumin-containing Lp A-I subfraction. Biochim Biophys Acta 1995; 1255:31–8

60. Kunitake ST, Jarvis MR, Hamilton RL, et al. Binding of transition metals by apolipoprotein A-I-containing plasma lipoproteins: inhibition of oxidation of low density lipoproteins. Proc Natl Acad Sci USA 1992; 89:6993–7

61. Klimov AN, Gurevich VS, Nikiforova AA, et al. Antioxidative activity of high density lipoproteins in vivo. Atherosclerosis 1993; 100:13–18

62. Mackness MI, Arrol S, Abbott C, et al. Protection of low-density lipoprotein against oxidative modification by high-density lipoprotein associated paraoxonase. Atherosclerosis 1993; 104:129–35

63. Mackness MI, Arrol S, Durrington PN. Paraoxonase prevents accumulation of lipoperoxides in low-density lipoprotein. FEBS Lett 1991; 286:152–4

64. Watson AD, Berliner JA, Hama SY, et al. Protective effect of high density lipoprotein associated paraoxonase. Inhibition of the biological activity of minimally oxidized low density lipoprotein. J Clin Invest 1995; 96:2882–91

65. Garner B, Waldeck AR, Witting PK, et al. Oxidation of high density lipoproteins. II. Evidence for direct reduction of lipid hydroperoxides by methionine residues of apolipoproteins AI and AII. J Biol Chem 1998; 273:6088–95

66. Cockerill GW, Rye KA, Gamble JR, et al. High-density lipoproteins inhibit cytokine-induced expression of endothelial cell adhesion molecules. Arterioscler Thromb Vasc Biol 1995; 15:1987–94

67. Xia P, Vadas MA, Rye KA, et al. High density lipoproteins (HDL) interrupt the sphingosine kinase signaling pathway. A possible mechanism for protection against atherosclerosis by HDL. J Biol Chem 1999; 274:33143–7

68. Calabresi L, Gomaraschi M, Villa B, et al. Elevated soluble cellular adhesion molecules in subjects with low HDL-cholesterol. Arterioscler Thromb Vasc Biol 2002; 22:656–61

69. O'Connell BJ, Genest J Jr. High-density lipoproteins and endothelial function. Circulation 2001; 104: 1978–83

70. Yuhanna IS, Zhu Y, Cox BE, et al. High-density lipoprotein binding to scavenger receptor-BI activates endothelial nitric oxide synthase. Nat Med 2001; 7:853–7

71. Spieker LE, Sudano I, Hurlimann D, et al. High-density lipoprotein restores endothelial function in hypercholesterolemic men. Circulation 2002; 105:1399–402

72. Badimon JJ, Badimon L, Fuster V. Regression of atherosclerotic lesions by high density lipoprotein plasma fraction in the cholesterol-fed rabbit. J Clin Invest 1990; 85:1234–41

73. Chiesa G, Monteggia E, Marchesi M, et al. Recombinant apolipoprotein A-I Milano infusion into rabbit carotid artery rapidly removes lipid from fatty streaks. Circ Res 2002; 90:974–80

74. Tangirala RK, Tsukamoto K, Chun SH, et al. Regression of atherosclerosis induced by liver-directed gene transfer of apolipoprotein A-I in mice. Circulation 1999; 100:1816–22

75. Liu AC, Lawn RM, Verstuyft JG, et al. Human apolipoprotein A-I prevents atherosclerosis associated with apolipoprotein[a] in transgenic mice. J Lipid Res 1994; 35:2263–7

76. Schultz JR, Verstuyft JG, Gong EL, et al. Protein composition determines the anti-atherogenic properties of HDL in transgenic mice. Nature 1993; 365:762–4

77. Tailleux A, Bouly M, Luc G, et al. Decreased susceptibility to diet-induced atherosclerosis in human apolipoprotein A-II transgenic mice. Arterioscler Thromb Vasc Biol 2000; 20:2453–8

78. Warden CH, Hedrick CC, Qiao JH, et al. Atherosclerosis in transgenic mice overexpressing apolipoprotein A-II. Science 1993; 261:469–72

79. The Lipid Research Clinics Coronary Primary Prevention Trial results. I. Reduction in incidence of coronary heart disease. JAMA 1984; 251:351–64

80. Pedersen TR, Olsson AG, Faergeman O, et al. Lipoprotein changes and reduction in the incidence of major coronary heart disease events in the

Scandinavian Simvastatin Survival Study (4S). Circulation. 1998; 97:1453–60

81. Manninen V, Tenkanen L, Koskinen P, et al. Joint effects of serum triglyceride and LDL cholesterol and HDL cholesterol concentrations on coronary heart disease risk in the Helsinki Heart Study. Implications for treatment. Circulation 1992; 85:37–45

82. Nissen SE, Tsunoda T, Tuzcu EM, et al. Effect of recombinant ApoA-I Milano on coronary atherosclerosis in patients with acute coronary syndromes: a randomized controlled trial. JAMA 2003; 290:2292–300

83. Fruchart J-C, Staels B, Duriez P. The role of fibric acids in atherosclerosis. Curr Athero Rep 2001; 3:83–92

84. Staels B, Dallongeville J, Auwerx J, et al. Mechanism of action of fibrates on lipid and lipoprotein metabolism. Circulation 1998; 98:2088–93

85. Martin G, Duez H, Blanquart C, et al. Statin-induced inhibition of the Rho-signaling pathway activates PPARalpha and induces HDL apoA-I. J Clin Invest 2001; 107:1423–32

86. McPherson R. Comparative effects of simvastatin and cholestyramine on plasma lipoproteins and CETP in humans. Can J Clin Pharmacol 1999; 6:85–90

LXR as a therapeutic target for atherosclerosis

9

I.G. Schulman and R.A. Heyman

BACKGROUND: NUCLEAR RECEPTORS AS REGULATORS OF METABOLISM

Nuclear receptors comprise a superfamily of ligand-dependent transcription factors that regulate genetic networks controlling cell growth, development and metabolism. Consisting of over 100 different proteins (48 in the human genome), the superfamily includes the well-known receptors for steroids, thyroid hormones and vitamins.[1] Members of the nuclear receptor superfamily are characterized by a conserved structural and functional organization (Figure 1) consisting of a heterogeneous amino terminal domain, a highly conserved central DNA binding domain (DBD) and a functionally complex carboxy terminal ligand-binding domain (LBD). The LBD mediates ligand binding, receptor homo- and heterodimerization, repression of transcription in the absence of ligand and ligand-dependent activation of transcription when agonist ligands are bound (for review, see reference 2).

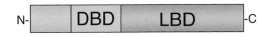

Figure 1 Structural organization of nuclear receptors. The DNA-binding domain (DBD) and the ligand-binding domain (LBD) are highlighted

Crystal structures of several LBDs support molecular and biochemical studies indicating that ligand binding promotes a conformational change in receptor structure. What appears to be a relatively flexible conserved helix near the carboxy terminus (helix 12) occupies unique positions when structures of unliganded, agonist-occupied and antagonist-occupied LBDs are compared (for review, see references 3, 4). Importantly, mutagenesis experiments indicate that helix 12, referred to as activation function 2 (AF-2), is necessary for ligand-dependent transactivation by nuclear receptors. Recent work indicates the AF-2 helix contributes an essential surface to the formation of an agonist-dependent hydrophobic pocket that serves as a binding site for co-activators. The alternative positions occupied by helix 12 in the unliganded or antagonist-occupied conformations preclude the formation of this binding pocket (for review, see references 5, 6).

Numerous experiments have defined the effects of glucocorticoids and thyroid hormone on metabolic control and provided the foundation for the endocrine regulation of metabolism (for review, see references 7, 8). More recently, studies have identified the peroxisome proliferator activated receptors (PPAR-α, PPAR-δ and PPAR-γ), liver X receptors (LXRα and LXRβ) and the farnesoid X receptor (FXR) as direct sensors of metabolic status. The PPARs, LXRs and FXR directly bind fatty acids and cholesterol derivatives and regulate target genes that control the transport and ultimate metabolic fate of the cognate ligand.[9–14] Thus these receptors are poised to sense and respond to small changes in the flux through the metabolic pathways that they control. Importantly, these fatty-acid- and cholesterol-derived natural ligands bind to receptors with dissociation constants close to the physiological concentrations known to exist for these metabolites.[11,12,15–18] The identification of the thiazolidinedione class of insulin sensitizers as synthetic ligands for PPAR-γ[19,20] served to validate the idea that these metabolic sensors can be therapeutic targets for the treatment of human disease.

REGULATION OF HEPATIC LIPID METABOLISM BY LXR

The LXR subgroup of the nuclear receptor superfamily is comprised of two isotypes, LXRα and LXRβ, that are encoded by separate genes. The founding member of the subgroup LXRα was originally cloned from a liver cDNA library, hence the name liver X receptor, using the DNA binding of the retinoic acid receptor as a probe, and found to be highly expressed in the liver, kidney and intestine.[21] In contrast, LXRβ is more ubiquitously expressed.[22] Both LXRs bind to DNA and regulate transcription as heterodimers with retinoid X receptors serving as the common heterodimeric partner.[21,22] The first link between LXR and lipid metabolism came from the identification of cholesterol derivatives including 22(R)-hydroxycholesterol, 24(S)-hydroxycholesterol and 24(S),25-epoxy-cholesterol as ligands that directly bind to both LXR-α and LXR-β and increase their transcriptional activity.[16–18)] More recent studies have also demonstrated that 27-hydroxycholesterol and cholestenoic acid are LXR ligands.[23,24] The identification of hydroxycholesterols as natural LXR ligands dovetailed nicely with the characterization of LXR-α knockout mice. While apparently normal under standard laboratory conditions, when challenged with a diet rich in cholesterol LXR-α[−/−] mice accumulate massive amounts of cholesterol in the liver. Molecular analysis uncovered aberrant regulation of several genes involved in lipid and cholesterol metabolism including *Cyp7a*, which encodes cholesterol 7α hydroxylase, the rate-limiting enzyme in the conversion of cholesterol to bile acids.[25] Subsequently, the ATP-binding cassette transporters (ABC) ABCG5 and ABCG8, which move cholesterol out of the liver and into the intestine, were identified as LXR target genes.[26,27] Thus an increase in cholesterol levels is predicted to lead to an elevation in the concentration of cholesterol-derived LXR ligands resulting in the catabolism of cholesterol to bile acid and the excretion of cholesterol out of the liver (Figure 2). Importantly, Cyp7a, ABCG5 and ABCG8 all appear to be directly regulated by LXR[18,26] although the binding site for LXR present in the murine Cyp7a gene is not conserved in the human gene.[18]

Along with effects on cholesterol metabolism, activation of LXR agonists also increases expression of genes involved in fatty acid metabolism including the master transcriptional regulator of fatty acid synthesis, the

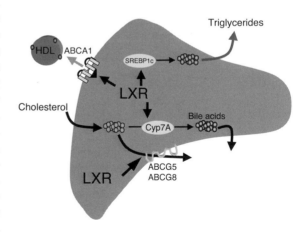

Figure 2 Hepatic activity of LXR. Activation of LXR in the liver results in upregulation of the genes encoding cholesterol 7 hydroxylase (Cyp7a), the rate-limiting enzyme in the catabolism of cholesterol to bile acids, the half ABC transporters ABCG5 and ABCG8 that function together to excrete cholesterol from the liver into the intestine and ABCA1, which promotes the efflux of cholesterol to HDL. LXR also regulates expression of SREBP1c, a master transcriptional regulator of genes involved in fatty acid and triglyceride synthesis. See text for details

sterol response element binding protein 1c (SREBP1c)[28,29] (Figure 2). Additionally, several of the genes encoding the enzymes involved in fatty acid metabolism, including fatty acid synthase (FAS) and stearoyl CoA desaturase 1 (SCD-1), are regulated directly or indirectly by LXR.[30–32] The coordinated upregulation of fatty acid synthesis with reverse cholesterol transport is most likely to provide lipids for the transport and storage of cholesterol. In contrast to the agonist activity of cholesterol metabolites, however, fatty acids act as antagonists of LXR transcriptional activity, suggesting the possibility of a negative feedback loop whereby the metabolic end product inhibits the inducer.[33]

REGULATION OF REVERSE CHOLESTEROL TRANSPORT BY LXR

Based on the defined role for LXR in hepatic cholesterol catabolism and excretion, one might have expected that synthetic LXR agonists would lower plasma cholesterol levels. Quite surprisingly, however, treatment of animals with LXR agonists significantly elevates HDL-cholesterol.[29] Gene expression analysis in the livers and intestines of LXR-agonist-treated mice identified *ABCA1* as a direct LXR gene and this discovery stimulated great interest in the therapeutic potential of LXR agonists given the links between ABCA1, HDL metabolism and atherosclerosis.[34–36] ABCA1 is required for the process of reverse cholesterol transport, whereby cells efflux internal cholesterol to acceptor proteins on pre-β-HDL particles. Loss of functional ABCA1 results in Tangier disease, a condition in which patients have extremely low levels of circulating HDL and an increased risk for developing atherosclerosis. Examination of fibroblasts isolated from subjects with Tangier disease reveals that ABCA1-defective cells are unable to efflux cholesterol, suggesting that the low HDL levels and increased risk of atherosclerosis result from a loss of reverse cholesterol transport. Historically, Tangier disease patients present with large accumulations of cholesterol-laden macrophages in their

lymph tissues, highlighting the role of ABCA1 and reverse cholesterol transport in macrophage cholesterol homeostasis (for review, see references 37–39). Importantly, accumulation of oxidized LDL-cholesterol by macrophages in the arterial wall is an initiating step in the development of atherosclerotic lesions (for review, see reference 40) and recent studies with mouse knockouts of ABCA1 further support a link between reverse cholesterol transport and atherosclerosis.[41–43] In support of the role of LXR as a direct regulator of ABCA1 expression and activity, treatment of primary macrophages or cell lines with LXR agonists results in induction of the ABCA1 gene, increased levels of ABCA1 protein and an increase in cholesterol efflux.[34,36,44] A binding site for LXR–RXR heterodimers in the ABCA1 promoter has also been described.[34] Subsequent studies identified other proteins involved in the reverse cholesterol transport including ABCG1, ABCG4 and apolipoprotein E (apoE) as direct LXR target genes.[44–47] Thus activation of LXR results in the mobilization of cholesterol in the periphery (Figure 3) and

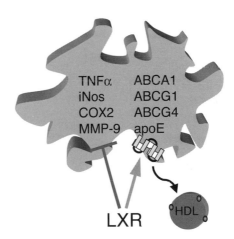

Figure 3 Activity of LXR in macrophages. Activation of LXR in macrophages results in the upregulation of genes encoding proteins that participate in reverse cholesterol transport including ABCA1, ABCG1, ABCG4 and apoE. LXR agonists can also induce reverse cholesterol transport in other tissues such as skeletal muscle.[61] Additionally, LXR also mediates an anti-inflammatory effect by repressing the ability of NFκB to induce proinflammatory genes. See text for details

stimulates the catabolism and excretion of cholesterol when it arrives in the liver (Figure 2). Interesting genetic deletion of LXR activity in mice (LXRαβ[-/-]) results in the accumulation of cholesterol-laden macrophages and spleno-megaly similar to that observed in Tangier disease patients.[48,49]

The accumulation of oxidized LDL-cholesterol by macrophages in blood vessel walls is an early event in the pathogenesis of atherosclerosis and it had long been suggested that reversing this process by pumping cholesterol out of macrophage foam cells would have an inhibitory effect on the progression of atherosclerosis (for review, see reference 40). The ability of LXR to directly regulate reverse cholesterol transport in macrophages allowed two experiments to be carried out to test this hypothesis. First, transplantation of lethally irradiated apoE[-/-] and LDL receptor knockout (LDLR[-/-]) mice with bone marrow from LXRαβ[+/+] or LXRαβ[-/-] mice demonstrated that genetic deletion of LXR leads to an increase in atherosclerosis is these well-established mouse models.[49] Second, treatment of apoE[-/-] and LDLR[-/-] mice with synthetic LXR agonists leads to a reduction in atherosclerosis.[50,51] Together the combination of genetic analysis and pharmacology clearly demonstrated the anti-atherogenic activity of LXR. Not surprisingly, the mRNA levels for LXR target genes including ABCA1 and apoE are elevated in the atherosclerotic lesions of mice treated with LXR agonists.[51] Subsequent studies in our laboratory combining bone marrow transplantation with the administration of synthetic LXR agonists have demonstrated that LXR activity in macrophages is necessary for the anti-atherogenic effect of LXR ligands.[52]

ANTI-INFLAMMATORY ACTIVITY OF LXR

It was certainly easy to assume that the ability of LXR to regulate lipid metabolism and reverse cholesterol transport provides the mechanistic basis for the anti-atherogenic activity of LXR.[49-51] Recent studies in macrophages, however, also demonstrate that LXR agonists can inhibit the expression of several pro-inflammatory genes including iNOS, COX-2, and MMP-9 and these compounds are effective in a murine model of irritant contact dermatitis.[53,54] Additionally, studies in our laboratory have shown that LXR agonists can inhibit LPS-dependent induction of TNF-α levels in vivo and this effect of LXR agonists is absent in LXR-αβ[-/-] mice (I. Schulman, personal observation). Molecular studies indicate that activation of LXR decreases the transcriptional activity of NFκB,[54] although the mechanistic basis for this inhibition has not yet been determined.

Since atherosclerosis is considered an inflammatory disease (for review, see reference 40) the question remains whether LXR mediates its anti-atherogenic via control of reverse cholesterol transport, by limiting the inflammatory response, or both. Future studies that combine genetically altered macrophages (i.e. ABCA1[-/-]) introduced by bone marrow transplantation along with the administration of LXR agonists can be used to define the individual contributions of reverse cholesterol transport and anti-inflammatory activity to therapeutic effects of LXR ligands. Additionally, studies with the glucocorticoid receptor have shown that it is possible to identify nuclear receptor ligands that repress inflammatory genes but do not activate positively regulated glucocorticoid receptor target genes.[55,56] One expects that such dissociated ligands will also be identified for LXR.

A number of studies have suggested a link between viral or bacterial infections and atherosclerosis (for review, see reference 57) and enhanced expression of Toll-like receptors (TLR), which mediate the rapid innate immunity to invading pathogens via stimulation of pro-inflammatory pathways, has been detected in human atherosclerotic lesions.[58] Interestingly, recent studies by Castrillo et al[59] indicate that activation of TLR4 inhibits the transcriptional activity of LXR and the ability of macrophages to efflux cholesterol. The cross-talk between TLR4 signalling and LXR activity suggests one potential mechanistic basis for the impact of infectious agents on cardiovascular disease.

LXR AND DIABETES

Treatment of experimental animals with LXR agonists leads to increases in hepatic fatty acid synthesis and plasma triglyceride levels.[28,29] Since elevations in fatty acids have been linked to insulin resistance and type II diabetes, several investigators have examined the cross-talk between LXR activity and glucose metabolism. Interestingly, along with upregulating fatty acid synthesis, activation of LXR also represses expression of the genes encoding the enzymes of gluconeogenesis including phosphoenolpyruvate carboxy kinase (PEPCK) and glucose 6-phosphatase[60,61] and induces expression of GLUT4 in adipose tissue.[60] Thus, in many ways, activation of LXR mimics treatment with insulin. Perhaps not surprisingly in light of this 'insulin-like' activity, LXR ligands decrease hepatic glucose output and lower blood glucose levels in animal models of type 2 diabetes.[60,61] The observation, however, that LXR ligands can behave as insulin sensitizers, even in the face of relatively large increases in plasma triglyceride levels, suggests the possibility of a broader role for LXR in regulating glucose homeostasis. Indeed, the observation that LXRs are also active in skeletal muscle[62] and that LXR-αβ[-/-] mice are resistant to diet-induced obesity (I. Schulman, personal observation) supports a role for the LXRs as important co-ordinators of energy metabolism.

THERAPEUTIC POTENTIAL OF LXR LIGANDS

The anti-atherogenic, anti-inflammatory and anti-diabetic activities of LXR agonists in animal models have highlighted the therapeutic potential of LXR-α and LXR-β. Nevertheless, the link between LXR activity and triglyceride metabolism has clearly dampened the enthusiasm surrounding this target class. Treatment of

mice and hamsters with synthetic LXR agonists results in a significant increase in plasma triglyceride levels,[29] although the kinetics and magnitude of the triglyceride elevation vary depending on the specific LXR ligand under study (I. Schulman and R. Heyman, personal observations). Treatment of patients with cardiovascular disease or metabolic syndrome with a drug that raises triglycerides, however, is not a viable option and approaches to separate the beneficial activities of LXR ligands from unwanted side-effects need to be explored. Furthermore, studies in human cells have shown that LXR agonists also increase expression of the gene encoding the cholesterol ester transfer protein (CETP).[63] CETP functions to transfer cholesterol esters from HDL to apolipoprotein-B-containing lipoprotein particles and CETP activity has been shown to inversely correlate with atherosclerosis.[64–66] Indeed CETP inhibitors are currently being explored for the treatment of atherosclerosis.[65]

Interestingly, defects in hepatic cholesterol metabolism are detected in LXR-α[-/-] single knockout mice, indicating that LXR-β is not functionally redundant with LXR-α.[25] In contrast, cholesterol and triglyceride levels appear normal in LXR-β[-/-] mice, suggesting that LXR-α mediates most, if not all, of the effects of LXR ligands on triglyceride metabolism.[67] The relatively low level of LXR-β in the liver most likely accounts for lack of functional redundancy in this tissue. Nevertheless, in macrophages either LXR-α or LXR-β alone appears to be sufficient to mediate the effects of LXR ligands on reverse cholesterol transport and inflammatory gene expression (I. Schulman, personal observation). Taken together these observations have led several investigators to suggest that LXR-β-selective ligands may provide a mechanistic basis for identification of LXR ligands with improved therapeutic profiles.[68] The enthusiasm for LXR-β-selective ligands must be tempered with the realization that the spectrum of activities measured in the complete absence of LXR-α activity may differ when an isotype selective synthetic ligand is used. Additionally, the observation that ligand-binding pockets of

LXR-α and LXR-β defined by crystallography[69–72] differ by only one amino acid suggests that identification of selective ligands may not be simple.

While the therapeutic activity of LXR-β-selective ligands is still an open question, it has been possible to identify ligands for other nuclear receptors that exhibit a restricted set of activities and therefore allow the separation of beneficial therapeutic activities from unwanted side-effects. Perhaps the best examples of such compounds are the selective oestrogen receptor modulators such as roloxifene that function as oestrogen receptor agonists in some tissues and oestrogen receptor antagonists in others (for review, see reference 73). More recently, synthetic ligands for PPAR-γ have been identified that appear to separate the insulin-sensitizing activity of PPAR-γ from unwanted effects on weight gain.[74,75] A common feature of all these selective receptor modulators is that they appear to function as partial or weak agonists when characterized in vitro. When bound to receptors, selective modulators produce unique conformational changes that cannot be achieved by more typical agonists (for review, see references 3, 4). The outcome of these unique conformations is an alteration in interactions between receptors and the downstream co-regulator proteins that mediate the transcriptional response leading to ligand-specific effects on gene expression.[73,76] Since the LXRs function in multiple tissues to mediate effects on lipid metabolism, glucose homoeostasis and inflammation we expect that the identification of selective LXR modulators will yield compounds with beneficial therapeutic activities.

References

1. Maglich JM, Sluder A, Guan X, et al. Comparison of complete nuclear receptor sets from the human, *Caenorhabditis elegans* and *Drosophila* genomes. Genome Biol 2001; 2:RESEARCH0029:1–7

2. Mangelsdorf DJ, Thummel C, Beato M, et al. The nuclear receptor superfamily: the second decade. Cell 1995; 83:835–9

3. Steinmetz AC, Renaud JP, Moras D. Binding of ligands and activation of transcription by nuclear receptors. Annu Rev Biophys Biomol Struct 2001; 30:329–59

4. Greschik H, Moras D. Structure–activity relationship of nuclear receptor–ligand interactions. Curr Top Med Chem 2003; 3:1573–99

5. McKenna NJ, O'Malley BW. Combinatorial control of gene expression by nuclear receptors and coregulators. Cell 2002; 108:465–74

6. Westin S, Rosenfeld MG, Glass CK. Nuclear receptor coactivators. Adv Pharmacol 2000; 47:89–112

7. Yen PM. Physiological and molecular basis of thyroid hormone action. Physiol Rev 2001; 81:1097–142

8. Schacke H, Docke WD, Asadullah K. Mechanisms involved in the side effects of glucocorticoids. Pharmacol Ther 2002; 96:23–43

9. Chawla A, Repa JJ, Evans RM, et al. Nuclear receptors and lipid physiology: opening the X-files. Science 2001; 294:1866–70

10. Edwards PA, Kast HR, Anisfeld AM. BAREing it all. The adoption of lxr and fxr and their roles in lipid homeostasis. J Lipid Res 2002; 43:2–12

11. Forman BM, Chen J, Evans RM. Hypolipidemic drugs, polyunsaturated fatty acids, and eicosanoids are ligands for peroxisome proliferator-activated receptors alpha and delta. Proc Natl Acad Sci USA 1997; 94:4312–7

12. Kliewer SA, Sundseth SS, Jones SA, et al. Fatty acids and eicosanoids regulate gene expression through direct interactions with peroxisome proliferator-activated receptors alpha and gamma. Proc Natl Acad Sci USA 1997; 94:4318–23

13. Lee CH, Olson P, Evans RM. Minireview: lipid metabolism, metabolic diseases, and peroxisome proliferator-activated receptors. Endocrinology 2003; 144:2201–7

14. Repa JJ, Mangelsdorf DJ. Nuclear receptor regulation of cholesterol and bile acid metabolism. Curr Opin Biotechnol 1999; 10:557–63

15. Forman BM, Ruan B, Chen J, et al. The orphan nuclear receptor LXRalpha is positively and negatively regulated by distinct products of mevalonate metabolism. Proc Natl Acad Sci USA 1997; 94:10588–93

16. Janowski BA, Grogan MJ, Jones SA, et al. Structural requirements of ligands for the oxysterol liver X receptors LXRalpha and LXRbeta. Proc Natl Acad Sci USA 1999; 96:266–71

17. Janowski BA, Willy PJ, Devi TR, et al. An oxysterol signalling pathway mediated by the nuclear receptor LXRα. Nature 1996; 383:728–31

18. Lehmann JM, Kliewer SA, Moore LB, et al. Activation of the nuclear receptor LXR by oxysterols defines a new hormone response pathway. J Biol Chem 1997; 272:3137–40

19. Lehmann JM, Moore LB, Smith-Oliver TA, et al. An antidiabetic thiazolidinedione is a high affinity ligand for peroxisome proliferator-activated receptor gamma (PPAR gamma). J Biol Chem 1995; 270: 12953–6

20. Forman BM, Tontonoz P, Chen J, et al. 15-Deoxy-delta 12, 14-prostaglandin J2 is a ligand for the adipocyte determination factor PPAR gamma. Cell 1995; 83:803–12

21. Willy PJ, Umesono K, Ong ES, et al. LXR, a nuclear receptor that defines a distinct retinoid response pathway. Genes Devel 1995; 9:1033–45

22. Shinar DM, Endo N, Rutledge SJ, et al. NER, a new member of the gene family encoding the human steroid hormone nuclear receptor. Gene 1994; 147:273–6

23. Song C, Liao S. Cholestenoic acid is a naturally occurring ligand for liver X receptor alpha. Endocrinology 2000; 141:4180–4

24. Fu X, Menke JG, Chen Y, et al. 27-hydroxycholesterol is an endogenous ligand for liver X receptor in cholesterol-loaded cells. J Biol Chem 2001; 276: 38378–87

25. Peet DJ, Turley SD, Ma W, et al. Cholesterol and bile acid metabolism are impaired in mice lacking the nuclear oxysterol receptor LXRα. Cell 1998; 93:693–704

26. Repa JJ, Berge KE, Pomajzl C, et al. Regulation of ATP-binding cassette sterol transporters ABCG5 and ABCG8 by the liver X receptors alpha and beta. J Biol Chem 2002; 277:18793–800

27. Berge KE, Tian H, Graf GA, et al. Accumulation of dietary cholesterol in sitosterolemia caused by mutations in adjacent ABC transporters. Science 2000; 290:1771–5

28. Repa JJ, Liang G, Ou J, et al. Regulation of mouse sterol regulatory element-binding protein-1c gene (SREBP-1c) by oxysterol receptors, LXRalpha and LXRbeta. Genes Dev 2000; 14:2819–30

29. Schultz JR, Tu H, Luk A, et al. Role of LXRs in control of lipogenesis. Genes Dev 2000; 14:2831–8

30. Zhang Y, Repa JJ, Gauthier K, et al. Regulation of lipoprotein lipase by the oxysterol receptors, LXRalpha and LXRbeta. J Biol Chem 2001; 276:43018–24

31. Wang Y, Kurdi-Haidar B, Oram JF. LXR-mediated activation of macrophage stearoyl-CoA desaturase generates unsaturated fatty acids that destabilize ABCA1. J Lipid Res 2004; 45:972–80

32. Joseph SB, Laffitte BA, Patel PH, et al. Direct and indirect mechanisms for regulation of fatty acid synthase gene expression by LXRs. J Biol Chem 2002; 277:11019–25

33. Ou J, Tu H, Shan B, et al. Unsaturated fatty acids inhibit transcription of the sterol regulatory element-binding protein-1c (SREBP-1c) gene by antagonizing ligand-dependent activation of the LXR. Proc Natl Acad Sci USA 2001; 98:6027–32

34. Costet P, Luo Y, Wang N, et al. Sterol-dependent transactivation of the ABC1 promoter by the liver X receptor/retinoid X receptor. J Biol Chem 2000; 275:28240–5

35. Repa JJ, Turley SD, Lobaccaro JA, et al. Regulation of absorption and ABC1–mediated efflux of cholesterol by RXR heterodimers. Science 2000; 289:1524–9

36. Venkateswaran A, Laffitte BA, Joseph SB, et al. Control of cellular cholesterol efflux by the nuclear oxysterol receptor LXR alpha. Proc Natl Acad Sci USA 2000; 97:12097–102

37. Hayden MR, Clee SM, Brooks-Wilson A, et al. Cholesterol efflux regulatory protein, Tangier disease and familial high-density lipoprotein deficiency. Curr Opin Lipidol 2000; 11:117–22

38. Hobbs HH, Rader DJ. ABC1: connecting yellow tonsils, neuropathy, and very low HDL. J Clin Invest 1999; 104:1015–17

39. Oram JF, Lawn RM. ABCA1. The gatekeeper for eliminating excess tissue cholesterol. J Lipid Res 2001; 42:1173–9

40. Glass CK, Witztum JL. Atherosclerosis. The road ahead. Cell 2001; 104:503–16

41. Aiello RJ, Brees D, Francone OL. ABCA1–deficient mice: insights into the role of monocyte lipid efflux in HDL formation and inflammation. Arterioscler Thromb Vasc Biol 2003; 23:972–80

42. Singaraja RR, Fievet C, Castro G, et al. Increased ABCA1 activity protects against atherosclerosis. J Clin Invest 2002; 110:35–42

43. Joyce CW, Amar MJ, Lambert G, et al. The ATP binding cassette transporter A1 (ABCA1) modulates the development of aortic atherosclerosis in C57BL/6 and apoE-knockout mice. Proc Natl Acad Sci USA 2002; 99:407–12

44. Wagner BL, Valledor AF, Shao G, et al. Promoter-specific roles for liver X receptor/corepressor complexes in the regulation of ABCA1 and SREBP1 gene expression. Mol Cell Biol 2003; 23:5780–9

45. Kennedy MA, Venkateswaran A, Tarr PT, et al. Characterization of the human ABCG1 gene: liver X receptor activates an internal promoter that produces a novel transcript encoding an alternative form of the protein. J Biol Chem 2001; 276:39438–47

46. Laffitte BA, Repa JJ, Joseph SB, et al. LXRs control lipid-inducible expression of the apolipoprotein E gene in macrophages and adipocytes. Proc Natl Acad Sci USA 2001; 98:507–12

47. Wang N, Lan D, Chen W, et al. ATP-binding cassette transporters G1 and G4 mediate cellular cholesterol efflux to high-density lipoproteins. Proc Natl Acad Sci USA 2004; 101:9774–9

48. Schuster GU, Parini P, Wang L, et al. Accumulation of foam cells in liver X receptor-deficient mice. Circulation 2002; 106:1147–53

49. Tangirala RK, Bischoff ED, Joseph SB, et al. Identification of macrophage liver X receptors as

inhibitors of atherosclerosis. Proc Natl Acad Sci USA 2002; 99:11896–901

50. Terasaka N, Hiroshima A, Koieyama T, et al. T-0901317, a synthetic liver X receptor ligand, inhibits development of atherosclerosis in LDL receptor-deficient mice. FEBS Lett 2003; 536:6–11

51. Joseph SB, McKilligin E, Pei L, et al. Synthetic LXR ligand inhibits the development of atherosclerosis in mice. Proc Natl Acad Sci USA 2002; 99:7604–9

52. Lenin N, Bischoff ED, Daige Dl et al. Macrophage liver X receptor is required for antiatherogenic activity of LXR agonists. Arterioscler Thromb Vasc Biol 2005; 25(1):135–42

53. Fowler AJ, Sheu MY, Schmuth M, et al. Liver X receptor activators display anti-inflammatory activity in irritant and allergic contact dermatitis models: liver-X-receptor-specific inhibition of inflammation and primary cytokine production. J Invest Dermatol 2003; 120:246–55

54. Joseph SB, Castrillo A, Laffitte BA, et al. Reciprocal regulation of inflammation and lipid metabolism by liver X receptors. Nat Med 2003; 9:213–9

55. Miner JN. Designer glucocorticoids. Biochem Pharmacol 2002; 64:355–61

56. Coghlan MJ, Jacobson PB, Lane B, et al. A novel anti-inflammatory maintains glucocorticoid efficacy with reduced side effects. Mol Endocrinol 2003; 17:860–9

57. Buja LM. Does atherosclerosis have an infectious etiology? Circulation 1996; 94:872–3

58. Edfeldt K, Swedenborg J, Hansson GK, et al. Expression of toll-like receptors in human atherosclerotic lesions: a possible pathway for plaque activation. Circulation 2002; 105:1158–61

59. Castrillo A, Joseph SB, Vaidya SA, et al. Crosstalk between LXR and toll-like receptor signaling mediates bacterial and viral antagonism of cholesterol metabolism. Mol Cell 2003; 12:805–16

60. Laffitte BA, Chao LC, Li J, et al. Activation of liver X receptor improves glucose tolerance through coordinate regulation of glucose metabolism in liver and adipose tissue. Proc Natl Acad Sci USA 2003; 100:5419–24

61. Cao G, Liang Y, Broderick CL, et al. Antidiabetic action of a liver x receptor agonist mediated by inhibition of hepatic gluconeogenesis. J Biol Chem 2003; 278:1131–6

62. Muscat GE, Wagner BL, Hou J, et al. Regulation of cholesterol homeostasis and lipid metabolism in skeletal muscle by liver X receptors. J Biol Chem 2002; 277:40722–8

63. Luo Y, Tall AR. Sterol upregulation of human CETP expression in vitro and in transgenic mice by an LXR element. J Clin Invest 2000; 105:513–20

64. de Grooth GJ, Smilde TJ, Van Wissen S, et al. The relationship between cholesteryl ester transfer protein levels and risk factor profile in patients with familial hypercholesterolemia. Atherosclerosis 2004; 173:261–7

65. Brousseau ME, Schaefer EJ, Wolfe ML, et al. Effects of an inhibitor of cholesteryl ester transfer protein on HDL cholesterol. N Engl J Med 2004; 350:1505–15

66. Klerkx AH, de Grooth GJ, Zwinderman AH, et al. Cholesteryl ester transfer protein concentration is associated with progression of atherosclerosis and response to pravastatin in men with coronary artery disease (REGRESS). Eur J Clin Invest 2004; 34:21–8

67. Alberti S, Schuster G, Parini P, et al. Hepatic cholesterol metabolism and resistance to dietary cholesterol in LXRbeta-deficient mice. J Clin Invest 2001; 107:565–73

68. Lund EG, Menke JG, Sparrow CP. Liver X receptor agonists as potential therapeutic agents for dyslipidemia and atherosclerosis. Arterioscler Thromb Vasc Biol 2003; 23:1169–77

69. Hoerer S, Schmid A, Heckel A, et al. Crystal structure of the human liver X receptor beta ligand-binding domain in complex with a synthetic agonist. J Mol Biol 2003; 334:853–61

70. Farnegardh M, Bonn T, Sun S, et al. The three-dimensional structure of the liver X receptor beta reveals a flexible ligand-binding pocket that can accommodate fundamentally different ligands. J Biol Chem 2003; 278:38821–8

71. Williams S, Bledsoe RK, Collins JL, et al. X-ray crystal structure of the liver X receptor beta ligand binding domain: regulation by a histidine–tryptophan switch. J Biol Chem 2003; 278:27138–43

72. Svensson S, Ostberg T, Jacobsson M, et al. Crystal structure of the heterodimeric complex of LXRalpha and RXRbeta ligand-binding domains in a fully agonistic conformation. Embo J 2003; 22:4625–33

73. McDonnell DP, Connor CE, Wijayaratne A, et al. Definition of the molecular and cellular mechanisms underlying the tissue-selective agonist/antagonist activities of selective estrogen receptor modulators. Recent Prog Horm Res 2002; 57:295–316

74. Oberfield JL, Collins JL, Holmes CP, et al. A peroxisome proliferator-activated receptor gamma ligand inhibits adipocyte differentiation. Proc Natl Acad Sci USA 1999; 96:6102–6

75. Rocchi S, Picard F, Vamecq J, et al. A unique PPARgamma ligand with potent insulin-sensitizing yet weak adipogenic activity. Mol Cell 2002; 8:737–47

76. Schulman IG, Heyman RA. The flip side: identifying small molecule regulators of nuclear receptors. Chem Biol 2004; 11:639–46

Endothelial lipase and the regulation of HDL metabolism

10

K.O. Badellino and W. Jin

INTRODUCTION

Since the initial report of an inverse relationship between high density lipoprotein (HDL) levels and cardiovascular risk,[1] plasma HDL levels have been a clinically important target for prevention of atherosclerosis. With the discovery of the role of ABCA1[2–4] in the vascular efflux of cholesterol to form nascent HDL particles and SR-B1[5–7] in the hepatic uptake of cholesterol from HDL came heightened interest in identifying novel genes in regulating plasma HDL levels.

With its discovery in 1999,[8,9] endothelial lipase joined lipoprotein lipase (LPL) and hepatic lipase (HL) as important plasma regulators of lipoprotein cholesterol levels. Although each of these enzymes is capable of hydrolysing triglycerides and phospholipids, there are differences in their substrate preferences. While LPL and, to a lesser extent, HL are predominantly triglyceride lipases, endothelial lipase (EL) is predominantly a phospholipase.[10] EL is also unique in its expression by endothelial cells.[8,9] EL, like LPL and HL, is secreted and then binds to heparan sulphate proteoglycans on the endothelial surface. There it interacts with HDL, hydrolysing HDL phospholipids and generating free fatty acids at the local tissue site. The ability of EL to profoundly decrease HDL levels in mice has stimulated significant interest in its relevance to human HDL metabolism. The focus of this chapter will be recent reports of both in vitro and in vivo function of endothelial lipase.

STRUCTURE AND FUNCTION OF ENDOTHELIAL LIPASE

Endothelial lipase is a 500-amino-acid protein with a predicted molecular weight of 55 kDa. Immunoblot analysis of EL expressed in 293 HEK cells, using an anti-human EL polyclonal antibody, reveals bands of apparent molecular weight 68 kDa, 40 kDa and 28 kDa. Amino terminal sequencing demonstrated that the 40 kDa and 28 kDa forms were proteolytic cleavage products of the full-length protein. Based on a preliminary analysis with glycosidases, the 68 kDa protein is probably the fully glycosylated monomer (unpublished data).

Two alternatively spliced products of the EL (LIPG) gene were recently reported by Ishida et al.[11] These isoforms, labelled EL2a and EL2b, were 480 amino acids and 346 amino acids, respectively. EL2a and EL2b have exon I while the original full-length form contains exon II, which encodes the aminoterminal sequence with the signal peptide. EL2b lacks exon VI, which encodes the catalytic aspartic acid residue and a portion of the lid region. EL2a and EL2b were localized to the cytosol and lacked enzymatic activity.

By comparison of their primary amino acid sequences, endothelial lipase has 45% homology with LPL and 40% homology with HL.[8] As displayed in Figure 1, the location of the 10 cysteine residues is conserved. The same catalytic residues, [149]serine, [173]aspartic acid and [254]histidine, assign this enzyme to the triglyceride lipase family. The GXSXG lipase motif

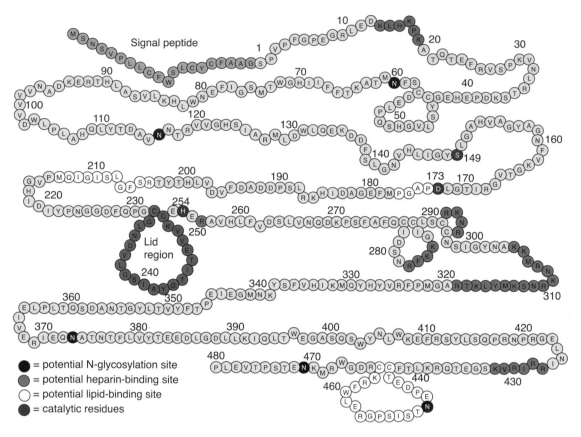

Figure 1   A model of endothelial lipase was developed, based on the crystal structure of pancreatic lipase and a published molecular model of LPL. The locations of cysteine residues, heparin-binding sites and the catalytic triad residues are conserved

surrounding the active site serine, common among other members of the lipase family, is also found in endothelial lipase.

An examination of the EL sequence also shows five areas that may represent N-linked glycosylation sites. Two potential lipid-binding regions have been identified by comparison to the crystal structure of pancreatic lipase:[12,13] [170]GLDPAGP[177] and [204]RSFGLSIGIQM[214]. EL also has four regions of positively charged residues that resemble heparin-binding sites: [14]KLHKPK[19], [282]RFKK[285] and [292]RKNR[295], [304]KKMRNKR[310] and [427]RRIRVK[432]. These potential heparin-binding, or proteoglycan-binding, sites are similar to regions found in LPL.[14,15] Endothelial lipase also has a 19-amino-acid putative lid region with a significantly

different sequence from the same regions in LPL and HL. This lid region may be important in determining the more predominant phospholipase activity of EL.

The phospholipid preference of EL was noted in both initial reports of the discovery of EL.[8,9] Jaye et al[8] also reported that EL hydrolysed a radiolabelled triolein substrate at a low level. McCoy et al[10] more definitively characterized EL lipolytic activity and compared it to HL and LPL. In the absence of serum as a source of apolipoprotein CII (apoC-II), EL hydrolysis of tributyrin, a 3-carbon acyl chain substrate, and triolein, an unsaturated octadecenoic acid, was similar to that of HL and LPL. The addition of heat-inactivated serum completely inhibited the ability of EL to

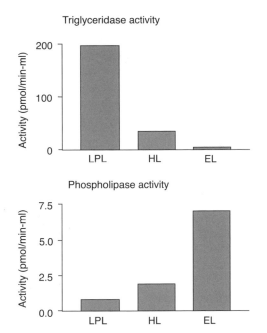

Figure 2 McCoy et al[10] compared the triglyceride lipase and phospholipase activities of LPL, HL and endothelial lipase. Culture medium from COS cells infected with adenoviruses containing the respective cDNAs was used. Used with permission from Journal of Lipid Research 2002; 43:921–9

hydrolyse both triolein and phospholipids. Addition of the same amount of serum had the expected effect of potentiating LPL hydrolysis of the triolein substrate. The addition of purified apoC-II also potentiated LPL. In contrast to the effect of serum, apoC-II had no effect on EL hydrolysis of either triolein or phospholipids.

McCoy et al also compared the triglyceride lipase to phospholipase activity ratio of EL to HL and LPL. Using lipases expressed by adenoviral gene transfer into COS cells, the triglyceride lipase to phospholipase activity ratio was determined to be 0.65 for EL, 24 for HL and 140 for LPL (plus serum) (Figure 2). These ratios demonstrate the preference of EL for phospholipids, versus the preference of both HL and LPL for triolein substrates.

While synthetic substrates can be used to characterize the lipase activity of these enzymes, their ability to hydrolyse naturally occurring lipoproteins more accurately displays their in vivo activity. McCoy et al isolated lipoproteins from non-fasted hyperlipaemic subjects. Lipoprotein fractions containing 1.25 mM phospholipids were incubated with either EL-, LPL- or HL-conditioned medium. A comparison of the free fatty acids released per reaction showed that, while EL hydrolyses triglyceride-containing lipoproteins, it is more active in hydrolysing HDL than either HL or LPL.

Duong et al[16] explored the influence of the phospholipid composition of recombinant spherical HDL on the ability of HL and EL to hydrolyse both phospholipid and triglyceride. For a comparison of phospholipid substrates, they created recombinant HDL (rHDL) with palmitic acid at sn-1 and that differed only in their phospholipid composition at the sn-2 position. They found that the V_{max} was greatest for EL hydrolysis of phospholipid with the longer chain docosodecanoic acid in the sn-2 position (PDPC), while HL preferred oleic acid at the sn-2 position (POPC). In contrast, for both EL and HL, triglyceride hydrolysis was modulated by the type of phospholipid included in triolein-containing rHDL. While EL is an extremely poor triglyceride lipase, the V_{max} for triolein in rHDL containing only arachidonic acid was highest, 41.4 nmol free fatty acid ml^{-1}h^{-1}, slightly increased over the rate for PDPC. HL was most active with linoleic acid in the sn-2 position, slightly increased over the V_{max} for POPC. The phospholipid content of HDL varies with the source of dietary fat. As noted by Duong et al, a diet rich in fish would enrich HDL with PDPC, making them better substrates for EL. Rye et al[17] found that a longer, more unsaturated, phospholipid content of HDL promotes the formation of the lipid-poor apoA-I particles involved in reverse cholesterol transport. Together, these findings suggest that EL hydrolysis of phospholipids may interfere with reverse cholesterol transport and promote the development of atherosclerosis.

In contrast, Gauster et al[18] studied the effect of EL modification of HDL on both SR-B1 and ABCA1-mediated free cholesterol efflux. HDL isolated from human plasma was incubated with COS7 cells infected with adenovirus encoding human EL. This HDL was found to be depleted in phosphatidylcholine and enriched in non-esterified fatty acids, with an increase in negative charge. EL-modified HDL had impaired ability to promote ^{3}H-cholesterol efflux from Chinese hamster ovary cells overexpressing SR-B1. There was no impairment of cholesterol efflux from ABCA1-expressing cells, however. These findings suggest that EL may promote reverse cholesterol transport by hydrolysing HDL phospholipid and modifying its surface charge.

TISSUE EXPRESSION OF ENDOTHELIAL LIPASE

The gene encoding endothelial lipase was first cloned in 1999 by two different groups[8,9] using two different strategies. Jaye et al[8] treated a monocyte cell line, THP-1, with phorbol 12-myristate 13 acetate, then exposed the cells to oxidized LDL-cholesterol. An RNA amplification product, found in the LDL-treated cells but not in untreated cells, was used to probe a human placental cDNA library. The clone obtained had significant homology to HL, pancreatic lipase and LPL. By Northern blot, they found EL is expressed in placenta, lung, liver, kidney, testis and thyroid in both mouse and human tissues (Figure 3). By Western blot, they showed that EL is constitutively and uniquely expressed by human coronary artery endothelial cells and human umbilical vein endothelial cells. Similarly, Hirata et al[9] identified EL as a gene upregulated in endothelial cells undergoing tube formation. They found a similar pattern of tissue expression.

Yu et al[19] examined mouse and rat tissues to discern whether EL is expressed exclusively by endothelial cells or whether it is first expressed by other cells such as hepatocytes and then

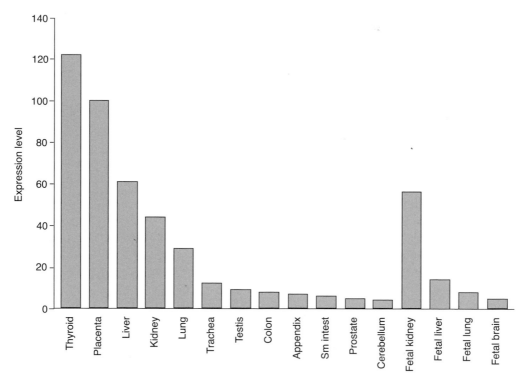

Figure 3   Relative expression of endothelial lipase mRNA in human tissues. Figure courtesy of M. Jaye

translocates to the endothelial surface. By immunostaining, they found that EL is expressed only by endothelial cells in liver, large vessels of the thyroid, the lung and adrenal glands.

The physiological role of EL in the placenta, thyroid, lung and adrenal gland is as yet unknown. Fetal HDL is apoE-rich, but has the same phospholipid content as adult HDL.[20] It is interesting to note that Yu et al[19] found that EL expression was decreased in the liver of apoE knockout mice, but increased in their aorta. This suggests a potential regulatory role of apoE in EL expression.

Thyroid hormone is known to decrease HL activity.[21] Its effect on EL expression and activity has yet to be examined. It is tempting to speculate that EL is involved in local vascular lipid metabolism, especially in certain endocrine tissues such as the thyroid and adrenal gland. This may be true in the lung as well. In their initial report of EL, Hirata et al[9] suggested that EL co-localizes with type II epithelial cells and may be involved in surfactant metabolism.

REGULATION OF ENDOTHELIAL LIPASE EXPRESSION

Both acute and chronic inflammatory diseases are associated with decreased HDL levels.[22,23] Two groups have shown that two early phase pro-inflammatory cytokines, tumour necrotic factor alpha (TNF-α) and interleukin-1 beta (IL-1β), both markedly increase the expression of EL mRNA in several lines of primary endothelial cells (Figure 4),[24,25] which is in sharp contradiction to their effects on HL and LPL.[26,27] The secretion of EL protein was induced by IL-1β and TNF-α in a dose- and time-dependent manner, and was the major source of extracellular lipase activity in endothelial cells after cytokine treatment.[25] In the presence of SN50 (a P50 inhibitor), the induction of EL by these two cytokines was partially blunted, indicating that the NF-κB pathway might be involved in the regulation of EL. In addition, two forms of mechanical force involved in vascular diseases, fluid shear stress and cyclic stretch, also upregulated EL mRNA expression in endothelial cells.[24] All these data suggest the possibility that

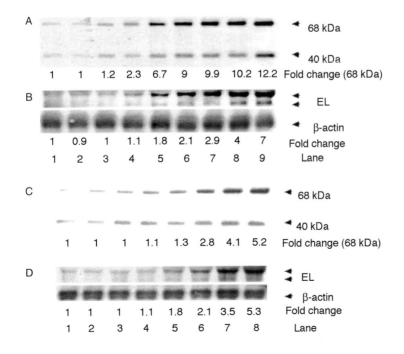

Figure 4 Effect of cytokine stimulation on endothelial lipase protein and mRNA expression in HUVEC. In panel A, protein expression and in panel B, mRNA expression in response to (1–9): 0, 1, 3, 10, 30, 100, 300, 1000 and 3000 pg/ml IL-1β. In panel C, protein expression and in panel D, mRNA expression in response to (1–8): 0, 10 pg, 30 pg, 100 pg, 300 pg, 1 ng, 3 ng, and 10 ng/ml TNFα. Fold change in EL protein is based on the 68 kDa form only. Reproduced with permission from Jin W et al.[25] Endothelial cells secrete triglyceride lipase and phospholipase activities in response to cytokines as a result of endothelial lipase. Circulation Research 2003; 92:644–50

inflammation-induced upregulation of EL could be a causal factor in reducing HDL levels seen in inflammatory conditions.

When fed with a high-fat diet, apoE[-/-] mice are susceptible to development of atherosclerosis, which is increasingly considered an inflammatory state. Yu et al measured EL mRNA by real-time PCR and Western blotting. Aortic EL mRNA and protein expression were higher than that in wild-type mice, whereas its hepatic expression was significantly decreased.[19] Cholesterol feeding alone, or with added saturated fat, further reduced hepatic EL mRNA expression. However, aortic EL mRNA was not regulated by these different diets. Interestingly, addition of cholic acid, which may induce hepatic inflammation, significant increased EL mRNA expression.[28] Together these data suggest a tissue-specific manner of regulation of EL. In human non-atherosclerotic coronary arteries, Azumi et al found that EL was expressed in endothelial cells and medial smooth muscle cells. However, in atherosclerotic coronary arteries, EL was expressed in macrophages within atheromatous plaques as well as endothelial and smooth muscle cells.[28] Thus, additional EL supplied by infiltrating macrophages may further strengthen its local effects on HDL at the site of atherosclerotic lesions. Under acute inflammatory conditions, upregulation of EL in endothelial cells at local sites of inflammation may be part of innate defence responses. Generated free fatty acids from HDL may be utilized by local tissues, including possibly the endothelial cells themselves, as an energy source. While initially potentially beneficial, the change of HDL by EL may be proatherogenic if present for an extended period.

MECHANISMS BY WHICH EL AFFECTS HDL METABOLISM

The lipolytic activity of EL against phospholipids of HDL is thought to play a major role in reducing HDL-cholesterol (HDL-C) levels. When overexpressed in HepG2 cells, EL effectively hydrolysed phospholipids from HDL and liberated fatty acids, which were then incorporated into cellular phospholipids and triglycerides. This leads to an increase in the amount of cellular lipids and suppressed the rate of fatty acid synthesis. In the presence of CD36, more fatty acids were incorporated into cellular lipids.[29] Maugeais et al demonstrated that, when overexpressed in mice, EL resulted in a dose-dependent increase in post-heparin plasma phospholipase activity. Kinetic studies demonstrated a dose-dependent acceleration of HDL-apolipoprotein catabolism, which was highly correlated to post-heparin plasma phospholipase activity ($r = 0.89$, $p < 0.01$). This effect was not the sole result of the reduction in HDL pool size.[30] Conversely, inhibition of EL activity caused a 21% slower fractional catabolic rate (FCR) of phospholipids in HDL particles (0.42 ± 0.03 vs 0.53 ± 0.02 pool per hour).[31] Post-heparin plasma phospholipase activity was dramatically reduced in EL[-/-] mice.[32] All these data suggest that the phospholipase activity of EL may directly modulate the phospholipid content of HDL and subsequently affect its turnover.

Independent of its lipolytic activity, EL can serve as a ligand to enhance binding and cellular processing of HDL particles via heparan sulphate proteoglycan-mediated pathways. Fuki et al[33] found, in in vitro studies using cultured cells expressing EL, that 70% of the surface-bound HDL was released back into the medium, and only 30% of HDL holoparticles were processed intracellularly. In addition, Strauss et al showed that the selective uptake of HDL-associated cholesterol esters was markedly elevated in EL-expressing cells and independent of SR-BI.[34] Broedl et al showed that, in vivo, a catalytic inactive EL mutant, ELS[149A], led to an intermediate reduction of HDL-C in HL[-/-] mice compared to catalytic active EL, but not in wild-type and apoA-I transgenic mice.[35] Thus, both lipolytic and non-lipolytic effects of EL may contribute to accelerate the catabolism of HDL-C. Indeed, Maugeais et al noted that the uptake of HDL particles was increased up to 158% and 189% by liver and kidney, respectively, in EL-expressing mice as assessed using [^{125}I]-tyramine-cellobiose-labelled HDL.[30] On the other hand,

Ma et al reported that the FCR of cholesteryl ester-labelled HDL was delayed in their kinetic study in EL[-/-] mice (2.22 ± 0.28 vs 3.04 ± 0.31 pool per hour).[36]

EFFECTS OF EL ON HDL METABOLISM IN MICE

Our understanding of the physiological role of EL in HDL metabolism is greatly advanced from several studies performed in mice. Hepatic EL overexpression, using an adenoviral vector encoding a human EL cDNA, first shed light on its effects on HDL metabolism in wild-type and human apoA-I transgenic mice. Three days after vector injection, overexpression of EL resulted in barely detectable plasma HDL-C and apoA-I levels. Impressively, these extremely low levels of HDL-C and apoA-I were sustained during the 28-day experimental course, although human EL protein is expected to have diminished to an almost undetectable level at day 28 post-injection.[8] A decreased HDL size was seen in EL-expressing mice as shown by gel filtration and non-denaturing gradient gel electrophoresis.[31] In line with these results, analysis of BAC-human EL-transgenic mice revealed an approximate 20% decrease in the plasma concentration of HDL-C, a 26% decrease in apoA-I but otherwise similar composition of their HDL particles. Of note, these mice expressed human EL transcript in brain, aorta, heart, lung, kidney and spleen, but not liver.[33]

Loss of function studies of EL in mice further established that EL is a major genetic modulator of HDL levels. A bolus injection of a neutralizing IgG specific for murine EL resulted in a 25–60% increased HDL-C in wild-type, apoA-I transgenic and HL[-/-] mice, with the peak HDL-C levels occurring at 48 hours after injection. In addition, acute inhibition of EL in HL[-/-] mice generated larger HDL particles.[32] Examination of two EL[-/-] mouse lines generated by two different laboratories demonstrated ~57% increase and ~25% increase of HDL-C levels in homozygous and heterozygous EL[-/-] mice, respectively.[33,36] Ishita

et al[33] also showed both male and female EL[-/-] mice had similar changes of HDL levels and its composition was not altered, suggesting an increased number of HDL particles. Ma et al[36] reported that EL[-/-] mice displayed higher levels of HDL even with high-cholesterol diet feeding. NMR analysis showed that EL[-/-] mice have an abundance of large HDL particles. Furthermore, EL[-/-] mice intercrossed onto a SR-BI[-/-] background showed a stepwise change in HDL-C levels, suggesting that the effects of EL on HDL levels are independent of SR-BI. All these data demonstrated that EL inversely regulates plasma HDL particle sizes and levels.

GENETIC STUDIES IN HUMANS

The relevance of studies of EL in cultured cells and mouse models to human cholesterol metabolism was first examined by deLemos et al.[37] They asked whether elevated HDL-C levels may be a result of functional polymorphisms and mutations in the EL gene. They sequenced 1200 base pairs of the promoter and all exons of the EL gene in 20 individuals with HDL-C levels greater than the 90th percentile for age, sex and race. They identified and confirmed 17 polymorphic sites in these individuals (Table 1). Six of these were potentially functional. Four polymorphisms resulted in amino acid changes: Gly26Ser, Thr111Ile, Thr298Ser and Asn396Ser. Two were in the promoter (−303A/C and −410C/G). The genotypic frequencies of each variant were measured in 176 black controls, 165 white controls and 123 whites with high HDL-C. The Thr111Ile polymorphism occurred in 32.6% of white subjects with high HDL-C, 31.2% of control white subjects and 10.3% of control black subjects. There was no association between HDL-C levels and the presence of this polymorphism. Three variants, Gly26Ser, Thr298Ser and -303A/C, were found in the cohort of high HDL-C whites and in blacks but not in the control white population.

Ma et al[36] examined 372 members of the Lipoprotein and Coronary Atherosclerosis Study for the presence of the single nucleotide

Table 1 Single nucleotide polymorphisms identified in the endothelial lipase gene summary of results from deLemos et al,[37] Yamakawa-Kobayashi et al[38] (in italics) and Mank-Seymour et al[39] (in bold)

Polymorphism	Amino acid change	Reference	Frequency				
			Black	White (high HDL white)	Japanese	Hispanic	Asian
–410 C/G		37	0	0.3			
–303 A/C		37	1.8	0 (0.4)			
328 G/A	Gly26Ser	37	5.7	0 (0.8)			
1145C/G	Thr298Ser	37	2.3	0 (0.4)			
1439A/G	Asn396Ser	37	0.6	1.2 (2.4)			
584C/T	Thr111Ile	37, *38*, **39**	10.3, **9**	31.2, **30** (32.6)		**23**	**34**
229T/G 5'UTR		37, **39**	12	35		**31**	**35**
51C/T Int1		37					
55C/G Int1		37					
98C/A Int4		37, **39**	12	22		**11**	**12**
264C/A	Ser4Ser	37, **39**	0	14		**0**	**0**
315C/T	Ser21Ser	37					
1922T/C Int2		37, **39**	7	18		**21**	**26**
42C/T Int5		37, **39**	16	48		**58**	**65**
840A/G Int7			53	42		**42**	**62**
2725T/C Int8		37					
2237A/G 3'UTR		37, *38*			*13.8*		
63C/T	Arg54Cys	**39**					
–384A/C		*38*, **39**			*2.1*		
2037T/C		*38*			*7.7*		
2842T/A		*38*			*6.2*		
3082T/C		*38*			*6.5*		

The following were found in reference 39 only:

–50G	2742A/G Int1	2884G/T Int1	5781C/A Int4	83G/A Int5	38C/G Ala277Ala	669T/G Int6	33G/A Int8
120A/T Int8	3600G/A Int9	304C/T 3'UTR					

polymorphism (SNP) 584C/T, which produces the Thr[111]Ile variant. They found a significant univariate association between the 584C/T allele and mean plasma levels of HDL-C. They found an allele-dependent variation with the rank order TT>CT>CC for both HDL-C and apoA-I/apoB ratios. They followed these individuals for 2.5 years and found no difference between genotypes in progression or regression of disease.

These studies were extended to a population of 340 Japanese children between the ages of 9 and 15 years without known lipid abnormalities.[38] Yamakawa-Kobayashi et al identified two new polymorphisms, –384A/C and 2237G/A. Using multiple linear regression with sex, age

and body mass index as co-variates, they found significant associations between the –384A/C polymorphism and serum HDL-C and apoA-I levels, and between the 2237G/A polymorphism and serum HDL-C levels.

An additional 13 polymorphisms were identified in genomic DNA from immortalized B-lymphocyte cell lines from 93 subjects of varying ethnic backgrounds in the Gennaissance Index Repository.[39] DNA from two cohorts of individuals with high and low HDL, derived from subjects enrolled in the ACCESS study, was examined for the seven polymorphisms which were found at greater than 5% frequency. The T229G exon 1 and C53T exon3 polymorphisms, as well as four intronic polymorphisms, were found to significantly associate with HDL levels. Two polymorphisms were found to be potentially protective for myocardial infraction, the C53T (Thr111Ile) and G98A Intron4. They found that the contribution of EL gene variation to overall variation in HDL-C was only 1–3%.

INHIBITION OF EL AS A PHARMACOLOGICAL MEANS OF ELEVATING HDL LEVELS

Collectively, studies that have examined the influence of EL on HDL particles confirm that EL is able to modulate the lipid contents of HDL and its function. Studies using mouse models of EL overexpression or, conversely, EL gene deletion or inhibition, strongly support the conclusion that EL is a significant enzyme in controlling the catabolism of HDL. Hence, pharmacological inhibition of EL expression or activity may provide a novel way to raise HDL levels.

If cytokine-induced upregulation of EL is a causal factor in reducing HDL levels seen in inflammatory conditions, one potential approach to the management of low HDL-C levels under these conditions might be inhibition of EL expression through the use of anti-inflammatory agents. These agents may also be useful to elevate HDL levels in patients with atherosclerosis since it is increasingly being recognized as a chronic inflammatory process.

The findings of Broedl et al[40] must be considered when entertaining the use of agents that would target EL for inhibition. They examined the effect of EL overexpression in three mouse models of elevated apoB-containing lipoproteins: apoE$^{-/-}$, LDL-receptor$^{-/-}$ and human apoB transgenics. They found that hepatic expression of EL resulted in markedly decreased levels of VLDL/LDL cholesterol, phospholipid and apoB, with increased catabolism of apoB-containing lipoproteins. This suggests that inhibition of EL might result in elevated levels of atherogenic lipoproteins and VLDL and LDL-C levels as well as HDL-C.

Extensive study of the mass and activity of EL in human subjects will be necessary to determine the applicability of these findings to human cholesterol metabolism. The associations between HDL levels and certain polymorphisms in the EL gene suggest that EL may be quite relevant to human HDL metabolism. Extending these studies to examine associations between EL gene variants and LDL levels will be essential to determining the risk/benefit balance of EL inhibition.

References

1. Gordon T, Castelli WP, Hjortland MC, et al. High density lipoprotein as a protective factor against coronary heart disease. The Framingham Study. Am J Med 1977; 62:707–14
2. Brooks-Wilson A, Marcil M, Clee SM, et al. Mutations in ABC1 in Tangier disease and familial high-density lipoprotein deficiency. Nat Genet 1999; 22:336–45
3. Bodzioch M, Orso E, Klucken J, et al. The gene encoding ATP-binding cassette transporter 1 is mutated in Tangier disease. Nat Genet 1999; 22:347–51
4. Rust S, Rosier M, Funke H, et al. Tangier disease is caused by mutations in the gene encoding ATP-binding cassette transporter 1. Nat Genet 1999; 22:352–5
5. Calvo D, Vega MA. Identification, primary structure, and distribution of CLA-1, a novel member of the CD36/LIMPII gene family. J Biol Chem 1993; 268:18929–35
6. Acton SL, Scherer PE, Lodish HF, et al. Expression cloning of SR-BI, a CD36–related class B scavenger receptor. J Biol Chem 1994; 269:21003–9
7. Acton S, Rigotti A, Landschulz KT, et al. Identification of scavenger receptor SR-BI as a high density lipoprotein receptor. Science 1996; 271:518–20
8. Jaye M, Lynch KJ, Krawiec J, et al. A novel endothelial-derived lipase that modulates HDL metabolism. Nat Genet 1999; 21:424–8
9. Hirata K, Dichek HL, Cioffi JA, et al. Cloning of a unique lipase from endothelial cells extends the lipase gene family. J Biol Chem 1999; 274:14170–5
10. McCoy MG, Sun GS, Marchadier D, et al.

Characterization of the lipolytic activity of endothelial lipase. J Lipid Res 2002; 43:921–9

11. Ishida T, Zheng Z, Dichek HL, et al. Molecular cloning of nonsecreted endothelial cell-derived lipase isoforms. Genomics 2004; 83:24–33

12. Bourne Y, Martinez C, Kerfelec B, 2004. Horse pancreatic lipase. The crystal structure refined at 2.3 A resolution. J Mol Biol 1994; 238:709–32

13. van Tilbeurgh H, Roussel A, Lalouel JM, et al. Lipoprotein lipase. Molecular model based on the pancreatic lipase x-ray structure: consequences for heparin binding and catalysis. J Biol Chem 1994; 269:4626–33

14. Hata A, Ridinger DN, Sutherland S, et al. Binding of lipoprotein lipase to heparin. Identification of five critical residues in two distinct segments of the amino-terminal domain. J Biol Chem 1993; 268:8447–57

15. Lookene A, Nielsen MS, Gliemann J, et al. Contribution of the carboxy-terminal domain of lipoprotein lipase to interaction with heparin and lipoproteins. Biochem Biophys Res Commun 2000; 271:15–21

16. Duong M, Psaltis M, Rader DJ, et al. Evidence that hepatic lipase and endothelial lipase have different substrate specificities for high-density lipoprotein phospholipids. Biochemistry 2003; 42:13778–85

17. Rye KA, Duong M, Psaltis MK, et al. Evidence that phospholipids play a key role in pre-beta apoA-I formation and high-density lipoprotein remodeling. Biochemistry 2002; 41:12538–45

18. Gauster M, Oskolkova OV, Innerlohinger J, et al. Endothelial lipase-modified high-density lipoprotein exhibits diminished ability to mediate SR-BI (scavenger receptor B type I)-dependent free-cholesterol efflux. Biochem J 2004; 382:75–82

19. Yu KCWDC, Kadambi SJ, Stahl A, et al. Endothelial lipase is synthesized by hepatic and aorta endothelial cells and its expression is altered in apoE-deficient mice. J Lipid Res 2004; 45:1614–23

20. Nagasaka H, Chiba H, Kikuta H, et al. Unique character and metabolism of high density lipoprotein (HDL) in fetus. Atherosclerosis 2002; 161:215–23

21. Tan KC, Shiu SW, Kung AW. Effect of thyroid dysfunction on high-density lipoprotein subfraction metabolism: roles of hepatic lipase and cholesteryl ester transfer protein. J Clin Endocrinol Metab 1998; 83:2921–4

22. Bausserman LL, Bernier DN, McAdam KP, et al. Serum amyloid A and high density lipoproteins during the acute phase response. Eur J Clin Invest 1988; 18:619–26

23. Barter P. Effects of inflammation on high-density lipoproteins. Arterioscler Thromb Vasc Biol 2002; 22:1062–3

24. Hirata K, Ishida T, Matsushita H, et al. Regulated expression of endothelial cell-derived lipase. Biochem Biophys Res Commun 2000; 272:90–3

25. Jin W, Sun GS, Marchadier D, et al. Endothelial cells secrete triglyceride lipase and phospholipase activities in response to cytokines as a result of endothelial lipase. Circ Res 2003; 92:644–50

26. Feingold KR, Marshall M, Gulli R, et al. Effect of endotoxin and cytokines on lipoprotein lipase activity in mice. Arterioscler Thromb 1994; 14:1866–72

27. Feingold KR, Memon RA, Moser AH, et al. Endotoxin and interleukin-1 decrease hepatic lipase mRNA levels. Atherosclerosis 1999; 142:379–87

28. Azumi H, Hirata K, Ishida T, et al. Immunohistochemical localization of endothelial cell-derived lipase in atherosclerotic human coronary arteries. Cardiovasc Res 2003; 58:647–54

29. Strauss JG, Hayn M, Zechner R, et al. Fatty acids liberated from high-density lipoprotein phospholipids by endothelial-derived lipase are incorporated into lipids in HepG2 cells. Biochem J 2003; 371:981–8

30. Maugeais C, Tietge UJ, Broedl UC, et al. Dose-dependent acceleration of high-density lipoprotein catabolism by endothelial lipase. Circulation 2003; 108:2121–6

31. Jin W, Millar JS, Broedl U, et al. Inhibition of endothelial lipase causes increased HDL cholesterol levels in vivo. J Clin Invest 2003; 111:357–62

32. Ishida T, Choi S, Kundu RK, et al. Endothelial lipase is a major determinant of HDL level. J Clin Invest 2003; 111:347–55

33. Fuki IV, Blanchard N, Jin W, et al. Endogenously produced endothelial lipase enhances binding and cellular processing of plasma lipoproteins via heparan sulfate proteoglycan-mediated pathway. J Biol Chem 2003; 278:34331–8

34. Strauss JG, Zimmermann R, Hrzenjak A, et al. Endothelial cell-derived lipase mediates uptake and binding of high-density lipoprotein (HDL) particles and the selective uptake of HDL-associated cholesterol esters independent of its enzymic activity. Biochem J 2002; 368:69–79

35. Broedl UC, Maugeais C, Marchadier D, et al. Effects of nonlipolytic ligand function of endothelial lipase on high density lipoprotein metabolism in vivo. J Biol Chem 2003; 278:40688–93

36. Ma K, Cilingiroglu M, Otvos JD, et al. Endothelial lipase is a major genetic determinant for high-density lipoprotein concentration, structure, and metabolism. Proc Natl Acad Sci USA 2003; 100:2748–53

37. deLemos AS, Wolfe ML, Long CJ, et al. Identification of genetic variants in endothelial lipase in persons with elevated high-density lipoprotein cholesterol. Circulation 2002; 106:1321–6

38. Yamakawa-Kobayashi K, Yanagi H, Endo K, et al. Relationship between serum HDL-C levels and common genetic variants of the endothelial lipase gene in Japanese school-aged children. Hum Genet 2003; 113:311–15

39. Mank-Seymour AR, Durham KL, Thompson JF, et al. Association between single-nucleotide polymorphisms in the endothelial lipase (LIPG) gene and high-density lipoprotein cholesterol levels. Biochim Biophys Acta 2004; 1636:40–6

40. Broedl UC, Maugeais C, Millar JS, et al. Endothelial lipase promotes the catabolism of ApoB-containing lipoproteins. Circ Res 2004; 94:1554–61

Cholesteryl ester transfer protein (CETP) inhibition as a therapeutic strategy for raising HDL-cholesterol levels and reducing atherosclerosis

11

D.J. Rader

INTRODUCTION

The risk of atherosclerotic cardiovascular disease (ASCVD) is strongly associated with plasma levels of both atherogenic and anti-atherogenic lipoproteins. Low density lipoproteins (LDLs) are the paradigm of the atherogenic lipoprotein. After modification, they are taken up by macrophages within the arterial intima and promote the generation of foam cells, the classic cell type of the atherosclerotic lesion. Therapy to reduce LDL cholesterol levels is proven to reduce the risk of ASCVD clinical events by about one third over 5 years.[1] A low level of HDL cholesterol (HDL-C) on statin therapy is an independent predictor of future cardiovascular events.[2] Therefore, HDL-C is a major target for the development of new therapies designed to raise HDL-C levels.[3] The cholesteryl ester transfer protein (CETP) transfers cholesteryl esters from HDL to apoB-containing lipoproteins such as LDL. Pharmacological inhibition of CETP raises HDL-C levels in animals and humans and reduces atherosclerosis in animals; it is currently being studied for its ability to reduce atherosclerosis in humans. Here we review the physiology of CETP and the issues around its inhibition as a novel therapeutic strategy to raise HDL-C.

THE PHYSIOLOGY OF CETP

Lipoproteins contain a core of hydrophobic lipids (triglycerides and cholesteryl esters) surrounded by phospholipids and apolipoproteins. Very low density lipoproteins (VLDLs) have as their major protein apoB-100. They are secreted by the liver, their core triglycerides are hydrolysed by lipoprotein lipase in muscle and adipose and they are eventually converted to LDL. LDL also contains the same apoB-100 protein, which binds to the LDL receptor and mediates its uptake by the liver. HDL and its major protein apoA-I are secreted by the intestine and the liver. Lipid-poor apoA-I acquires phospholipids and unesterified cholesterol from tissues through efflux mediated by ATP-binding cassette transporter proteins such as ABCA1. The enzyme lecithin:cholesterol acyltransferase (LCAT) converts unesterified cholesterol on HDL to cholesteryl ester (CE).

HDL cholesteryl ester has several possible routes of metabolism. One is direct selective uptake into steroidogenic tissues and the liver mediated by the cell-surface receptor SR-BI. Another is transfer via CETP to apoB-containing lipoproteins such as VLDL and LDL. CETP promotes exchange of cholesteryl esters from HDL to apoB-containing lipoproteins in exchange for triglyceride which moves from apoB-containing lipoproteins to HDL. The action of CETP therefore influences lipoprotein metabolism in a variety of ways. It increases the CE content of apoB-containing lipoproteins and promotes the generation of small, dense LDL. It results in depletion of CE and enrichment of TG in HDL, making HDL a better substrate for lipases such as hepatic lipase (HL) and resulting in the generation of smaller, denser HDL particles that are more rapidly catabolized via the kidney.[4] Rodents lack CETP and the SR-BI pathway for selective uptake of HDL CE into the liver is very active. In species that have CETP (such as rabbits and primates), the CETP pathway appears to be the major route of metabolism of HDL CE and the importance of the SR-BI pathway is uncertain.

One of the major questions about the physiology of CETP in humans regards its role in reverse cholesterol transport. In rabbits the CETP pathway accounts for a major amount of the clearance of HDL CE.[5] Schwartz and colleagues have done most detailed work in humans regarding the pathways of HDL-C metabolism. Studies in healthy human volunteers in which HDL was labelled with cholesteryl ester ex vivo and reinjected, followed by multiple sampling of plasma and continuous collection of bile for 6 days, revealed that the vast majority of tracer that appeared in bile was derived after transfer to apoB-containing lipoproteins,[6] presumably by CETP. Thus, transfer of HDL CE to apoB-containing lipoproteins may be a major route of delivery of HDL CE to the liver, suggesting that inhibiting CETP could potentially slow that pathway. However, about 30% of cholesterol in HDL is unesterified, and studies by Schwartz and colleagues demonstrated that the majority of HDL unesterified cholesterol gets to the liver and bile via direct transfer from HDL.[6,7] Thus, substantial RCT could theoretically occur via direct transport by HDL of unesterified cholesterol to the liver, a pathway for which CETP is not required. Indeed, both CETP deficiency and CETP inhibition are associated with absolute increases in HDL free cholesterol.

GENETIC DEFICIENCY OF AND VARIATION IN CETP IN HUMANS: INSIGHT INTO THE ROLE OF CETP IN HUMAN LIPOPROTEIN METABOLISM AND ATHEROSCLEROSIS

Japanese subjects with extremely elevated levels of HDL-C were found to have markely reduced CETP activity in plasma and subsequently found to have mutations in the CETP gene that were the cause of the low CETP activity.[8,9] The initial CETP mutations included a splice site mutation of intron 14 and an aspartic acid to glycine substitution at the 442 position of exon 15.[10] Homozygotes for the intron 14 mutation have no measurable CETP mass or activity in their plasma. In contrast, homozygosity for the D442G mutation results in partial CETP deficiency. Other mutations in CETP causing deficiency have subsequently been described. Heterozygotes for loss-of-function mutations in the CETP gene usually have slightly more than half of the CETP activity of normal controls and generally have only a modest increase in HDL-C levels. The finding that CETP deficiency causes very high HDL-C levels led directly to the concept that pharmacological inhibition of CETP could be a novel strategy for raising HDL-C levels.

Kinetic studies in patients with homozygous CETP deficiency have demonstrated that the turnover of apoA-I is significantly reduced in CETP-deficient subjects, as is the turnover of the second most abundant HDL apolipoprotein, apoA-II.[11] Even though CETP-deficient LDL had delayed catabolism in normal subjects (consistent with decreased LDL receptor affinity), there was increased catabolism of LDL apoB in CETP-deficient subjects, consistent with endogenous upregulation of the LDL-receptor.[12]

There is no consensus about whether homozygous CETP-deficient subjects are at reduced risk of cardiovascular disease compared with the normal population; indeed, one group in Japan believes they may be at increased risk. In the Omigari region of Japan, of 201 patients with HDL-C levels >100 mg/dl,

29 were homozygotes or compound heterozygotes for CETP deficiency. One of these subjects had clinical coronary heart disease (CHD),[13] but was also found to have substantially reduced hepatic lipase activity.[14] Given the relatively small number of homozygous CETP-deficient subjects in Japan, the issue of their cardiovascular risk relative to the general population may not be easily resolved. There are considerably greater numbers of heterozygous CETP-deficient subjects for addressing this question. In the same series of 201 Japanese patients from the Omigari region with HDL-C levels >100 mg/dl described above, 52 were heterozygotes for CETP deficiency and eight had clinical CHD.[13] However, all had reduced hepatic lipase activity, suggesting that markedly elevated HDL-C in the setting of heterozygous CETP deficiency and reduced hepatic lipase may not necessarily afford protection from CHD. In a population-based study of 104 505 persons in the Omigari region of Japan, there was found to be an increased prevalence of ECG changes in subjects with very high HDL-C levels,[15] but the number of documented heterozygous subjects was low. In contrast, in another study among Japanese subjects with HDL-C >80 mg/dl and a low risk of cardiovascular disease, heterozygous CETP gene mutations were identified in about one quarter of the subjects,[16] suggesting a possible protective effect.

The Honolulu Heart Study (which includes many subjects of Japanese origin) initially reported in a cross-sectional study that heterozygous D442G carriers with normal HDL-C concentrations of 40–60 mg/dl had an apparent increase in CHD compared with controls in the same HDL range.[17] However, a recent prospective analysis reported after a 7-year follow-up that, after adjustment for other CV risk factors, heterozygotes with the CETP D442G mutation had no evidence of increased CHD risk at any HDL-C strata and, in fact, had the lowest rates of CHD (although this was not statistically significant).[18] Therefore, the issue of whether heterozygous CETP deficiency is associated with altered cardiovascular risk has not been resolved.

Insights into the relationship between CETP and cardiovascular disease may also be provided by studies of common polymorphisms in the human CETP gene. The Taq1B RFLP in intron 1 of the human CETP gene is the most extensively studied CETP polymorphism. Subjects from the Framingham Offspring Study carrying the Taq1B B2 allele had lower CETP levels and higher HDL-C levels and a reduced risk of CHD (in men) compared with homozygotes for the B1 allele.[19] The VA-HIT study in men with CHD and low HDL showed a similar result.[20] The common SNP resulting in conversion of the isoleucine at postion 405 to valine (I405V) has also been studied extensively. CHD risk was higher in those with the VV genotype among men in the Honolulu Heart Study[21] and carriers of I405V SNP has been associated with increased HDL-C and increased risk of CHD in women in the Copenhagen City Heart Study.[22] In a case-control study of Ashkenazi Jews with exceptional longevity, probands had a nearly 3-fold increased frequency of homozygosity for the CETP 405V allele compared with controls, and also had larger HDL and LDL particle size.[23] A formal meta-analysis of the Taq1B and I405V SNPs suggested that the Taq1B B2 allele was significantly associated with reduced CETP mass and activity and increased HDL-C levels and the B2B2 genotype with possibly reduced cardiovascular disease, but suggested that there was no convincing evidence that the I405V was associated with altered risk of cardiovascular disease.[24] Two additional CETP-coding SNPs, A373P and R451Q, are in linkage disequilibrium. In one study, carriers of the rarer 373P/451Q haplotype had reduced levels of HDL-C and a lower CHD risk.[25] Common promoter SNPs in the CETP gene, including −629A/C and a variable number tandem repeat (VNTR) 1946 upstream of the transcription initiation site, are associated with variation in CETP mass and HDL-C levels,[26,27] but not with CHD. The human CETP gene divides into two linkage disequilibrium groups, a 5' block and a 3' block.[27,28] The 5' haplotype block, which contains the promoter polymorphisms and the Taq1B SNP, has a significant association with CETP mass and HDL-C levels, whereas the 3' haplotype block does not. Neither haplotype block has been shown to have an unequivocal association with cardiovascular risk. Thus, the relationship between CETP SNPs and atherosclerosis is variable and does not provide major insight into the relationship of CETP and ASCVD.

OBSERVATIONAL STUDIES OF PLASMA CETP LEVELS AND CARDIOVASCULAR RISK

It is surprising that there have been relatively few observational studies of the association of plasma CETP levels (mass or activity) with cardiovascular outcomes. Patients with lower CETP mass had more rapid progression of carotid intimal medial thickness[29] and angiographic coronary disease.[30] A small coronary angiographic study in Japanese patients found no correlation of CETP mass levels with extent of coronary atherosclerosis.[31] Another small case-control study in Chinese patients found that subjects with MI or stroke had higher CETP mass and activity compared to controls.[32] A small case-control study found no difference between CETP activity levels in CHD cases and controls.[33] The largest observational study of plasma CETP levels and cardiovascular risk was the EPIC-Norfolk cohort study, in which CETP mass was measured in 755 originally healthy individuals who developed CAD during follow-up and 1400 matched controls who remained free of CAD.[34] CETP levels were inversely related to HDL-C levels and directly related to LDL-C levels. Mean CETP levels were not significantly different in cases and controls; however, subjects in the highest quintile of CETP mass had a 1.5-fold increased risk of CAD compared to those in the lowest quintile after adjusting for several cardiovascular risk factors but not lipids. Furthermore, a stratified analysis in subjects above or below the median (non-fasting) triglyceride level showed a significant positive association for those above the TG median but no association of CETP levels and CAD in those below the TG median.

CETP INHIBITION IN ANIMAL MODELS: EFFECTS ON LIPIDS AND ATHEROSCLEROSIS

Rodents

Rodents such as mice and rats are naturally deficient in CETP, and thus they cannot be used as models for addressing the effects of CETP inhibition on atherosclerosis. Studies in which the CETP gene was introduced transgenically into these species have uniformly demonstrated reduction in HDL-C levels, but have provided mixed results with regard to effects on atherosclerosis. Expression of CETP in C57BL/6 mice fed an atherogenic diet,[35] apoE knockout mice fed a chow diet,[36] LDL-receptor knockout mice fed an atherogenic diet[36] and Dahl salt-sensitive hypertensive rats fed an atherogenic diet[37] all resulted in increased atherosclerosis, suggesting that CETP is pro-atherogenic in rodents. However, expression of CETP in human apoC-III transgenic mice, in diabetic mice and in LPL-deficient mice reduced atherosclerosis[38] and expression of CETP in LCAT transgenic mice also reduced atherosclerosis.[39] Overall, the reasons for these discrepant results are unclear, but may relate to the effects of CETP on the cholesterol content in atherogenic VLDL remnant particles. In any case, it is difficult to extrapolate from these studies in rodents to the potential effects of inhibiting CETP in humans with regard to effects on atherogenesis.

Rabbits

Rabbits have high levels of CETP, approximately four times those found in human plasma. Several approaches to CETP inhibition have been utilized in rabbits. Reduction of CETP expression by injection of anti-sense oligodeoxynucleotides in rabbits resulted in an increase in HDL-C and a reduction in aortic cholesterol content as a marker of atherosclerosis.[40] Immunization of rabbits with a peptide based on the CETP sequence generated auto-antibodies against CETP, resulting in reduced plasma CETP activity, increased HDL-C and reduced aortic atherosclerosis.[41] Treatment of rabbits for 6 months with the small-molecule CETP inhibitor JTT-705 reduced CETP activity, increased HDL-C by 90% and reduced aortic atherosclerosis by 70%.[42] However, the interpretation of this study was confounded by the fact that JTT-705 decreased non-HDL-C levels substantially, and another control group administered simvastatin had a similar reduction in non-HDL-C without a change in HDL-C and also had significant reduction in atherosclerosis. In another study in which rabbits were made even more severely hypercholesterolaemic, 3 months of treatment with JTT-705 did not reduce non-HDL-C levels and, although it raised HDL-C levels, it failed to reduce atherosclerosis.[43] Finally, a study in rabbits with the small molecule CETP inhibitor torcetrapib showed increased HDL-C without reduction in non-HDL-C and nevertheless demonstrated significant reduction in atherosclerosis.[44] Thus, CETP inhibition in rabbits reduces atherosclerosis. Although the rabbit has much higher levels of CETP than humans, these data are among the most encouraging that CETP inhibition may reduce atherosclerosis in humans.

CETP INHIBITION IN HUMANS: EFFECTS ON LIPIDS AND LIPOPROTEIN METABOLISM

A phase I clinical trial of a CETP peptide immunization approach in 36 subjects reported that one subject who received a single injection of the CETP peptide at the highest dose developed anti-CETP antibodies.[45] In an extension study of 15 subjects who received a second injection of the active vaccine, eight developed anti-CETP antibodies. There were no changes in HDL-C levels in this phase I study.

Two small molecule inhibitors of CETP, JTT-705 and torcetrapib, have been studied in humans and some of the data have been published. In a phase II study of three doses of JTT-705 (300, 600 and 900 mg) in 198 healthy volunteers with modest hyperlipidaemia, JTT-705 900 mg for 4 weeks reduced CETP activity by 37%, decreased LDL-C by 7% and increased

HDL-C by 34%.[46] JTT-705 also increased apoA-I levels modestly but significantly compared with placebo at each dose.

In a phase I study in healthy volunteers, torcetrapib was administered at doses of 10, 30, 60 and 120 mg daily and 120 mg twice daily for 14 days.[47] CETP inhibition ranged from 12% at the 30 mg dose to 80% at the 120 mg bid dose. There was also a dose-dependent increase in HDL-C, ranging from 16% to 91%. There was also a dose-dependent reduction in non-HDL-C, with 8% reduction in LDL-C at the 60 mg dose and 42% reduction of LDL-C at the highest dose.

Finally, a small phase II study designed to address the effects of torcetrapib on lipoprotein metabolism in subjects with low HDL-C (<40 mg/dl) has been published.[48] Subjects with LDL-C levels >160 mg/dl were initially treated with 20 mg of atorvastatin daily for reduction in LDL-C (nine subjects) and the remaining subjects were on no statin therapy (10 subjects). All subjects received placebo for 4 weeks, then 120 mg of torcetrapib daily for 4 weeks; a subgroup of the subjects not taking atorvastatin went on to receive 120 mg of torcetrapib twice daily for another 4 weeks. Plasma lipids and lipoprotein kinetic studies were performed at the end of each 4-week period. Torcetrapib resulted in a 46% increase in HDL-C when given at 120 mg daily without atorvastatin, a 61% increase in HDL-C when given at 120 mg with atorvastatin and a 106% increase in HDL-C when given at 120 mg twice daily without atorvastatin. Corresponding increases in apoA-I were 16%, 13% and 36%. Torcetrapib elevated all types of HDL particles, but increased the large, more buoyant HDL_2 particles to a greater extent than the smaller and denser HDL_3 particles. Torcetrapib also reduced LDL-C and apoB by about 14–17% when administered with atorvastatin. Finally, torcetrapib significantly altered the distribution of cholesterol among HDL and LDL subclasses, resulting in increases in the mean particle size of HDL and LDL in each cohort. Kinetic studies of HDL apolipoprotein metabolism using endogenous labelling with deuterated leucine demonstrated slower catabolism of apoA-I after torcetrapib administration.[49]

SUMMARY

It is now clear that pharmacological inhibition of CETP in humans substantially increases HDL-C levels. The question of whether CETP inhibition will reduce atherosclerosis burden and clinical cardiovascular events in humans is one of the most important and fascinating questions in the fields of translational lipidology and atherosclerosis. Arguments can be made on both sides. On one hand, CETP may indeed play an important role in reverse cholesterol transport, humans deficient in CETP are not obviously protected from atherosclerotic cardiovascular disease and the rodent studies are equivocal in their results regarding the effects of CETP expression on atherosclerosis. On the other hand, much RCT may occur as free cholesterol, HDL may inhibit atherosclerosis through a variety of properties unrelated to RCT, observational studies suggest elevated CETP levels are associated with increased cardiovascular risk and the rabbit studies of CETP inhibition indicate significant reduction in atherosclerosis. Large randomized clinical trials designed to assess the effects of CETP inhibition on atherosclerosis burden using imaging modalities as well as on hard clinical cardiovascular events are under way. It will be a fascinating chapter in the progress toward targeting HDL metabolism as a therapeutic approach against atherosclerotic cardiovascular disease.[50,51]

References

1. Expert Panel ATP-III. Executive Summary of The Third Report of The National Cholesterol Education Program (NCEP) Expert Panel on Detection, Evaluation, And Treatment of High Blood Cholesterol In Adults (Adult Treatment Panel III). JAMA 2001; 285:2486–97

2. Gordon DJ, Rifkind BM. High-density lipoprotein—the clinical implications of recent studies. N Engl J Med 1989; 321:1311–16

3. Sacks FM. The role of high-density lipoprotein (HDL) cholesterol in the prevention and treatment of coronary heart disease: expert group recommendations. Am J Cardiol 2002; 90:139–43

4. Rye K-A, Clay MA, Barter PJ. Remodelling of high density lipoproteins by plasma factors. Atherosclerosis 1999; 145:227–38

5. Goldberg DI, Beltz WF, Pittman RC. Evaluation of pathways for the cellular uptake of high density lipoprotein cholesteryl esters in rabbits. J Clin Invest 1991; 87:331–46

6. Schwartz CC, VandenBroek JM, Cooper PS. Lipoprotein cholesteryl ester production, transfer and output in vivo in humans. J Lipid Res 2004; 45:1594–607

7. Schwartz CC, Zech LA, VandenBroek JM, et al. Cholesterol kinetics in subjects with bile fistula. Positive relationship between size of the bile acid precursor pool and bile acid synthetic rate. J Clin Invest 1993; 91:923–38

8. Brown ML, Inazu A, Hesler CB, et al. Molecular basis of lipid transfer protein deficiency in a family with increased high-density lipoproteins. Nature 1989; 342:448–51

9. Inazu A, Brown ML, Hesler CB, et al. Increased high-density lipoprotein levels caused by a common cholesteryl-ester transfer protein gene mutation. N Engl J Med 1990; 323:1234–8

10. Inazu A, Jiang XC, Haraki T, et al. Genetic cholesteryl ester transfer protein deficiency caused by two prevalent mutations as a major determinant of increased levels of high density lipoprotein cholesterol. J Clin Invest 1994; 94:1872–82

11. Ikewaki K, Rader DJ, Sakamoto T, et al. Delayed catabolism of high density lipoprotein apolipoprotein A-I and A-II in human cholesteryl ester transfer protein deficiency. J Clin Invest 1993; 92:1650–8

12. Ikewaki K, Nishiwaki M, Sakamoto T, et al. Increased catabolic rate of low density lipoproteins in humans with cholesteryl ester transfer protein deficiency. J Clin Invest 1995; 96:1573–81

13. Hirano K, Yamashita S, Kuga Y, et al. Atherosclerotic disease in marked hyperalphalipoproteinemia: combined reduction of cholesteryl ester transfer protein and hepatic triglyceride lipase. Arterioscler Thromb Vasc Biol 1995; 15:1849–56

14. Sakai N, Yamashita S, Hirano K, et al. Frequency of exon 15 missense mutation (D442: G) in cholesteryl ester transfer protein gene in hyperalphalipoproteinemic Japanese subjects. Atherosclerosis 1995; 114:139–46

15. Hirano K, Yamashita S, Nakajima N, et al. Genetic cholesteryl ester transfer protein deficiency is extremely frequent in the Omagari area of Japan. Marked hyperalphalipoproteinemia caused by CETP gene mutation is not associated with longevity. Arterioscler Thromb Vasc Biol 1997; 17:1053–9

16. Moriyama Y, Okamura T, Inazu A, et al. A low prevalence of coronary heart disease among subjects with increased high density lipoprotein cholesterol levels, including those with plasma cholesteryl ester transfer protein deficiency. Prev Med 1998; 27:659–67

17. Zhong S, Sharp DS, Grove JS, et al. Increased coronary heart disease in Japanese-American men with mutation in the cholesteryl ester transfer protein gene despite increased HDL levels. J Clin Invest 1996; 97:2917–23

18. Curb JD, Abbott RD, Rodriguez BL, et al. A prospective study of HDL-C and cholesteryl ester transfer protein gene mutations and the risk of coronary heart disease in the elderly. J Lipid Res 2004; 45:948–53

19. Ordovas JM, Cupples LA, Corella D, et al. Association of cholesteryl ester transfer protein-TaqIB polymorphism with variations in lipoprotein subclasses and coronary heart disease risk. Arterioscler Thromb Vasc Biol 2000; 20:1323–9

20. Brousseau ME, O'Connor JJ Jr, Ordovas JM, et al. Cholesteryl ester transfer protein TaqI B2B2 genotype is associated with higher HDL cholesterol levels and lower risk of coronary heart disease end points in men with HDL deficiency: Veterans Affairs HDL Cholesterol Intervention Trial. Arterioscler Thromb Vasc Biol 2002; 22:1148–54

21. Bruce C, Sharp DS, Tall AR. Relationship of HDL and coronary heart disease to a common amino acid polymorphism in the cholesteryl ester transfer protein in men with and without hypertriglyceridemia. J Lipid Res 1998; 39:1071–8

22. Agerholm-Larsen B, Nordestgaard BG, Steffensen R, et al. Elevated HDL cholesterol is a risk factor for ischemic heart disease in white women when caused by a common mutation in the cholesteryl ester transfer protein gene. Circulation 2000; 101:1907–12

23. Barzilai N, Atzmon G, Schechter C, et al. Unique lipoprotein phenotype and genotype associated with exceptional longevity. JAMA 2003; 290:2030–40

24. Boekholdt SM, Thompson JF. Natural genetic variation as a tool in understanding the role of CETP in lipid levels and disease. J Lipid Res 2003; 44:1080–93

25. Agerholm-Larsen B, Tybjaerg-Hansen A, Schnohr P, et al. Common cholesteryl ester transfer protein mutations, decreased HDL cholesterol, and possible decreased risk of ischemic heart disease. The Copenhagen City Heart Study. Circulation 2000; 102:2197–203

26. Dachet C, Poirier O, Cambien F, et al. New functional promoter polymorphism, CETP/-629, in cholesteryl ester transfer protein (CETO) gene related to CETP mass and high density lipoprotein levels: role of Sp1/Sp3 in transcriptional regulation. Arterioscler Thromb Vasc Biol 2000; 20:507–15

27. Thompson JF, Lira ME, Durham LK, et al. Polymorphisms in the CETP gene and association with CETP mass and HDL levels. Atherosclerosis 2003; 167:195–204

28. Corbex M, Poirier O, Fumeron F, et al. Extensive association analysis between the CETP gene and coronary heart disease phenotypes reveals several putative functional polymorphisms and gene–environment interaction. Genet Epidemiol 2000; 19:64–80

29. de Grooth GJ, Smilde TJ, van Wissen S, et al. The relationship between cholesteryl ester transfer protein levels and risk factor profile in patients with familial hypercholesterolemia. Atherosclerosis 2004; 173:261–7

30. Klerkx AHEM, de Grooth GJ, Zwinderman AH, et al. Cholesteryl ester transfer protein concentration is associated with progression of atherosclerosis and response to pravastatin in men with coronary artery disease (REGRESS). Eur J Clin Invest 2004; 34:21–8

31. Goto A, Sasai K, Suzuki S, et al. Cholesteryl ester transfer protein and atherosclerosis in Japanese subjects: a study based on coronary angiography. Atherosclerosis 2001; 159:153–63

32. Zhuang Y, Wang J, Qiang H, et al. Cholesteryl ester transfer protein levels and gene deficiency in Chinese patients with cardio-cerebrovascular diseases. Chin Med J 2002; 115:371–4

33. Blankenberg S, Rupprecht HJ, Bickel C, et al. Common genetic variation of the cholesteryl ester transfer protein gene strongly predicts future cardiovascular death in patients with coronary artery disease. J Am Coll Cardiol 2003; 41:1983–9

34. Boekholdt SM, Kuivenhoven JA, Wareham NJ, et al. Plasma levels of cholesteryl ester transfer protein and the risk of future coronary artery disease in apparently healthy men and women; the prospective EPIC-Norfolk population study. Circulation 2004; 110:1418–23

35. Marotti KR, Castle CK, Boyle TP, et al. Severe atherosclerosis in transgenic mice expressing simian cholesteryl ester transfer protein. Nature 1993; 364:73 5

36. Plump AS, Masucci-Magoulas L, Bruce C, et al. Increased atherosclerosis in apoE and LDL receptor gene knock-out mice as a result of human cholesteryl ester transfer protein transgene expression. Arterioscler Thromb Vasc Biol 1999; 19:1105–10

37. Herrera VL, Makrides SC, Xie HX, et al. Spontaneous combined hyperlipidemia, coronary heart disease and decreased survival in Dahl salt-sensitive hypertensive rats transgenic for human cholesteryl ester transfer protein. Nat Med 1999; 5:1383–9

38. Hayek T, Masucci-Magoulas L, Jiang X, et al. Decreased early atherosclerotic lesions in hypertriglyceridemic mice expressing cholesteryl ester transfer protein transgene. J Clin Invest 1995; 96:2071–4

39. Foger B, Chase M, Amar MJ, et al. Cholesteryl ester transfer protein corrects dysfunctional high density lipoproteins and reduces aortic atherosclerosis in lecithin cholesterol acyltransferase transgenic mice. J Biol Chem 1999; 274:36912–20

40. Sugano M, Makino N, Sawada S, et al. Effect of antisense oligonucleotides against cholesteryl ester

transfer protein on the development of atherosclerosis in cholesterol-fed rabbits. J Biol Chem 1998; 273:5033–6

41. Rittershaus CW, Miller DP, Thomas LJ, et al. Vaccine-induced antibodies inhibit CETP activity in vivo and reduce aortic lesions in a rabbit model of atherosclerosis. Arterioscler Thromb Vasc Biol 2000; 20:2106–12

42. Okamoto H, Yonemori F, Wakitani K, et al. A cholesteryl ester transfer protein inhibitor attenuates atherosclerosis in rabbits. Nature 2000; 406:203–7

43. Huang Z, Inazu A, Nohara A, et al. Cholesteryl ester transfer protein inhibitor (JTT-705) and the development of atherosclerosis in rabbits with severe hypercholesterolemia. Clin Sci 2002; 103:587–94

44. Morehouse LA, Sugarman ED, Bourassa PA, et al. HDL elevation by the CETP-inhibitor torcetrapib prevents aortic atherosclerosis in rabbits. Circulation 2004; 110:III-243 (abstr)

45. Davidson MH, Maki K, Umporowicz D, et al. The safety and immunogenicity of a CETP vaccine in healthy adults. Atherosclerosis 2003; 169:113–20

46. de Grooth GJ, Kuivenhoven JA, Stalenhoef AF, et al. Efficacy and safety of a novel cholesteryl ester transfer protein inhibitor, JTT-705, in humans: a randomized phase II dose-response study. Circulation 2002; 105:2159–65

47. Clark RW, Sutfin TA, Ruggeri RB, et al. Raising high-density lipoprotein in humans through inhibition of cholesteryl ester transfer protein: an initial multidose study of torcetrapib. Arterioscler Thromb Vasc Biol 2004; 24:490–7

48. Brousseau ME, Schaefer EJ, Wolfe ML, et al. Effects of an inhibitor of cholesteryl ester transfer protein on HDL cholesterol. N Engl J Med 2004; 350:1505–15

49. Brousseau ME, Diffenderfer MR, Millar JS, et al. Effects of cholesteryl ester transfer protein inhibition on high-density lipoprotein subspecies and apolipoprotein A-I metabolism. Circulation 2004; 110:III-144 (abstr)

50. van der Steeg WA, Kuivenhoven JA, Klerkx AH, et al. Role of CETP inhibitors in the treatment of dyslipidemia. Curr Opin Lipidol 2004; 15:631–6

51. Rader DJ. High-density lipoproteins as an emerging therapeutic target for atherosclerosis. JAMA 2003; 290:2322–4

Overview of insulin resistance and the metabolic syndrome

12

N. Sattar and B. Mukhopadhyay

INTRODUCTION

The fundamental role of insulin is to facilitate cellular uptake of glucose in skeletal muscle; in addition, insulin suppresses hepatic gluconeogenesis, the other key determinant of steady-state plasma glucose levels. In the steady (or fasted) state the quantity of insulin required to maintain a plasma glucose level depends on muscle mass and hepatic glucose output. However, there is more than a 2-fold variation in the plasma insulin levels required to maintain identical plasma glucose levels in normal subjects.[1] This variation in insulin requirement for glucose disposal has been termed insulin resistance, whereby subjects needing higher amounts of insulin are 'insulin resistant' compared to those who need lesser amounts of insulin. Insulin response is a linear variable across populations; insulin resistance (or insulin sensitivity) is a relative concept in normal glucose-tolerant subjects, and there are no absolute cut-off values.

In pathogenic terms, insulin resistance is a principal feature of type 2 diabetes and precedes the clinical development of the disease by 10 to 20 years.[2] Insulin resistance is caused by the decreased ability of peripheral target tissues (muscle and liver) to respond properly to normal insulin levels. Initially, increasing pancreatic insulin secretion is able to counteract insulin resistance and thus normal glucose homoeostasis can be maintained. However, pancreatic reserve eventually diminishes in the face of increasing

peripheral demands and glucose concentrations rise, heralding a diagnosis of type 2 diabetes once plasma glucose concentrations go beyond universally agreed diagnostic cut-offs, whether fasting or post-glucose loading.

It would be important to mention at this point that there are eponymous syndromes of extreme insulin resistance which are due to molecular defects in either the insulin molecule, its receptor or in post-receptor signalling. Plasma insulin levels are extremely elevated in such circumstances.[3] These subjects often have morphological abnormalities and have a shortened life expectancy due to severe dysregulation of intermediary metabolism. For the purposes of this chapter, however, we shall use the term insulin resistance with regard to more subtle changes in plasma insulin levels, as happens across normal populations and subjects with impaired glucose tolerance, type 2 diabetes.

Insulin resistance is relevant not only to the pathogenesis of type 2 diabetes but also to atherogenesis and vascular disease. Although somewhat described earlier by others, the relationship between serum insulin levels and cardiovascular disease was perhaps best conceptualized by Gerald Reaven in his Banting lecture of 1988.[4] Reaven explained that insulin resistance and hyperinsulinaemia were associated not only with glucose intolerance but also with hypertriglyceridaemia, low HDL-cholesterol (HDL-C) and hypertension (Figure 1). He thus argued that insulin resistance may be causally related to the risk of

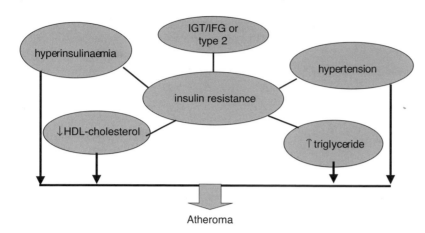

Figure 1   CHD risk factors linked to insulin resistance as initially proposed by Reaven[4]

coronary heart disease (CHD).[4] Similarly, others have suggested that both vascular disease and diabetes arise from a 'common soil'[5] and such hypotheses currently form the basis of our understanding of the central role that insulin resistance plays in the pathogenesis of diabetes and macrovascular disease.

This chapter will review recent advances in our understanding of the pathogenesis of insulin resistance, discuss its relevance to CHD and describe recent attempts to encapsulate insulin-resistance-associated vascular risk by the creation of metabolic syndrome criteria. Finally, therapeutic opportunities for tackling insulin resistance and metabolic syndrome will be briefly reviewed.

FACTORS INVOLVED IN THE PATHOGENESIS OF INSULIN RESISTANCE

Obesity

Obesity has long been considered the major risk factor for insulin resistance and type 2 diabetes. For example, in a recent 10-year follow-up of the Bruneck study,[6] the relative risk for new onset type 2 diabetes in non-diabetic individuals at baseline with BMI >30 kg/m^2 was 9.9 (95% CI 4.5 to 21.4) as compared to similar subjects with BMI <25 kg/m^2. In overweight subjects the relative risk for type 2 diabetes was 3.4-fold (95% CI 1.8

to 6.3). The rising prevalence of obesity worldwide is contributing to substantially increasing rates of type 2 diabetes. Indeed, the total number of people with diabetes is projected to rise from 171 million in 2000 to 366 million in 2030, an increase contributed to by both higher obesity rates and an aging population.[7] At the other end of the age spectrum, many recent cases of type 2 diabetes in children have been reported[8] and caused alarm in the UK and elsewhere.

But how does obesity increase the risk for diabetes? In a study of 42 obese and 36 non-obese subjects, Bonadonna and colleagues[9] demonstrated that in the physiological range of plasma insulin concentrations, the increase in total body glucose uptake and suppression of hepatic glucose output were both significantly impaired in the obese group. The glucose uptake and hepatic glucose output could be normalized by supraphysiological insulin levels in obese subjects. Moreover, both in the basal state and hyperglycaemic state, obese subjects were hyperinsulinaemic, which directly correlated with the degree of insulin resistance.[9] More recently, such findings have been corroborated in a study of 356 children aged 11 to 14 years.[10] In that study, body mass index directly correlated with fasting insulin and inversely with insulin sensitivity. There was also a clustering of conventional cardiovascular risk factors in those within the highest quartile of insulin resistance.[10]

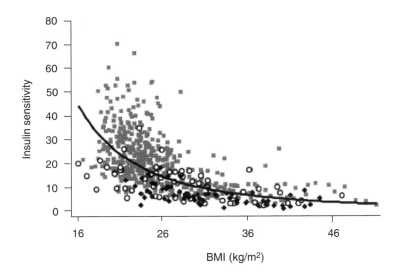

Figure 2 Inverse, curvilinear relationship between obesity (quantitated by BMI) and insulin sensitivity (in arbitrary units[11]) across different stages of glucose tolerance. Grey squares, NGT (n = 483); white circles, IGT (n = 71); black diamonds, type 2 diabetes (n = 65). Reproduced with permission from Stumvoll[99] with kind permission of Springer Science and Business Media.

At this stage it would therefore be safe to say that obese subjects are more insulin resistant than non-obese subjects across all age groups. However, the curvilinear relationship between BMI and insulin sensitivity is not precise. For example, by examining Figure 2 it can be seen that even within a normal glucose tolerance cohort, the variability of insulin sensitivity at any given BMI is substantial.[11] In this respect the relevance of fat distribution to insulin resistance beyond total adiposity (or BMI) deserves discussion.

Body fat location: visceral versus subcutaneous

Many, but not all, clinical investigators have noted that visceral adiposity is more strongly correlated with insulin resistance as compared to subcutaneous adiposity. Visceral adipose tissue is morphologically and functionally different from subcutaneous adipose tissue. Visceral fat originates from brown adipose tissue, has higher rates of lipolysis and glycolysis than subcutaneous fat and drains directly into the liver via the portal circulation.[12] It is thus argued to be more relevant to the development of insulin resistance than subcutaneous fat.

Wajchenberg et al[13] studied clinical characteristics and resistance to free fatty acid suppres-

sion in lean and obese non-diabetic women; obese subjects were further subdivided into two groups, based on normal or increased amount of visceral fat. As predicted, obese women (with normal visceral fat) had higher BMI, waist:hip ratio, blood pressure and resistance to free fatty acid (FFA) suppression during oral glucose tolerance test (OGTT) in comparison to the lean controls. However, when the two BMI-similar obese groups were compared, those with higher visceral fat were noted to have greater insulin resistance and higher plasma triglycerides. Subsequently correlation analysis showed that visceral fat contributed more to insulin resistance than subcutaneous fat.[13]

A recent elegant study provided further evidence for the relative importance of regional adiposity. Klein et al[14] studied 15 obese women before and 10 to 12 weeks after abdominal liposuction. Although liposuction decreased the volume of subcutaneous abdominal adipose tissue by significant amounts in both women with normal glucose tolerance and in those with diabetes, it did not significantly alter the insulin sensitivity of muscle, liver or adipose tissue. By contrast, in animal studies, the surgical removal of visceral adipose tissue resulted in marked and nearly immediate improvements in insulin resistance.[15] In line with these observations, Weiss et al have shown a near doubling of the visceral to subcutaneous fat ratio in obese children with impaired glucose tolerance compared to BMI-matched children with normal glucose tolerance.[16]

There are two main inferences that can be drawn from the above observations. First, visceral fat accumulation is significantly correlated to the development of insulin resistance. Second, body mass index is not an ideal obesity-related marker of insulin resistance since it gives an estimate of overall adiposity, not central (visceral) adiposity. As a result, a number of investigators have proposed waist circumference as a better marker of visceral fat and related metabolic complications.[17–19] In fact, the extent of evidence is sufficiently robust for waist circumference to be recommended as a simpler screening tool for health risks linked to obesity inclusive of cardiovascular disease and type 2 diabetes by the National Institute of Health and Scottish Intercollegiate Guidelines Network.

Free fatty acids

Of course, one of the major roles of adipocytes is to store fat as triacylglycerol. Lipolysis of stored fat releases FFAs into the circulation in the fasting state. Insulin suppresses lipolysis and promotes esterification. It is well accepted that elevations in FFAs can impair insulin-mediated glucose uptake by cells.[20,21] Moreover, FFAs might also impair beta cell function and release of insulin. In vivo studies have shown that acute rises in FFAs increase insulin secretion whereas prolonged elevation causes a reduction in glucose-stimulated insulin secretion from beta cells.[22] This effect may be more pronounced in genetically predisposed individuals, such as those with impaired glucose tolerance who are thus at risk of developing type 2 diabetes.[23] Elevated FFAs also impair insulin-mediated suppression of hepatic gluconeogenesis and augment glycogenolysis, thereby increasing glucose efflux from the liver.[24] Visceral body fat is positively associated with increased FFA levels and insulin resistance/type 2 diabetes.[25] Interestingly, FFA flux from visceral fat is relatively resistant to

suppression by insulin in obese type 2 diabetes patients compared to obese non-diabetic individuals.[26] Finally there is evidence to show that insulin clearance by the liver is impaired by circulating levels of FFAs.[27]

Overall, therefore, adiposity in general, and visceral adiposity in particular, can impart insulin resistance by decreasing cellular glucose uptake, increasing hepatic glucose output and possibly impairing insulin secretion; all these three effects mediated in part by excess FFAs released from visceral fat.

Muscle fat accumulation

In parallel with the growing interest in visceral adiposity as a mediator of insulin resistance, there is growing interest in the potential roles of hepatic and intramyocellular (IMCL) fat accumulation. Muscle is an important site of insulin action. The relationship between skeletal muscle triglyceride content and insulin resistance was first proposed in animal studies by Falholt.[28] Interestingly, this relationship was noted to be independent of obesity. Subsequently they demonstrated that insulin-resistant type 2 diabetes patients had higher triglycerides in rectus abdominis muscle compared to control subjects.[29]

From ensuing work by others, it is now clear that the degree of IMCL is inversely related to the extent of this organ's insulin sensitivity and positively related to the degree of visceral fat accumulation.[30] It has been speculated that elevated FFA delivery and/or impaired fatty acid (FA) oxidation result in IMCL fat accumulation of triacylglycerol and FA metabolites (diacylglycerol, long-chain acyl CoA), which are likely to induce defects in the insulin signalling cascade, causing insulin resistance.[30] In support of the relevance of IMCL fat, a recent elegant study from Schulman's group demonstrated a significantly higher IMCL fat content in parallel with 60% lower insulin sensitivity in offspring of diabetic parents relative to age- and body mass index (BMI)-matched healthy glucose tolerant controls.[31] Of additional interest, using magnetic resonance spectroscopy the authors were able to demonstrate that, whereas lowering of FFA post-glucose load was similar in both groups, the offspring of diabetic subjects had 30% lower mitochondrial oxidative phosphorylation, indicative of lower beta oxidative capacity. The authors speculated that offspring of diabetic subjects have a lower ratio of type 1 (mostly oxidative) to type II (mostly glycolytic) fibres, and thereby have an inherited reduction in mitochondrial content in muscle. These intriguing data clearly require confirmation in other cohorts. It should be noted that the 'insulin-resistant' offspring were generally of acceptable weight (mean BMI 23). An obvious interpretation is that individuals genetically prone to insulin resistance require lower increments in BMI to manifest adverse metabolic control. Put another way, such individuals should have far more incentive to maintain a healthy weight and remain physically active.

Hepatic fat accumulation

The role of the liver, and hepatic fat accumulation in particular, in the pathogenesis of type 2 diabetes has attracted recent interest. In a recent study,[32] liver fat content was shown to correlate with several features of insulin resistance in normal weight and moderately overweight subjects independent of BMI and intra-abdominal or overall obesity. Moreover, the surprisingly common condition of non-alcoholic fatty liver disease (NAFLD), prevalent in 5–20% of the population and up to 75% of obese individuals or those with type 2 diabetes, has been shown to be linked to insulin resistance.[33]

Why then does the liver accumulate fat? One possibility is simply excess flux of fatty acids to the liver from abdominal or visceral fat depots.[34] However, others suggest that increased liver fat content may relate better to dietary fat intake.[35] In this respect, a recent study in rats demonstrated that even short-term fat feeding can lead to ~3-fold increase in liver triglyceride and total fatty acyl-CoA content without any significant increase in visceral or skeletal muscle fat content.[36] Further possibili-

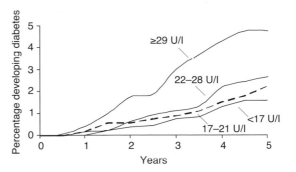

Figure 3 Association of ALT quartiles (U/L) with new onset diabetes in WOSCOPS (modified from reference 37)

ties for liver fat accumulation include excessive intravascular lipolysis of triglyceride-rich lipoproteins or indeed impaired FFA clearance. Whether acquired or genetic defects in hepatic β-oxidation are involved in liver fat accumulation, as they appear to be for IMCL fat accumulation, requires direct examination. Whatever the exact mechanism for fat accumulation, recent animal data indicate that this increase in hepatic fat leads to decreased insulin activation of glycogen synthase and increased gluconeogenesis by inducing defects in the insulin-signalling cascade.[36]

Interestingly, indirect estimates of liver fat (e.g. liver enzymes, in particular alanine aminotransferase (ALT)), are linked to hepatic insulin resistance and predict diabetes independent of other risk factors. Indeed, we recently demonstrated a graded association of higher ALTs with risk for new onset diabetes over a 4.9-year follow-up in the West of Scotland Coronary Prevention Study (WOSCOPS, Figure 3),[37] a finding extending prior observations from other groups.[38,39]

Thus, hepatic and muscle fat accumulation is highly relevant to the pathogenesis of insulin resistance and type 2 diabetes. Their place in the scheme of abnormalities contributing to type 2 diabetes and CHD is shown in Figure 4. Clearly, future studies aimed at improving our understanding of the mechanism(s) for such fat accumulation might lead to novel therapies to target insulin resistance.

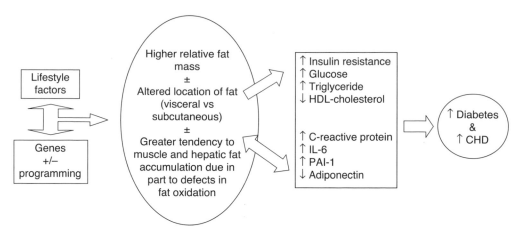

Figure 4 Individuals at risk for developing type 2 diabetes are likely to preferentially store fat in visceral stores and utilize fat less efficiently in muscle and liver, thereby accumulating fat in these organs. The consequences are greater insulin resistance and associated metabolic consequences for equivalent and even modest levels of total adiposity. Of course, if such individuals are able to stay lean by remaining active and adhering to good diet, they will protect themselves from such metabolic consequences as increasing obesity is germane to the expression of an underlying genetic potential towards insulin resistance

Inflammatory factors

Although considerable research has addressed the potential role of inflammatory mediators (e.g. C-reactive protein (CRP), interleukin-6, TNF-α) in the pathogenesis of coronary heart disease,[40] the relevance of this pathway to the pathogenesis of insulin resistance and type 2 diabetes has only recently attracted interest. It has now been shown in cross-sectional studies that circulating inflammatory marker levels correlate with obesity and insulin resistance and are elevated in groups at risk of type 2 diabetes, i.e. offspring of diabetics, women with polycystic ovary syndrome and subjects of South Asian origin.[41–43] The link between obesity and inflammation is intriguing and predominantly stems from the observation that adipocytes release IL-6 and TNF-α together with a range of 'adipokines', such as leptin, resistin and adiponectin, all of which have relevance to insulin action.[44]

Beyond cross-sectional findings, several prospective studies now indicate that C-reactive protein and white cell count, together with other acute phase markers, predict incident diabetes independently of established predic-

tors.[45–47] One of the best examples of such data comes from WOSCOPS.[45] In this study, we were able not only to show a graded relationship between baseline CRP and new onset diabetes (Figure 5) but also that such prediction was independent of several routinely measured parameters associated with diabetes risk, including fasting triglyceride, blood pressure, BMI and fasting glucose.[45]

In light of the foregoing associations, the search for mechanisms linking inflammation to insulin resistance and diabetes pathogenesis has become an important research avenue and several potential mechanisms (reviewed in reference 48), both direct and indirect, are summarized in Table 1. Many of these illustrate the intimate links between inflammatory and nutrient pathways, with dysregulation of one often leading to dysregulation of the other. For example, cytokines can accelerate adipocyte lipolysis and enhance hepatic fatty acid and triglyceride synthesis. Cytokines may therefore contribute to hepatic fat accumulation and insulin resistance by this mechanism.

It is important to note, however, that insulin has anti-inflammatory properties so that, rather

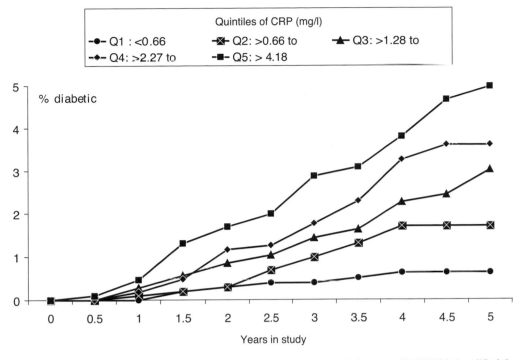

Figure 5 Association of baseline C-reactive protein (CRP) with new onset diabetes in WOSCOPS (modified from reference 45)

Table 1 Potential mechanisms linking inflammation to diabetes development

Levels of acute phase mediators may reflect parallel release of other adipocyte products that cause insulin resistance

Direct effects of cytokines on insulin-signalling cascade

Pro-inflammatory cytokine-mediated lipolytic effects and hepatic de novo fatty acid synthesis

Pro-inflammatory cytokine-mediated endothelial dysfunction

Impaired anti-inflammatory cytokine (IL-10) release and thus potentially impaired endothelial function and insulin signalling

IL-6-mediated increased glucocorticoid receptor density and responsiveness

than inflammation causing insulin resistance, the reverse may also be true.[49] Further studies are required to disentangle causal pathways and the advent of specific cytokine blockers may help in this respect.

Adiponectin

Adiponectin is perhaps the most relevant of the spectrum of adipokines to the pathogenesis of insulin resistance. It is a recently identified adipose-tissue-derived protein with important metabolic effects.[50] It is a 244-amino-acid protein, which, despite being solely derived from adipose tissue, is paradoxically reduced in obesity.[50] Adiponectin enhances hepatic and muscle fatty acid oxidation and thereby lessens fat accumulation in these organs. It does so by enhancing AMP-activated protein kinase (AMPK) activity.[51] In line with this and previously discussed observations on the relevance of IMCL and hepatic fat accumulation, high adiponectin concentrations correlate with greater insulin sensitivity and independently predict a reduced risk of type 2 diabetes.[52] Moreover, recombinant adiponectin increases insulin sensitivity and improves glucose tolerance in various animal models.[53] Therefore, low adiponectin may contribute to the decrease in whole-body insulin sensitivity that accompanies obesity in humans and reversal or alleviation of hypoadiponectinaemia may represent a target for development of drugs improving insulin sensitivity and glucose tolerance. It is also relevant that adiponectin is strongly anti-inflammatory, acting through the NFκB pathway,[54] and downregulates adhesion molecule expression on endothelial cells.[55] Recent data have linked low circulating adiponectin to the subsequent occurrence of vascular events, independently of traditional markers of CHD, but additional studies are required to confirm this.[56]

Plasminogen activator inhibitor 1

Increased plasminogen activator inhibitor 1 (PAI-1) has been linked not only to thrombosis and fibrosis, but also to obesity and insulin resistance. Recent data suggest increased PAI-1 levels predict diabetes independently of obesity, insulin levels and indeed inflammatory proteins.[57] Furthermore, recent animal studies have reported enhanced insulin sensitivity in PAI-1$^{-/-}$ mice relative to wild type on a high-fat and high-carbohydrate diet.[58] Although direct causal mechanisms can presently only be speculated, the authors argued that inhibition of PAI-1 might provide a novel anti-obesity and anti-insulin resistance treatment.[58]

Endothelial dysfunction

The endothelium plays an important role in regulating blood flow and thus glucose uptake in insulin-sensitive tissues.[59] Although the physiological importance of the latter mechanism remains controversial, circulating factors that impede endothelial-dependent vasodilatation (such as FFAs or cytokines) may reduce glucose uptake in response to insulin.[59,60] In support of the relevance of this pathway is a recent nested case-control analysis of the Nurses' Health Study examining plasma levels of biomarkers reflecting endothelial dysfunction (adhesion molecules) as predictors of new-onset diabetes.[61] Meigs and colleagues

noted that baseline levels of several adhesion molecules were significantly higher among cases than among controls. More importantly, elevated E-selectin and ICAM-1 levels predicted incident diabetes in logistic regression models adjusted for BMI, family history of diabetes, smoking, diet score, alcohol intake, activity index and post-menopausal hormone use. Further adjustment for waist circumference instead of BMI or for baseline levels of CRP, fasting insulin and haemoglobin A(1c) did not alter these associations.[61]

Relevance of insulin resistance to coronary heart disease

From the foregoing discussion, it is patently clear that insulin resistance must be relevant to the pathogenesis of CHD; the associated elevated triglyceride, blood pressure and lower HDL-C are themselves sufficient to implicate insulin resistance in CHD pathogenesis, as elegantly described by Reaven.[4] Additionally, it is now clear that many other parameters correlated with insulin resistance and potentially relevant to its pathogenesis might also play a critical role in atherogenesis (e.g. inflammatory mediators, adhesion molecules, PAI-1, adiponectin).

Several studies have directly associated insulin resistance with CHD events. For example, the Verona Diabetes study[62] showed that, along with sex, age, smoking, HDL/total cholesterol ratio and hypertension, HOMA-IR (see below) was an independent predictor of both prevalent and incident CHD. A 1-unit increase in (log)HOMA-IR value was associated with an odds ratio for incident CHD during follow-up of 1.56 (95% CI 1.14–2.12, $p < 0.001$). Similarly, hyperinsulinaemia predicted CHD risk in Helsinki policemen over the 22-year follow-up, and to a large extent independently of other CHD risk factors.[63]

Measurement of insulin resistance

For clinical and study purposes, measurement of insulin resistance needs a reliable and reproducible method. The choice of technique varies among investigators. The following are the commonly employed techniques in the experimental situation:

- Euglycaemic hyperinsulinaemic clamp. This procedure measures glucose disposal under hyperinsulinaemic conditions, insulin being infused at a constant rate and 20% glucose at a variable rate to give a constant (clamped) plasma glucose level. This remains the gold standard test for assessment of whole-body insulin sensitivity.[64]
- HOMA. Homeostatic model assessment considers fasting glucose and insulin levels: easier to perform and gives an estimate of mainly hepatic insulin resistance.[65]
- Intravenous glucose tolerance test. One of the earlier techniques, insulin resistance is estimated from the insulin response to glucose load and fractional glucose removal; it has been largely superseded by the above methods.[66]
- Fasting insulin resistance index (FIRI). Similar to HOMA, insulin resistance is assessed from fasting insulin and glucose values; it correlates well with the euglycaemic clamp technique.[67]
- Finally, the quantitative insulin sensitivity check index (QUICKI) is derived from logarithmic-transformed fasting plasma glucose (FPG) and insulin levels[68] and is a useful index of insulin resistance in comparison with clamp-IR.

Advent of metabolic syndrome criteria

Clearly, many of the techniques needed to measure insulin resistance are complex and most require insulin measurements. Samples for fasting insulin measurement need to be centrifuged and plasma separated rapidly (recommended 30 minutes). Such requirements limit the use of many of these techniques for clinical application and epidemiological research. Thus, researchers have attempted to define sets of criteria to approximate the dysfunctional metabolism associated with insulin resistance. Several different names have been applied to such criteria but 'metabolic syndrome' is now the

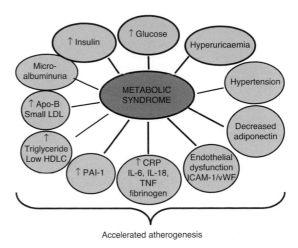

Figure 6 Expanded list of parameters correlated with insulin resistance (by no means comprehensive)

favoured term. While many more factors, such as small, dense LDL, C-reactive protein, plasminogen activator inhibitor-1, adiponectin, etc., have now been added to the list of risk factors linked to metabolic syndrome and insulin resistance (Figure 6), the core clinical drivers to identify individuals with metabolic syndrome continue to be obesity, dyslipidaemia, hypertension and markers of glucose dysregulation.

The first formal attempt to define the metabolic syndrome was made by the World Health Organization (WHO).[69] However, this definition focuses on patients with existing evidence of glucose dysregulation, at which stage the risk of conversion to diabetes is already high (Table 2). The modified WHO criteria allow metabolic syndrome to be diagnosed in individuals with normal glucose tolerance but the criteria are more complex and prescriptive, requiring documented evidence of insulin resistance or at least a surrogate measure such as fasting insulin. As mentioned above, the difficulties involved in obtaining these data will preclude widespread clinical use of these criteria.

In 2001 the Adult Treatment Panel (ATP) III of the National Cholesterol Education Program (NCEP)[70] proposed a new definition

Table 2   Definitions of the metabolic syndrome derived from the NCEP and WHO criteria

NCEP* definition of metabolic syndrome in men	WHO* definition of metabolic syndrome in men
Presence of **at least three** (≥3) of the following: • Fasting plasma glucose ≥110 mg/dl (6.1 mmol/l) • Serum triglyceride ≥150 mg/dl (1.7 mmol/l) • Serum HDL-cholesterol <40 mg/dl (1.04 mmol/l) • Blood pressure† ≥130 systolic or ≥85 diastolic or on medication • Abdominal obesity waist girth >102 cm	Presence of **at least one** (≥1) of the following: • Fasting plasma glucose ≥110 mg/dl (6.1 mmol/l) • Hyperinsulinaemia (upper quartile of fasting insulin in non-diabetic population) • Diabetes or impaired glucose tolerance **and** Presence of **at least two** (≥2) of the following: • Hyperlipidaemia: serum triglyceride ≥150 mg/dl (1.7 mmol/l) or serum HDL-C <35 mg/dl (0.9 mmol/l) • Blood pressure†: ≥140 systolic or ≥90 diastolic or on medication • Obesity: waist/hip ratio >0.90 or BMI ≥30 kg/m²

*NCEP, National Cholesterol Education Programme; WHO, World Health Organization
† Blood pressure is measured in mm/Hg

of the metabolic syndrome using thresholds for five easily measured variables linked to insulin resistance: waist circumference, triglyceride, HDL-C, fasting plasma glucose concentration and blood pressure (Table 2). It is triggered when pre-defined limits of any three criteria are exceeded and, therefore, many such individuals will have normal fasting glucose concentrations. This definition allows population data to be more easily gathered.

There are now numerous studies using these criteria. The first four published studies examined the prevalence of metabolic syndrome in middle-aged men and women using the NCEP criteria as shown in Table 3. Three of these[71–74] suggested that around a quarter of men and women aged 50–55 years have metabolic syndrome, and others have since confirmed this incidence. When these data were combined with US census data, it was estimated that 47 million adults had the metabolic syndrome.[75]

Of course, the most important criterion for definitions of metabolic syndrome is whether they have any clinical utility. Several studies have demonstrated that the NCEP criteria predict vascular events or mortality[71–74] (Table 3). Moreover, such prediction appears to be independent of classical risk factors in a small number of studies thus far examined. This is probably because the classification incorporates variables such as BMI, triglyceride, glucose and diastolic BP that are not included in current risk factor stratification. In addition, where examined,[72] the NCEP definition was more strikingly correlated with diabetes than with CHD risk (Table 3), a valuable benefit since predictive charts for diabetes are generally lacking. This is despite the fact that the vast majority of men diagnosed with metabolic syndrome had 'normal' glucose levels at baseline. This point is particularly important since, by the time impaired glucose tolerance has appeared, the conversion rate to frank diabetes is very high and opportunity for successful intervention is limited.

It should be noted that metabolic syndrome as defined by NCEP is only modestly correlated with directly measured insulin resistance.[76] Thus, whether individual clinicians will incorporate the NCEP definition of metabolic syndrome into clinical practice remains uncertain. There is no doubt that the NCEP definitions could be useful for recruiting individuals into intervention trials, and indeed are being used for this purpose. Lifestyle measures have already been shown to reduce diabetes risk by 58% in subjects at high risk for diabetes[77,78] and metformin[77] and acarbose[79] also have beneficial effects, although these studies were conducted

Table 3 Prevalence and predictive ability of metabolic syndrome using recent definitions

Investigators	Criteria	Population studied	Mean age at baseline	Average follow-up period	Prevalence of metabolic syndrome at baseline	Notable features	RR (95% CI) for incident CHD events/mortality or diabetes in subjects with metabolic syndrome
Ford et al[74]	NCEP	8814 men and women 20 years or older	–	–	24% men 23% women	Higher incidence in Hispanic men and especially Hispanic women Higher incidence by age	–
Ridker et al[71]	NCEP*	14 719 healthy women >45 years	54 years	8 years	24.4%	CRP levels higher in those with metabolic syndrome	CHD events 2.3 (1.6–3.3) to 4.0 (3.0–5.4) for CRP above and below 3 mg/l
Sattar et al[72]	NCEP*	6447 men with high cholesterol	55 years	4.9 years	26.2%	90% with FBG <6.1 mmol/l CRP levels higher in those with metabolic syndrome	CHD events 1.8 (1.4–2.2) to 1.3 (1.0–1.7)† Diabetes: 3.5 (3.5 to 4.9)
Lakka et al[74]	WHO NCEP	1209 healthy men aged 42–60 years	52 years	11.6 years	WHO 14.2% NCEP 8.8%	Unclear why incidence lower, but lipids levels appeared superior to other groups	CHD mortality WHO: 2.9 (1.2–6.8)** NCEP: 4.2 (1.6–10.8)**

WHO, World Health Organization; NCEP, National Cholesterol Education Program; CRP, C-reactive protein

*Studies used a BMI cut-off in place of the waist threshold

†Adjusted for age, SBP, cholesterol to HDL ratio and smoking

**Adjusted for age, examination year, LDL-cholesterol, smoking, family history of CHD

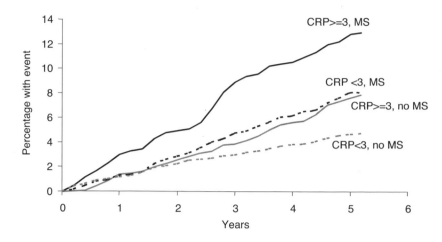

Figure 7 Risk of CHD events in relation to metabolic syndrome (MS) and elevated C-reactive protein (CRP) in WOSCOPS (modified from reference 72)

in obese subjects who already had impaired glucose tolerance, in whom much of the cardiovascular risk associated with metabolic dysfunction had already been accrued.

Clearly, there is considerable potential for further refinement of metabolic syndrome definitions. For example, two trials have noted higher CRP levels in men and women with the metabolic syndrome.[71,72] Moreover, CRP retained its independence as a predictor of CHD events in women with or without the metabolic syndrome[71,72] (Figure 7). Further data demonstrated slightly improved prediction of CHD and diabetes following reduction of the glucose cut-off from 6.1 mmol/l to 5.5 mmol/l.[72] These data are clearly not comprehensive but demonstrate the potential for refining the NCEP definition to increase the predictive value for CHD and/or diabetes. In other words, current metabolic syndrome criteria should be considered to be 'works in progress'.[73]

TREATMENTS FOR METABOLIC SYNDROME

Downstream targets

Of course, current clinical practice is predominantly geared towards treating the downstream consequences of insulin resistance by individually targeting the dyslipidaemia (lipid-lowering agents), blood pressure (anti-hypertensives),

elevated glucose (oral hypoglycaemic agents) and pro-thrombotic (anti-platelet agents) aspects of metabolic syndrome (Figure 8). However, it makes sense to consider treatments aimed at the upstream cause of metabolic syndrome, namely insulin resistance. There is some preliminary evidence that specific anti-hypertensive agents (ACE inhibitors and angiotensin receptor blockers) may also lessen the risk for type 2 diabetes.[80] Similarly, there are plentiful data to suggest statins and ACE inhibitors exert anti-inflammatory properties, but the clinical relevance of these effects remain to be fully elucidated.

Upstream targets

Lifestyle changes

Ideally, to treat metabolic syndrome, one should target the precursor causes. This would involve increased physical activity combined with dietary improvement both in terms of reduced caloric intake and altered composition of diet. Such measures would result in weight loss and there are plentiful data to demonstrate improvements in a range of metabolic parameters secondary to lifestyle changes[81,82] (Table 4). Of note, increasing physical activity levels alone, i.e. without necessarily altering diet or losing weight, can improve several metabolic-syndrome-related

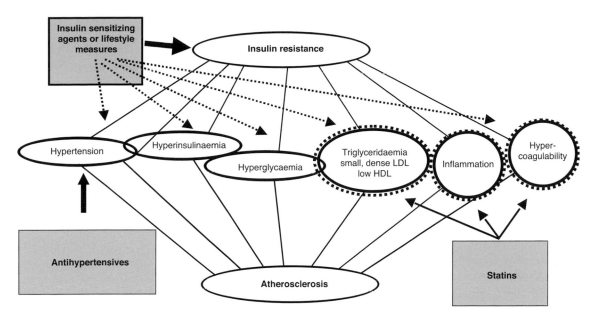

Figure 8 Upstream (insulin sensitizing) vs downstream (e.g. anti-hypertensive, lipid-lowering) targeting of metabolic syndrome

Table 4 Summary of metabolic and clinical effects of insulin sensitizing modalities

Agent	Primary mode of action	Other metabolic benefits	Clinical trial data	Ongoing studies
Physical activity and weight loss	Improve insulin sensitivity	Improved lipid profile Lower inflammatory levels Improved vascular and haemostatic function Lower blood pressure	Lower risk for diabetes Reduce risk of vascular events post-infarct as compared to CABG	To determine levels of exercise needed to lessen CHD risk Best mechanisms to promote increased physical activity (e.g. use of pedometers, etc.)
Metformin	Improve insulin sensitivity Lower weight	Improved lipid profile Improved haemostatic function Some suggestion of decreased hepatic steatosis	Lower risks for type 2 diabetes Lower risk of CHD events in type 2 diabetes	Studies in subjects with metabolic syndrome Ongoing work in polycystic ovary syndrome, a condition in young women linked to insulin resistance, elevated risk for type 2 diabetes and CHD
PPAR-γ agonists	Improve insulin sensitivity Weight unchanged or slightly increased	Improved lipid profile Lower inflammatory levels Improved vascular and haemostatic function Lower blood pressure Decreased hepatic steatosis	Reduce stent restenosis Reduced carotid IMT Improved endothelial function	Vascular endpoint studies in type 2 diabetes and in subjects with metabolic syndrome Studies in inflammatory conditions

parameters.[83] Moreover, other evidence suggests physical activity may be more important to vascular risk than initially appreciated. As an example, a recent randomized study to compare the effects of exercise training versus standard percutaneous coronary intervention with stenting on clinical symptoms and clinical vascular endpoints demonstrated significantly superior event-free survival in those randomized to exercise.[84]

Insulin sensitizing agents: metformin

Metformin is an effective anti-diabetic drug that lowers blood glucose concentrations by decreasing hepatic glucose production and increasing glucose disposal in skeletal muscle; however, the molecular site of metformin action has only recently received attention. Recent studies suggest that, similar to the endogenously synthesized adiponectin, metformin increases AMPK activity.[85,86] AMPK has been implicated in the stimulation of glucose uptake into skeletal muscle and the inhibition of liver gluconeogenesis. In addition, via the increase in APMK, metformin might also increase hepatic fatty acid oxidation and may thus lessen hepatic fat accumulation as reported in one recent study,[87] although a more recent trial did not show an effect of metformin on liver fat content.[88] Interestingly, exercise also increases AMPK activity.

In terms of metformin's metabolic effects outwith glucose lowering, there are data to suggest it improves lipids (variably reduces triglyceride, LDL-C, apo B, remnants concentrations and elevates HDL-C), decreases coagualibility/thrombosis (in particular lowers PAI-1 and t-PA levels), and preliminary data suggest it reduces some inflammation-related molecules (CAMs, CRP).[89,90] More impressive are metformin's effects in reducing risk for diabetes[77] and emerging evidence for its CHD events risk reduction in diabetes subjects as compared to non-insulin-sensitizing therapies.[91,92]

Metformin does not provoke hyperinsulinaemia and it has a good clinical track record. It is now recommended as first-line therapy in overweight patients with diabetes by most leading clinical associations (e.g. SIGN guidelines, Diabetes UK).

Insulin sensitizing agents: peroxisome proliferator activated receptors

Peroxisome proliferator activated receptors (PPARs) are members of a superfamily of nuclear hormone receptors. PPARs are ligand-activated transcription factors and have a subfamily of three different isoforms: PPAR-α, PPAR-γ and PPAR-β/δ. All isoforms heterodimerize with the 9-cis-retinoic acid receptor RXR and play an important part in the regulation of several metabolic pathways, including adipocyte metabolism, lipid biosynthesis and glucose metabolism.[93] They are discussed in greater detail in Chapter 13.

In terms of evidence presented previously in this chapter, it is relevant that a major mechanism of action of PPAR-γ agonists is to involve the alteration of the tissue distribution of FFA uptake and utilization. Indeed, PPAR-γ agonists induce the differentiation of pre-adipocytes into adipocytes and stimulate triglyceride storage in expanded 'safe' subcutaneous but not visceral fat depots.[94] Moreover, they lessen hepatic and IMCL fat accumulation by enhancing β-oxidation, an action that may be due to their ability to significantly enhance adiponectin concentrations. Such effects in turn promote glucose utilization. They increase HDL-C and are also potently anti-inflammatory, acting to lower cytokine synthesis in adipocyte and other tissues.[95]

Thiazolidinediones are activators of PPAR-γ and are now used as hypoglycaemic, muscle insulin-sensitizing agents in type 2 diabetes. They are far more potent insulin sensitizers than metformin. They have also been shown to exert anti-proliferative effects, and to antagonize angiotensin II actions in vivo and in vitro.[96] The latter actions may help to explain evidence of clinically relevant blood pressure lowering by the thiazolidinediones, rosiglitazone and pioglitazone, whereas metformin does not appear to lessen blood pressure significantly. Given the excellent spectrum of favourable metabolic actions of thiazolidine-diones, they are prime agents to be tested in individuals with metabolic syndrome. Morcover, their relative efficacy in reducing CHD risk factors and vascular events, in comparison with conventional anti-diabetic agents, is of significant interest and relevant studies are ongoing.[97,98]

CONCLUSION

There is now a major interest in insulin resistance as a candidate pathway in the pathogenesis of vascular disease. Part of this interest stems from the rapidly increasing rates of obesity worldwide which fuel insulin resistance, particularly in susceptible 'at risk' individuals. Insulin resistance is associated with a plethora of metabolic perturbances (as summarized

herein) and many of these can directly or indirectly accelerate the atherogenic process. There is thus great clinical interest in assessing the degree of insulin resistance in subjects at risk for vascular disease or type 2 diabetes. Direct measurements of insulin resistance are generally unsuitable for widespread clinical use. Rather simple criteria based on readily measured factors associated with it have been proposed under the broader term of metabolic syndrome. Abundant data to suggest such metabolic syndrome criteria predict CHD events and more strongly risk for type 2 diabetes now exist. However, ongoing work is required to refine the existing criteria to predict CHD events and scrutinize clinical application. In parallel, ongoing clinical trials will determine the role of lifestyle factors and insulin-sensitizing agents in reducing risk of disease in such high-risk subjects.

References

1. Hollenbeck C, Reaven GM. Variations in insulin-stimulated glucose uptake in healthy individuals with normal glucose tolerance. J Clin Endocrinol Metab 1987; 64:1169–73

2. Warram JH, Martin BC, Krolewski AS, et al. Slow glucose removal rate and hyperinsulinemia precede the development of type II diabetes in the offspring of diabetic parents. Ann Intern Med 1990; 113:909–15

3. Taylor SI. Lilly lecture: molecular mechanisms of insulin resistance: lessons from patients with mutations in the insulin-receptor gene. Diabetes 1992; 41:1473–90

4. Reaven GM. Banting lecture 1988. Role of insulin resistance in human disease. Diabetes 1988; 37:1595–607

5. Stern MP. Diabetes and cardiovascular disease. The 'common soil' hypothesis. Diabetes 1995; 44:369–74

6. Bonora E, Formentini G, Calcaterra F, et al. HOMA-estimated insulin resistance is an independent predictor of cardiovascular disease in type 2 diabetic subjects: prospective data from the Verona Diabetes Complications Study. Diabetes Care 2002; 25:1135–41

7. Wild S, Roglic G, Green A, et al. Global prevalence of diabetes: estimates for the year 2000 and projections for 2030. Diabetes Care 2004; 27:1047–53

8. Ehtisham S, Hattersley AT, Dunger DB, et al. British Society for Paediatric Endocrinology and Diabetes Clinical Trials Group. First UK survey of paediatric type 2 diabetes and MODY. Arch Dis Child 2004; 89:526–9

9. Bonadonna RC, Groop L, Kraemer N, et al. Obesity and insulin resistance in humans: a dose-response study. Metabolism 1990; 39:452–9

10. Sinaiko AR, Jacobs DR Jr, Steinberger J, et al. Insulin resistance syndrome in childhood: associations of the euglycemic insulin clamp and fasting insulin with fatness and other risk factors. J Pediatr 2001; 139: 700–7

11. Matsuda M, DeFronzo RA. Insulin sensitivity indices obtained from oral glucose tolerance testing: comparison with the euglycemic insulin clamp. Diabetes Care 1999; 22:1462–70

12. Montague CT, O'Rahilly S. The perils of portliness: causes and consequences of visceral adiposity. Diabetes 2000; 49:883–8

13. Wajchenberg BL, Giannella-Neto D, da Silva ME, et al. Depot-specific hormonal characteristics of subcutaneous and visceral adipose tissue and their relation to the metabolic syndrome. Horm Metab Res 2002; 34:616–21

14. Klein S, Fontana L, Young VL, et al. Absence of an effect of liposuction on insulin action and risk factors for coronary heart disease. N Engl J Med 2004; 350:2549–57

15. Gabriely I, Ma XH, Yang XM, et al. Removal of visceral fat prevents insulin resistance and glucose

intolerance of aging: an adipokine-mediated process? Diabetes 2002; 51:2951–8

16. Weiss R, Dufour S, Taksali SE, et al. Prediabetes in obese youth: a syndrome of impaired glucose tolerance, severe insulin resistance, and altered myocellular and abdominal fat partitioning. Lancet 2003; 362:951–7

17. Han TS, van Leer EM, Seidell JC, et al. Waist circumference action levels in the identification of cardiovascular risk factors: prevalence study in a random sample. BMJ 1995; 311:1401–5

18. Sattar N, Tan CE, Han TS, et al. Associations of indices of adiposity with atherogenic lipoprotein subfractions. Int J Obes Relat Metab Disord 1998; 22:432–9

19. Rexrode KM, Carey VJ, Hennekens CH, et al. Abdominal adiposity and coronary heart disease in women. JAMA 1998; 280:1843–8

20. Boden G, Jadali F, White J, et al. Effects of fat on insulin stimulated carbohydrate metabolism in normal men. J Clin Invest 1991; 88:960–6

21. Dresner A, Laurent D, Marcucci M, et al. Effects of free fatty acids on glucose transport and IRS-1-associated phosphatidylinositol 3–kinase activity. J Clin Invest 1999; 103:253–9

22. Carpentier A, Mittelman SD, Lamarche B, et al. Acute enhancement of insulin secretion by FFA in humans is lost with prolonged FFA elevation. Am J Physiol 1999; 276:E1055–66

23. Storgaard H, Jensen CB, Vaag AA, et al. Insulin secretion after short- and long-term low-grade free fatty acid infusion in men with increased risk of developing type 2 diabetes. Metab Clin Exp 2003; 52:885–94l

24. Chen X, Iqbal N, Boden G. The effects of free fatty acids on gluconeogenesis and glycogenolysis in normal subjects. J Clin Invest 1999; 103:365–72

25. Pouliot MC, Despres JP, Nadeau A, et al. Visceral obesity in men. Associations with glucose tolerance, plasma insulin, and lipoprotein levels. Diabetes 1992; 41:826–34

26. Basu A, Basu R, Shah P, et al. Systemic and regional free fatty acid metabolism in type 2 diabetes. Am J Physiol Endocrinol Metab 2001; 280:E1000–6

27. Wiesenthal S, Sandhu H, McCall R, et al. Free fatty acids impair hepatic insulin extraction in vivo. Diabetes 1999; 48:766–74

28. Falholt K, Cutfield R, Alejandro R, et al. The effects of hyperinsulinaemia on arterial wall and peripheral muscle metabolism in dogs. Metabolism 1985; 34:1146–9

29. Falholt K, Jensen I, Lindkaer JS, et al. Carbohydrate and lipid metabolism of skeletal muscle in type 2 diabetic patients. Diab Med 1988; 5:27–31

30. Petersen KF, Shulman GI. Pathogenesis of skeletal muscle insulin resistance in type 2 diabetes mellitus. Am J Cardiol 2002; 90:11G-18G

31. Petersen KF, Dufour S, Befroy D, et al. Impaired mitochondrial activity in the insulin-resistant offspring of patients with type 2 diabetes. N Engl J Med 2004; 350:664–71

32. Seppala-Lindroos A, Vehkavaara S, Hakkinen AM, et al. Fat accumulation in the liver is associated with defects in insulin suppression of glucose production and serum free fatty acids independent of obesity in normal men. J Clin Endocrinol Metab 2002; 87:3023–8

33. Medina J, Fernandez-Salazar LI, Garcia-Buey L, et al. Approach to the pathogenesis and treatment of nonalcoholic steatohepatitis. Diab Care 2004; 27:2057–66

34. Kelley DE, McKolanis TM, Hegazi RA, et al. Fatty liver in type 2 diabetes mellitus: relation to regional adiposity, fatty acids, and insulin resistance. Am J Physiol Endocrinol Metab 2003; 285:E906–16

35. Tiikkainen M, Bergholm R, Vehkavaara S, et al. Effects of identical weight loss on body composition and features of insulin resistance in obese women with high and low liver fat content. Diabetes 2003; 52:701–7

36. Samuel VT, Liu ZX, Qu X, et al. Mechanism of hepatic insulin resistance in non-alcoholic fatty liver disease. J Biol Chem 2004; 279:32345–53

37. Sattar N, Scherbakova O, Ford I, et al. Elevated alanine aminotransferase predicts new-onset type 2 diabetes independently of classical risk factors, metabolic syndrome and C-reactive protein in the West of Scotland Coronary Prevention Study. Diabetes 2004; 53:2855–60

38. Ohlson LO, Larsson B, Bjorntorp P, et al. Risk factors for type 2 (non-insulin-dependent) diabetes mellitus. Thirteen and one-half years of follow-up of the participants in a study of Swedish men born in 1913. Diabetologia 1988; 31:798–805

39. Vozarova B, Stefan N, Lindsay RS, et al. High alanine aminotransferase is associated with decreased hepatic insulin sensitivity and predicts the development of type 2 diabetes. Diabetes 2002; 51:1889–95

40. Willerson JT, Ridker PM. Inflammation as a cardiovascular risk factor. Circulation 2004; 109(Suppl 1):II2–10

41. Kelly CCJ, Lyall H, Petrie JR, et al. Low-grade chronic Inflammation in women with PCOS. J Clin Endocrinol Metab 2001; 86:2453–5

42. Forouhi NG, Sattar N, McKeigue P. Relation of C-reactive protein to cardiovascular risk factors in Europeans and South Asians. Int J Obesity 2001; 25:1327–31

43. Chambers JC, Eda S, Bassett P, et al. C-reactive protein, insulin resistance, central obesity, and coronary heart disease risk in Indian Asians from the United Kingdom compared with European whites. Circulation 2001; 104:145–50

44. Lehrke M, Lazar MA. Inflamed about obesity. Nat Med 2004; 10:126–7

45. Freeman DJ, Norrie J, Caslake MJ, et al. C-reactive protein is an independent predictor of risk for the development of diabetes in the West of Scotland Coronary Prevention Study. Diabetes 2002; 51:1596–600

46. Pradhan AD, Manson JE, Rifai N, et al. C-reactive protein, interleukin-6, and risk of developing type 2 diabetes mellitus. JAMA 2001; 286:327–34

47. Barzilay JI, Abraham L, Heckbert SR, et al. The relation of markers of inflammation to the development of glucose disorders in the elderly: the Cardiovascular Health Study. Diabetes 2001; 50:2384–9

48. Sattar N, Perry CG, Petrie JR. Type 2 diabetes as an inflammatory disorder. Br J Diabet Vasc Dis 2003; 3:36–41

49. Dandona P, Aljada A, Dhindsa S, et al. Insulin as an anti-inflammatory and antiatherosclerotic hormone. Clin Cornerstone 2003; (Suppl 4):S13–20

50. Weyer C, Funahashi T, Tanaka S, et al. Hypoadiponectinemia in obesity and type 2 diabetes: close association with insulin resistance and hyperinsulinemia. J Clin Endocrinol Metab 2001; 86:1930–5

51. Yamauchi T, Kamon J, Minokoshi Y, et al. Adiponectin stimulates glucose utilization and fatty-acid oxidation by activating AMP-activated protein kinase. Nat Med 2002; 8:1288–95

52. Lindsay RS, Funahashi T, Matsuzawa Y, et al. Adiponectin protects against development of type 2 diabetes in the Pima Indian population. Lancet 2002; 360:57–8

53. Yamauchi T, Kamon J, Waki H, et al. The fat-derived hormone adiponectin reverses insulin resistance associated with both lipoatrophy and obesity. Nat Med 2001; 7:941–6

54. Ouchi N, Kihara S, Arita Y, et al. Adiponectin, an adipocyte-derived plasma protein, inhibits endothelial NF-kappaB signaling through a cAMP-dependent pathway. Circulation 2000; 102:1296–301

55. Ouchi N, Kihara S, Arita Y, et al. Novel modulator for endothelial adhesion molecules: adipocyte-derived plasma protein adiponectin. Circulation 1999; 100:2473–6

56. Pischon T, Girman CJ, Hotamisligil GS, et al. Plasma adiponectin levels and risk of myocardial infarction in men. JAMA 2004; 291:1730–7

57. Festa A, D'Agostino R Jr, Tracy RP, et al. Insulin Resistance Atherosclerosis Study. Elevated levels of acute-phase proteins and plasminogen activator inhibitor-1 predict the development of type 2 diabetes: the insulin resistance atherosclerosis study. Diabetes 2003; 51:1131–7

58. Ma LJ, Mao SL, Taylor KL, et al. Prevention of obesity and insulin resistance in mice lacking plasminogen activator inhibitor 1. Diabetes 2004; 53:336–46

59. Steinberg HO, Baron AD, Steinberg H, et al. Vascular function, insulin resistance and fatty acids. Diabetologia 2002; 45:623–34

60. Sattar N. Inflammation and endothelial dysfunction: intimate companions in the pathogenesis of vascular disease? Clin Sci (Lond) 2004; 106:443–5

61. Meigs JB, Hu FB, Rifai N, et al. Biomarkers of endothelial dysfunction and risk of type 2 diabetes mellitus. JAMA 2004; 291:1978–86

62. Bonora E, Formentini G, Calcaterra F, et al. HOMA-estimated insulin resistance is an independent predictor of cardiovascular disease in type 2 diabetic subjects: prospective data from the Verona Diabetes Complications Study. Diabetes Care 2002; 25:1135–41

63. Pyorala M, Miettinen H, Laakso M, et al. Hyperinsulinemia predicts coronary heart disease risk in healthy middle-aged men: the 22–year follow-up results of the Helsinki Policemen Study. Circulation 1998; 98:398–404

64. DeFronzo R, Tobin J, Andres R. Glucose clamp technique: a method for quantifying insulin secretion and resistance. Am J Physiol 1979; 237:E214–23

65. Mathews D, Hosker J, Rudenski A, et al. Homeostasis model assessment: insulin resistance and β-cell function from plasma fasting glucose and insulin concentrations in man. Diabetologia 1985; 28:412–19

66. Reaven GM, Olefsky JM. Relationship between insulin response during the intravenous glucose tolerance test, rate of fractional glucose removal and the degree of insulin resistance in normal adults. Diabetes 1974; 23:454–9

67. Cleland S, Petrie J, Morris A, et al. FIRI: a fair insulin resistance index? Lancet 1996; 347:770

68. Katz A, Nambi SS, Mather K, et al. Quantitative insulin sensitivity check index: a simple, accurate method for assessing insulin sensitivity in humans. J Clin Endocrinol Metab 2000; 85:2402–10

69. Alberti KG, Zimmet PZ. Definition, diagnosis and classification of diabetes mellitus and its complications. Part 1: diagnosis and classification of diabetes mellitus provisional report of a WHO consultation. Diabet Med 1998; 15:539–53

70. Expert Panel on Detection, Evaluation, and Treatment of High Blood Cholesterol in Adults. Executive Summary of The Third Report of The National Cholesterol Education Program (NCEP) Expert Panel on Detection, Evaluation, And Treatment of High Blood Cholesterol In Adults (Adult Treatment Panel III). JAMA 2001; 285:2486–97

71. Ridker PM, Buring JE, Cook NR, et al. C-reactive protein, the metabolic syndrome, and risk of incident cardiovascular events: an 8-year follow-up of 14 719 initially healthy American women. Circulation 2003; 107:391–7

72. Sattar N, Gaw A, Scherbakova O, et al. Metabolic syndrome with and without CRP as a predictor of CHD and diabetes in West of Scotland Coronary Prevention Study. Circulation 2003; 108:414–9

73. Sattar N, Forouhi NG. Metabolic syndrome criteria: ready for clinical prime time or work in progress? Eur Heart J 2005 Apr 13 [Epub ahead of print]

74. Lakka HM, Laaksonen DE, Lakka TA, et al. The metabolic syndrome and total and cardiovascular disease mortality in middle-aged men. JAMA 2002; 288:2709–16

75. Ford ES, Giles WH, Dietz WH. Prevalence of the metabolic syndrome among US adults: findings from

the third National Health and Nutrition Examination Survey. JAMA 2002; 16:356–9

76. Cheal KL, Abbasi F, Lamendola C, et al. Relationship to insulin resistance of the adult treatment panel III diagnostic criteria for identification of the metabolic syndrome. Diabetes 2004; 53:1195–200

77. Knowler WC, Barrett-Connor E, Fowler SE, et al. Reduction in the incidence of type 2 diabetes with lifestyle intervention or metformin. N Engl J Med 2002; 346:393–403

78. Tuomilehto J, Lindström J, Erickson JG, et al, for the Finnish Diabetes Prevention Study Group. Prevention of type 2 diabetes mellitus by changes in lifestyle among subjects with impaired glucose tolerance. N Engl J Med 2001; 344:1343–50

79. Chiasson JL, Josse RG, Gomis R, et al. STOP-NIDDM Trial Research Group. Acarbose for prevention of type 2 diabetes mellitus: the STOP-NIDDM randomised trial. Lancet 2002; 359:2072–7

80. Teo K, Yusuf S, Anderson C, et al. ONTARGET/ TRANSCEND Investigators. Rationale, design, and baseline characteristics of 2 large, simple, random-ized trials evaluating telmisartan, ramipril, and their combination in high-risk patients: the Ongoing Telmisartan Alone and in Combination with Ramipril Global Endpoint Trial/Telmisartan Randomized Assessment Study in ACE Intolerant Subjects with Cardiovascular Disease (ONTARGET/TRANSCEND) trials. Am Heart J 2004; 148:52–61

81. Anderson JW, Kendall CW, Jenkins DJ. Importance of weight management in type 2 diabetes: review with meta-analysis of clinical studies. J Am Coll Nutr 2003; 22:331–9

82. Tuomilehto J. Reducing coronary heart disease associated with type 2 diabetes: lifestyle intervention and treatment of dyslipidaemia. Diabetes Res Clin Pract 2003; 61 (Suppl 1):S27–34

83. Wannamethee SG, Lowe GD, Whincup PH, et al. Physical activity and hemostatic and inflammatory variables in elderly men. Circulation 2002; 105:1785–90

84. Hambrecht R, Walther C, Mobius-Winkler S, et al. Percutaneous coronary angioplasty compared with exercise training in patients with stable coronary artery disease: a randomized trial. Circulation 2004; 109:1371–8

85. Musi N, Hirshman MF, Nygren J, et al. Metformin increases AMP-activated protein kinase activity in skeletal muscle of subjects with type 2 diabetes. Diabetes 2002; 51:2074–81

86. Zhou G, Myers R, Li Y, et al. Role of AMP-activated protein kinase in mechanism of metformin action. J Clin Invest 2001; 108:1167–74

87. Marchesini G, Brizi M, Bianchi G, et al. Metformin in non-alcoholic steatohepatitis. Lancet 2001; 358:893–4

88. Tiikkainen M, Hakkinen AM, Korsheninnikova E, et al. Effects of rosiglitazone and metformin on liver fat content, hepatic insulin resistance, insulin clearance, and gene expression in adipose tissue in patients with type 2 diabetes. Diabetes 2004; 53:2169–76

89. Shin JJ, Rothman J, Farag A, et al. Role of oral anti-diabetic agents in modifying cardiovascular risk factors. Minerva Med 2003; 94:401–8

90. Morin-Papunen L, Rautio K, Ruokonen A, et al. Metformin reduces serum C-reactive protein levels in women with polycystic ovary syndrome. J Clin Endocrinol Metab 2003; 88:4649–54

91. UK Prospective Diabetes Study (UKPDS) Group. Effect of intensive blood-glucose control with metformin on complications in overweight patients with type 2 diabetes (UKPDS 34). Lancet 1998; 352:854–65

92. Kao J, Tobis J, McClelland RL, et al. Investigators in the Prevention of Restenosis With Tranilast and Its Outcomes Trial. Relation of metformin treatment to clinical events in diabetic patients undergoing percu-taneous intervention. Am J Cardiol 2004; 93:1347–50

93. Evans RM, Barish GD, Wang YX. PPARs and the complex journey to obesity. Nat Med 2004; 10:355–61

94. Berthiaume M, Sell H, Lalonde J, et al. Actions of PPARgamma agonism on adipose tissue remodeling, insulin sensitivity and lipemia in absence of glucocor-ticoids. Am J Physiol Regul Integr Comp Physiol 2004; 287:R1116–23

95. Marx N, Duez H, Fruchart JC, et al. Peroxisome proliferator-activated receptors and atherogenesis: regulators of gene expression in vascular cells. Circ Res 2004; 94:1168–78

96. Schiffrin EL, Amiri F, Benkirane K, et al. Peroxisome proliferator-activated receptors: vascular and cardiac effects in hypertension. Hypertension 2003; 42:664–8

97. Charbonnel B, Dormandy J, Erdmann E, et al. PROactive Study Group. The prospective pioglita-zone clinical trial in macrovascular events (PROactive): can pioglitazone reduce cardiovascular events in diabetes? Study design and baseline charac-teristics of 5238 patients. Diabetes Care 2004; 27:1647–53

98. Viberti G, Kahn SE, Greene DA, et al. A diabetes outcome progression trial (ADOPT): an international multicenter study of the comparative efficacy of rosiglitazone, glyburide, and metformin in recently diagnosed type 2 diabetes. Diabetes Care 2002; 25:1737–43

99. Stumvoll M. Control of glycemia: from molecules to men. Minowski Lecture 2003. Diabetologia 2004; 47:770–81

Peroxisome proliferator activated receptors and energy metabolism

13

P. Gervois, J-C. Fruchart and B. Staels

INTRODUCTION

Carbohydrates and lipids constitute the main source of energy for eukaryote organisms. Optimal energy homeostasis depends on a fine control of lipid and carbohydrate metabolism and is influenced by a diversity of environmental and physiological conditions. Such regulation occurs in a co-ordinated fashion at several levels of metabolic pathways by different factors triggering an adapted modulation of metabolic parameters. Some factors may affect enzyme activities while others act at the level of gene transcription of proteins with key functions in anabolic or catabolic pathways. Several transcription factors play pivotal regulatory functions in lipid and carbohydrate metabolism. The sterol regulatory element binding proteins (SREBPs) regulate the expression of genes involved in cholesterol and fatty acid (FA) metabolism.[1] The nuclear receptors are a family of ligand-activated transcription factors involved in translating the effects of lipid-soluble signalling molecules, such as hormones, vitamins, FAs and various drugs, at the gene expression level. For instance, the liver X receptors (LXRs) are activated by cholesterol derivatives and control genes involved in cholesterol homeostasis.[2] In this chapter, we will focus on the role of peroxisome proliferator activated receptors (PPARs) in energy metabolism. PPARs are FA-activated nuclear receptors[3] that control lipid and glucose homeostasis via the modulation of gene expression of various proteins orchestrat-

ing lipid biosynthesis, degradation, uptake, extracellular and intracellular transport and storage. Dysfunctional regulation of these genes gives rise to metabolic disorders such as dyslipidaemia, glucose intolerance, hyperinsulinaemia and obesity that ultimately lead to the development of cardiovascular diseases. PPAR activity may also be modulated by synthetic ligands and as such this class of transcription factors offers interesting opportunities for therapeutic intervention.

MOLECULAR CHARACTERISTICS

Three distinct PPARs, α (NR1C1), $\beta(\delta)$, (NR1C2) and γ (NR1C3), each encoded by a separate gene and displaying different tissue[4–7] and developmental[4] expression patterns, have been identified. PPAR-α, the first identified PPAR family member, is principally expressed in tissues exhibiting high rates of fatty acid oxidation such as liver, kidney, heart and muscle. PPAR-γ, on the other hand, is expressed at high levels in brown and white adipose tissue, and the intestine. PPAR-β/δ is expressed in a wide range of tissues including heart, adipose tissue, brain, intestine, muscle, spleen, lung and adrenal glands.[8] All PPARs are also expressed, to variable extents, in the different cell types of the vascular wall, including endothelial cells, smooth muscle cells and monocytes/macrophages. Whereas PPAR-α and PPAR-β/δ modulate the transcription of genes implicated in lipid and lipoprotein

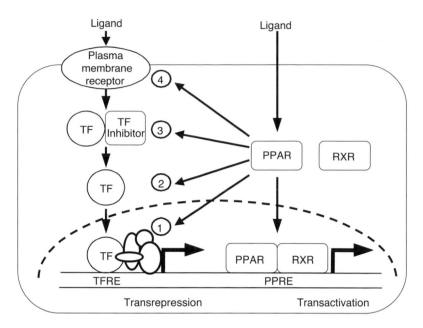

Figure 1 Mechanisms of transcriptional gene regulation by PPARs. Activated PPARs form a heterodimeric complex with the retinoic X receptor (RXR), which subsequently binds to a PPRE located within the regulatory sequence of target genes to modulate gene transcription (transactivation). PPARs negatively regulate gene transcription (transrepression) through several mechanism including (1) competition for co-factors, (2) protein–protein interaction between PPAR with the STATs, NF-κB, C/EBPs or Fos/Jun transcription factors, (3) induction of the expression of the NF-κB inhibitor IκB and (4) repression of membrane receptor expression. PPRE, peroxisome proliferator response element; TFRE, transcription factor response element

metabolism in liver and muscle,[9] PPAR-γ controls cellular differentiation, mediates adipogenesis and modulates insulin action.[10]

Following ligand binding, PPARs associate with the retinoic X receptor (RXR) to form a PPAR/RXR heterodimeric complex, capable of binding to a specific response element, termed peroxisome proliferator response element (PPRE), located in the promoter region of target genes (Figure 1). Although the majority of PPREs identified so far consist of a direct repeat (DR) of the canonical AGGTCA sequence spaced by one nucleotide (DR-1),[3] DR-2 elements may also function as PPRE.[11] PPARs regulate target genes through this DNA-binding-dependent mechanism termed transactivation. In addition, PPARs may repress gene transcription in a DNA-binding-independent manner via a transrepression mechanism. As such, PPARs interfere with other transcription factor pathways such as NF-κB, STAT, C/EBP and AP-1. The transrepression mediated by PPARs occurs at different levels of these signal transduction pathways including protein–protein interaction between PPARs and these transcription factors leading to the formation of inactive complexes,[12–18] competition for cofactors, induction of IκB, the major inhibitor of the NF-κB pathway, and down-regulation of plasma membrane receptor gene transcription (Figure 1).[11,19,20]

PPAR activity may be regulated at the transcriptional, post-transcriptional and protein level. In rats, PPAR-α expression is regulated by hormones, such as glucocorticoids, insulin and leptin, by physiological stimuli such as stress and fasting and follows a diurnal rhythm.[21–26] Although little is known about factors regulating PPAR-α expression in humans, the observation that PPAR-α expression in liver varies significantly among individuals[27,28] suggests that PPAR-α is also strongly regulated at the gene level in humans by genetic and environmental factors. The transcriptional regulation of PPAR-γ occurs via alternative promoters, which results both in rodents and humans[29,30] in the production of two distinct proteins, PPAR-γ1 and PPAR-γ2, with distinct activation capacities.[31] In addition, glucocorticoids are implicated in the regulation of PPAR-γ expression during differentiation of 3T3-L1 preadipocytes.[32] PPAR activity is also modulated at the protein level. Protein phosphorylation constitutes a common post-translational mechanism of regulation. Both PPAR-α and PPAR-γ activities depend on their phosphorylation status, that affects their transactivation potential and modulates their biological functions.[33–38] PPAR protein levels are also subject to regulation. PPAR-γ activators induce PPAR-γ receptor ubiquitination and subsequent degradation by the proteasome,[39] whereas PPAR-α activators inhibit PPAR-α ubiquitination and increase PPAR-α protein half-life.[40,41] The production of isoforms with repressive activity on the wild-type receptor represents another mechanism of regulation of PPAR signalling occurring at the protein level. Such an isoform, resulting from alternative splicing and giving rise to a truncated protein, has been identified for PPAR-α.[27,28] This variant acts in a ligand-independent manner and alters PPAR-α wild-type transcriptional capacity.

PPARs are activated by natural ligands derived from fatty acids (FAs), such as 8(S) hydroxyeicosatetraenoic acid, 8(S) hydroxy-eicosapentaenoic acid and leukotriene B4 for PPAR-α[42] and prostaglandin-J2 and components of oxidized low-density lipoprotein (oxLDL) for PPAR-γ.[42,43] Hypolipidaemic drugs of the fibrate class are synthetic agonists for PPAR-α and anti-diabetic glitazones are high-affinity synthetic ligands for PPAR-γ.[42] Natural and synthetic ligands have also been identified for PPAR-β/δ,[44,45] but these are not yet used in clinical practice. PPAR-β/δ ligands include natural polyunsaturated FAs and prostaglandins and synthetic ligands such as carbaprostacyclin and other potent, subtype-specific agonists.[46]

PPARS AND THE CONTROL OF ENERGY METABOLISM

PPAR-α and intracellular metabolism

PPAR-α plays a pivotal role in the regulation of intracellular lipid metabolism (Figure 2). A high level of PPAR-α expression is observed in tissues with elevated FA catabolism. PPREs have been identified in the promoter region of rodent genes coding for enzymes implicated in the peroxisomal β-oxidation pathway such as acyl-CoA oxidase (ACO), multi-functional

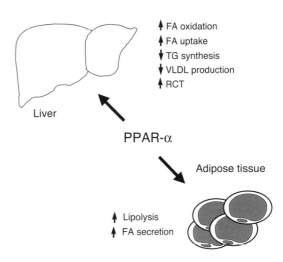

Figure 2   By modulating gene expression, PPAR-α directly or indirectly affects several regulatory processes that maintain lipid homeostasis: (1) Limitation of hepatic TG synthesis and VLDL production due to increased fatty acid (FA) uptake, enhanced FA catabolism and reduced FA synthesis. PPAR-α activation enhances FA β-oxidation and therefore diminishes the FA pool to be incorporated into triglyceride (TG)-rich lipoproteins. Consequently, PPAR-α stimulates lipid flux by controlling the FA flux from peripheral tissues such as adipose tissue to the liver. (2) Induction of lipoprotein lipolysis as a result of either an increase in intrinsic lipoprotein lipase activity or an increased accessibility of TG-rich lipoprotein particles for lipolysis due to reduced TG-rich lipoprotein apoC-III content and induction of ApoA-V. (3) Increase in HDL production and stimulation of reverse cholesterol transport. PPAR-α activators increase the production of apolipoprotein A-I and A-II in human liver, which leads to increased plasma HDL concentrations and enhanced reverse cholesterol transport (RCT)

enzyme and 3-ketoacyl-CoA thiolase,[3] linking PPAR-α to the regulation of FA catabolism. Interestingly, these enzymes are also involved in the biosynthesis of endogenous PPAR-α ligands.[47,48] PPAR-α also modulates genes involved in FA uptake, activation to acyl-CoA esters, mitochondrial β-oxidation and ketone body synthesis.[3,49] Intracellular FA concentrations are controlled, in part, by the activity of the FA transport protein-1 (FATP-1), which controls the entry of FAs through the cell membrane, and by acyl-CoA synthetase (ACS), which traps FAs inside the cells by their conversion to ester derivatives. PPAR-α activates FATP-1 expression in liver and intestine and ACS expression in liver and kidney.[50] The implication of PPAR-α in FA transport was further demonstrated by the lack of induction of FATP and FA translocase mRNA in liver by PPAR-α activators in PPAR-α-null mice.[51] FA metabolism is also tightly linked to the rate of mitochondrial FA uptake. PPAR-α has been demonstrated to affect FA import into mitochondria by upregulating the expression of the muscle-[52–54] and liver-type carnitine palmitoyltransferase I genes.[25] Interestingly, further inhibition of mitochondrial FA import in PPAR-α-null mice causes hepatic and cardiac lipid accumulation, hypoglycaemia and death in 100% of males and 25% of females.[55] Furthermore, PPAR-α-deficient mice fed a high-fat diet display a massive accumulation of lipids in liver,[25,56] highlighting the crucial role that PPAR-α plays in lipid metabolism. A concordant phenotype was observed in PPAR-α-deficient mice fasted for 24 hours who displayed hypoglycaemia, hypoketonaemia and elevated plasma FA levels.[25] Other studies revealed that PPAR-α might increase energy expenditure by upregulating the expression of uncoupling proteins (UCPs).[57–59] These data strongly argue in favour of a critical role for PPAR-α in lipid homeostasis. Through their effects on the expression of FA transporter and FA oxidation genes, PPAR-α directs the FA flux to the β-oxidation pathway and therefore diminishes the FA pool to be incorporated in triglyceride (TG)-rich lipoproteins. Consequently, PPAR-α maintains lipid homeostasis by controlling the FA flux from peripheral tissues, such as adipose tissue, to the liver (Figure 2).

PPAR-α and extracellular lipid metabolism

PPAR-α is an important regulator of extracellular lipid metabolism. The role of PPARs in TG metabolism is convincingly established.[3] The hypotriglyceridaemic effect of PPAR-α activators is the result of increased lipoprotein lipolysis and enhanced FA oxidation. The process of TG clearance is directly under the control of lipoprotein lipase (LPL) and apoC-III. PPAR-α activators repress apolipoprotein C-III (apoC-III) expression[60,61] and induce LPL in liver.[62] Moreover, PPAR-α enhances FA catabolic rate, which subsequently affects TG synthesis and VLDL production.[3] PPAR-α plays a central role in hepatic apoC-III gene regulation.[63] ApoC-III repression by PPAR-α occurs via PPAR-α-dependent induction of human and rat Rev-erbα, a nuclear orphan receptor that is a strong repressor of transcription.[11,64] The induction of Rev-erbα is mediated by PPAR-α, which interacts with a PPRE located within the human Rev-erbα promoter.[11] Such a mechanism is consistent with the observation that Rev-erbα-deficient mice exhibit increased plasma TG and apoC-III concentrations and elevated hepatic apoC-III mRNA levels.[65] Therefore, by upregulating Rev-erbα, PPAR-α indirectly modulates apoC-III expression, an effect that may contribute to the normolipaemic action of PPAR-α activators. Recently, a new apolipoprotein, apoA-V, has been identified to be an important determinant of plasma triglycerides.[66–68] Vu-Dac et al demonstrated that fibrates induce apoA-V expression in human hepatocytes.[69] These findings define a novel mechanism via which PPAR-α activators can influence triglyceride homeostasis.

Both apoA-I and HDL are inversely correlated with the incidence of coronary artery disease.[70] There is evidence supporting the protective role of HDL through the removal and the recycling of cholesterol excess from peripheral tissues to the liver. PPAR-α has important actions on HDL metabolism. PPAR-α activators affect HDL metabolism in an opposite manner in rodents and humans. Whereas fibrate treatment of rats lowers plasma HDL, an increase is generally observed in humans.[71-73] Such an increase in plasma HDL levels is related, at least in part, to changes in apoA-I and apoA-II gene expression in liver. The human apoA-I gene contains a PPRE that mediates upregulation by PPAR-α activators.[74,75] Studies on the regulation of hepatic apoA-I gene expression, carried out in human apoA-I transgenic mice, demonstrated an induction of plasma HDL and human apoA-I concentrations by PPAR-α activators.[74] PPAR-α also influences the expression of human apoA-II, the other major protein component of HDL.[76] Administration of fenofibrate to patients with coronary artery disease results in a marked increase in plasma apoA-II concentrations. This increase in plasma apoA-II is due to a direct effect on hepatic apoA-II production, since fibrates induce apoA-II mRNA levels both in primary cultures of human hepatocytes and in human hepatoblastoma HepG2 cells.[76] The induction of apoA-II mRNA levels is followed by an increase in apoA-II secretion in both cell culture systems. PPAR-α binds with high affinity to a PPRE located in the human apoA-II promoter, thereby activating apoA-II gene transcription. These data demonstrate that PPAR-α activators increase human apoA-II plasma levels by stimulating transcription of its gene through the interaction of activated PPAR-α with the apoA-II-PPRE.

The reverse cholesterol transport (RCT) pathway mediates the transport of cholesterol from peripheral tissues to the liver. Peripheral cell cholesterol is captured by HDL particles, which bring it back to the liver for direct elimination into the bile or, after metabolism, in bile acids. PPARs influence the RCT pathways by regulating macrophage cholesterol efflux, HDL transport in plasma and bile acid synthesis. Cholesterol efflux is the first step of the RCT that occurs either via passive diffusion or via transmembrane receptors such as the scavenger receptor (SR) class B type 1 (SR-B1/CLA-1) and the ATP-binding cassette A1 (ABCA1)

proteins. Murine scavenger receptor BI (SR-BI) and its human homologue CLA-1 have been identified as HDL receptors, which bind HDL with high affinity and mediate the selective uptake of cholesteryl esters in liver and steroidogenic tissues.[77,78] Interestingly, PPAR-α is expressed in human macrophages[79] and induces the expression of SR-B1/CLA-1[80] and ABCA1.[46,81,82] The induction of ABCA1 occurs via an indirect mechanism involving induction of LXR-α expression,[83] a major regulator of ABCA1. Increased ABCA1 expression results in a higher cholesterol efflux from macrophages. The major contribution of ABCA1 in the control of plasma HDL-cholesterol levels was highlighted by the identification of mutations in the ABCA1 gene in patients with familial HDL deficiency and Tangier disease.

In addition to influencing the transcription of HDL apolipoproteins and receptors regulating HDL metabolism, PPARs also affect the expression of enzymes involved in HDL metabolism. In rats, PPAR-α activators decrease the production of HDL-remodelling enzymes, such as hepatic lipase and lecithin:cholesterol acyltransferase (LCAT).[84,85] PPAR-α also induces the expression and activity of phospholipid transfer protein (PLTP),[86] an enzyme promoting the transfer of phospholipids from VLDL/LDL to HDL in mice. However, gene regulation studies on PLTP and LCAT by PPARs have been performed so far only in rodent models and need to be investigated in humans.

PPAR-α adiposity and steatosis

Although the expression of PPAR-α is very low in white adipose tissue, several arguments are in favour of a function of PPAR-α in the control of adiposity. PPAR-α may also play a role in adipose tissue as a mediator of leptin-induced lipolysis.[23] Indeed, hyperleptinaemia in rodents depletes adipocyte fat while upregulating FA oxidation enzymes, UCPs and PPAR-α, whose expression is normally low in white adipocytes. The essential role of PPAR-α in mediating the actions of leptin on lipid metabolism in liver and adipose tissue was shown by Lee et al.[87] More directly, PPAR-α activators reduce adiposity in rodent models of obesity.[88-90] Despite similar degrees of hyper-leptinaemia and reduction in food intake, epididymal fat was strongly reduced in wild-type but only weakly in PPAR-α-deficient mice. Accumulation of FAs in the liver is controlled by an equilibrium between hepatic lipid secretion and intracellular lipid metabolism pathways. Potentiation of FA oxidation prevents conversion into triglycerides and hepatic accumulation of lipids. PPAR-α exerts anti-steatotic actions in mice. PPAR-α plays a critical role in the cellular response to fasting. Upon short-term starvation, PPAR-α-deficient mice exhibit hepatic steatosis, myocardial lipid accumulation and hypoglycaemia with an inadequate ketogenic response.[56] Moreover, diet-induced liver triglyceride accumulation is decreased by PPAR-α activation in wild-type but not in PPAR-α-deficient mice that display severe steatohepatitis.[91] In addition, Chou et al performed similar investigations in a lipoat-rophic mouse model.[92] Activation of PPAR-α led to reduced triglyceride levels in liver and muscle, an effect attributed to an increased expression of FA oxidation enzymes rather than reduced lipogenesis or lipid uptake. These observations suggest that PPAR-α may modulate obesity-linked disorders such as steatosis, whether such effects also occur in humans awaits further studies.

PPAR-β/δ

As PPAR-β/δ is ubiquitously expressed, numerous and various functions have been attributed to this receptor. PPAR-β/δ was found to modulate tumorigenic pathways in the APC model of intestinal adenomatous polyposis.[93] PPAR-β/δ also influences blastocyst implantation.[94] PPAR-β/δ may also control cell proliferation in skin.[95] However, recent studies identified specific functions for this nuclear receptor in energy metabolism as well (Figure 3).

PPAR-β/δ and adiposity

PPAR-β/δ plays an important role in adipose tissue. Transgenic overexpression of a VP16-

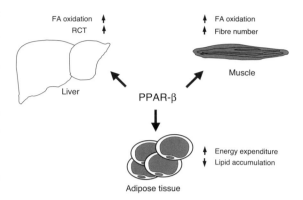

Figure 3 PPAR-β/δ functions in energy metabolism. PPAR-β/δ regulates the expression of genes implicated in β-oxidation, energy uncoupling and cholesterol efflux. Activation of PPAR-β/δ in muscle results in an increase in fibre number displaying high oxidative metabolism and improves exercise performance. In adipose tissue, PPAR-β/δ acts as a regulator of fat burning by co-ordinating FA oxidation and energy uncoupling. PPAR-β/δ stimulates cholesterol efflux from the cells, uptake by HDL and transport back to the liver. Although less expressed than PPAR-α, PPAR-β/δ may enhance β-oxidation in liver

PPAR-β/δ chimeric protein in adipocytes results in a reduction of body weight and adiposity.[96] Upon high-fat-diet feeding, these mice are resistant to weight gain, have a normal lipid profile, display no hypertrophy of white and brown adipose tissue and develop no fatty liver. Crossing these transgenic mice into the db/db background of a genetically predisposed mouse model results in a reversal of the obesity phenotype. In contrast, PPAR-β/δ-deficient mice fed a high-fat diet display reduced energy uncoupling and are prone to obesity.[96] In addition, pharmacological activation of PPAR-β/δ in db/db mice reduces the size of lipid droplets in brown fat and prevents lipid accumulation in liver due to enhanced FA oxidation. PPAR-β/δ treatment reversed the diet-induced obesity and insulin resistance in mice.[97] PPAR-β/δ can thus be considered as a regulator of fat burning by coordinating FA oxidation and energy uncoupling. However, the relevance of these findings in rodent models, that have substantial amounts of brown adipose tissue, cannot be easily extended to the human situation and investigation is required in other animal models such as the insulin-resistant monkeys.

PPAR-β/δ and lipid metabolism

Recently, in vitro and in vivo genetic and pharmacological studies firmly established a role for PPAR-β/δ in lipid metabolism. PPAR-β/δ regulates acyl-CoA synthetase 2 expression in rat brain cells[8] and promotes reverse cholesterol transport.[46] Moreover, incubation of skeletal and cardiac muscle cells with the PPAR-β/δ agonist GW501516 led to the modulation of genes implicated in β-oxidation, cholesterol efflux and energy uncoupling.[98,99] Since PPAR-α-deficient mice do not display a compromised β-oxidation in muscle during exercise and fasting, Muoio et al proposed a compensatory regulation by PPAR-β/δ.[100] Several studies corroborated this hypothesis. Indeed, overexpression of PPAR-β/δ in muscle resulted in an increase in fibre number displaying high oxidative metabolism, upregulation of CPT1b, UCP2 and m-FABP,[98,100–102] and in a reduction of fat. PPAR-β/δ acts as a mediator of the adaptative response to exercise in muscle and has a remodelling function through the increase of muscle fibre[101] that consequently improves exercise performance.

PPAR-β/δ also plays a role in lipoprotein metabolism. Treatment of obese rhesus monkeys with the PPAR-β/δ agonist GW501516 not only significantly increased HDL levels via a mechanism involving the induction of apoA-I and apoA-II, but also decreased plasma VLDL and the number of small dense LDL particles. These findings support a model in which PPAR-β/δ stimulates cholesterol efflux from the cells, capture by HDL and transport back to the liver. Evidence that PPAR-β/δ regulates cholesterol efflux was provided using PPAR-β/δ-selective agonists.[46,103] PPAR-β/δ activation increases ABCA1 expression and apoA-I mediated cholesterol efflux. However, a controversial role of PPAR-β/δ in macrophage lipid homeostasis is illustrated by the findings that PPAR-β/δ may promote VLDL-triglyceride and cholesterol loading and storage in macrophages via the

induction of the scavenger receptors CD36 and SRA, as well as ADRP and a/FABP expression.[103,104] Thus, the overall effect of PPAR-β/δ on macrophage cholesterol homeostasis needs further clarification.

Therefore, PPAR-β/δ constitutes a potential pharmacological target of interest for the metabolic syndrome.[46] Whether an improvement in the lipid profile is also observed in humans will remain elusive until specific agonists are being tested in clinical trials.

PPAR-γ

PPAR-γ and adipogenesis

Adipose tissue is the main site for lipid storage and plays a crucial role in the modulation of lipid levels in response to hormonal stimulation. Pharmacological activation of PPAR-γ improves insulin sensitivity.[105] PPAR-γ modulates lipid and glucose homeostasis through its function in adipose tissue, but also exerts indirect actions in liver and muscle (Figure 4). Several crucial genes for adipocyte differentiation and lipid uptake and storage contain a PPRE. Gene expression of CD36,[106] aP2,[107] phosphoenol pyruvate carboxykinase,[108]

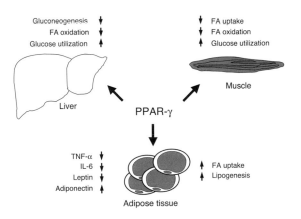

Figure 4 Activation of adipose PPAR-γ stimulates fatty acid (FA) and triglyceride flux toward the adipocyte and lipogenesis. Modulation of adipokines leads to indirect effects in other tissues. PPAR-γ action potentiates glucose utilization by muscle and liver to the detriment of fatty acid oxidation

ACS,[109,110] FAT[50] and LPL[62] are regulated by PPAR-γ. The induction of LPL promotes FA delivery to adipocytes while induction of FAT, FATP-1 and ACS results in enhanced FA storage by the adipocyte. Moreover, activation of PPAR-γ induces expression of glycerol kinase[111] that converts glycerol to glycerol-phosphate, allowing FA re-incorporation into triglycerides. Consequently, PPAR-γ activation prevents free FA release from the adipocyte, thus resulting in lower levels of circulating FA. These effects should result indirectly in a decrease in FA uptake and oxidation by the liver and the muscle. Thus, PPAR-γ action promotes glucose utilization in both tissues and consequently decreases gluconeogenesis in the liver and improves glucose oxidation in muscle. PPAR-γ also interferes with tumour necrosis factor alpha (TNF-α) signalling. TNF-α inhibits insulin signalling and promotes lipolysis in adipose tissue, enhancing the development of insulin resistance in muscle and liver. Inhibition of TNF-α signalling by PPAR-γ preserves normal glucose and lipid homeostasis. PPAR-γ also modulates the expression of adipokines such as leptin and adiponectin.[112-115] PPAR-γ inhibits leptin-induced lipolysis via repression of leptin gene expression. Adiponectin, strongly expressed in adipose tissue, is upregulated by PPAR-γ.[116] Adiponectin stimulates FA oxidation in muscle and decreases production of glucose by the liver. These actions lead to the lowering of circulating FA, triglycerides and glucose, and contribute to improved insulin sensitivity. Altogether, the actions of PPAR-γ preserve a mature, insulin-sensitive adipocyte phenotype and appear to be crucial for lipid and glucose homeostasis. As anti-diabetic agents, glitazones are primarily studied for their effect on glucose homeostasis. Nevertheless, these drugs exert hypotriglyceridaemic actions in rodents by increasing lipolysis and clearance of TG-rich lipoproteins.[117-122] This effect may be attributed, at least in part, to the induction of adipose tissue LPL expression.[62,123] However, whether these mechanisms are operative in humans is unclear.

PPAR-γ is expressed in human macrophages.[79] PPAR-γ affects the RCT in a manner similar to PPAR-α. PPAR-γ induces the expression of SR-B1/CLA-1[80] and ABCA1.[46,81,82] PPAR-γ-induced expression of LXR-α[83] results in ABCA1 expression.

PPAR–γ and steatosis

Although PPAR-α is the main PPAR isotype expressed in liver under normal conditions, PPAR-γ is induced in fatty livers. The roles of PPAR-γ and thiazolidinediones in liver have been investigated in various animal models. Herzig et al. showed that CREB-deficient mice develop a fatty liver phenotype and display elevated expression of PPAR-γ. The authors demonstrated that CREB inhibits hepatic PPAR-γ expression in the fasted state and proposed that PPAR-γ probably behaves as a pro-steatotic factor by a direct action in the liver.[124] Chronic treatment of obese (NZO × NON)F1 mice[125] or diabetic KKAy mice[126] with anti-diabetic thiazolidinediones led to severe hepatic steatosis, while normal mice were not affected. The function of liver PPAR-γ was also investigated in lipoatrophic A-ZIP/F-1 (AZIP) mice. In AZIP mice, ablation of liver PPAR-γ reduced hepatic steatosis and also abolished the hypoglycaemic and hypolipidaemic effects of rosiglitazone, demonstrating that, in the absence of adipose tissue, the liver is an important site of PPAR-γ action. Thus, in mice, liver PPAR-γ contributes to hepatic steatosis, but prevents triglyceride accumulation and insulin resistance in other tissues.[127] Interestingly, mice lacking PPAR-γ in adipose tissue displayed a marked increase in hepatic glucogenesis and insulin resistance and were significantly more susceptible to high-fat diet-induced steatosis.[128] Therefore, in mice, fasting or pathological conditions, such as obesity and diabetes, stimulate hepatic PPAR-γ expression and activity that consequently promotes hepatic steatosis.

In humans, by contrast, PPAR-γ activation appears to improve hepatic steatosis. Pathophysiological evaluation of patients with dominant-negative PPAR-γ mutations revealed not only all the features of the metabolic syndrome but also the existence of non-alcoholic steatohepatitis.[129] Moreover, treatment of type 2 diabetic patients with rosiglitazone or pioglitazone decreases liver fat content.[130–132] PPAR-γ activation also decreases liver fat content in subjects with non-alcoholic steato-hepatitis.[133,134] Therefore, PPAR-γ appears to play an important opposite role in hepatic steatosis in humans and rodents.

PPAR-γ in clinical practice

Several studies have tested the effects of glita-zone treatment on glucose homeostasis in diabetic and insulin-resistant patients.[135,136] Glitazone therapy lowers fasting and post-prandial glucose levels and improves insulin-stimulated glucose disposal. However, the effect of glitazones on the plasma lipid profile in humans depends on the molecule tested, and intervention trials assessing the influence of these compounds on the incidence of cardiovascular disease, are still lacking. Never-theless, glitazone treatment of patients with type 2 diabetes suggested that these drugs may inhibit early atherosclerotic lesion progres-sion.[135,136] In patients with type 2 diabetes, pioglitazone and rosiglitazone appear to have distinct effects on the plasma levels of triglyc-erides and LDL. Pioglitazone treatment lowers serum concentrations of LDL and triglycerides, whereas rosiglitazone treatment does not appear to lower triglycerides and increases the levels of LDL-cholesterol.[137–139] Although the mechanistic basis for these differences is unclear, one possible explanation may be that pioglitazone has, albeit limited, PPAR-α activ-ity.[140] Despite their atheroprotective proper-ties, certain glitazones may present a risk for heart failure in advanced diabetic patients. Thus, their clinical use should be carefully monitored.[141] The risk of heart failure with glitazones, which is probably due to plasma volume expansion, appears to be enhanced when they are used in combination therapy with insulin.[141] Troglitazone has been withdrawn worldwide because of its hepato-toxic effects. Such effects are not observed with other glitazones.

CONCLUSION

PPARs are activated by dietary fatty acids and eicosanoids, as well as by pharmacological drugs, such as fibrates for PPAR-α and glita-zones for PPAR-γ. PPAR-α and PPAR-β/δ are considered major regulators of intra- and extracellular lipid metabolism. PPAR-γ improves glucose metabolism via induction of key genes of adipocyte differentiation and function. As such, PPARs control plasma lipid and glucose levels, elevated levels of which are associated with diabetes and cardiovascular diseases. Recent investigations suggest that PPAR-α and PPAR-γ activation attenuates atherosclerosis progression, not only by correcting metabolic disorders but also through direct effects on the vascular wall. The intimate and causative relationships between lipid metabolism and coronary heart disease have stimulated research on the physiological functions of the lipid-activated transcription factors of the PPAR family. This research has resulted in the development and understand-ing of the action mechanism of drugs useful in the treatment of metabolic disorders predis-posing to atherosclerosis. It is now anticipated that future development of drugs exerting their activity via PPARs will focus not so much on the search of more potent activators but rather on selective receptor modulators in an attempt to separate desirable from unwanted side-effects. Finally, ongoing clinical studies with specific PPAR-α/PPAR-β/δ/PPAR-γ (co)activators should prove (or disprove) their activity in reducing coronary events and total mortality.

References

1. Brown MS, Goldstein JL. The SREBP pathway: regulation of cholesterol metabolism by proteolysis of a membrane-bound transcription factor. Cell 1997; 89:331–40

2. Peet D, Janowski B, Mangelsdorf D. The LXRs: a new class of oxysterol receptors. Curr Opin Genet Dev 1998; 8:571–5

3. Schoonjans K, Staels B, Auwerx J. The peroxisome proliferator activated receptors (PPARs) and their effects on lipid metabolism and adipocyte differentiation. Biochim Biophys Acta 1996; 1302:93–109

4. Braissant O, Wahli W. Differential expression of peroxisome proliferator-activated receptor-alpha, -beta, and -gamma during rat embryonic development. Endocrinology 1998; 139:2748–54

5. Auboeuf D, Rieusset J, Fajas L, et al. Tissue distribution and quantification of the expression of mRNAs of peroxisome proliferator-activated receptors and liver X receptor-alpha in humans: no alteration in adipose tissue of obese and NIDDM patients. Diabetes 1997; 46:1319–27

6. Cullingford TE, Bhakoo K, Peuchen S, et al. Distribution of mRNAs encoding the peroxisome proliferator-activated receptor alpha, beta, and gamma and the retinoid X receptor alpha, beta, and gamma in rat central nervous system. J Neurochem 1998; 70:1366–75

7. Dreyer C, Krey G, Keller H, et al. Control of the peroxisomal beta-oxidation pathway by a novel family of nuclear hormone receptors. Cell 1992; 68:879–87

8. Basu-Modak S, Braisssant O, Escher P, et al. Peroxisome proliferator-activated receptor beta regulates acyl-CoA synthetase 2 in reaggregated rat brain cell cultures. J Biol Chem 1999; 274:35881–8

9. Staels B, Dallongeville J, Auwerx J, et al. Mechanism of action of fibrates on lipid and lipoprotein metabolism. Circulation 1998; 98:2088–93

10. Spiegelman BM. PPAR-gamma: adipogenic regulator and thiazolidinedione receptor. Diabetes 1998; 47:507–14

11. Gervois P, Chopin-Delannoy S, Fadel A, et al. Fibrates increase human REV-ERBalpha expression in liver via a novel peroxisome proliferator-activated receptor response element. Mol Endocrinol 1999; 13:400–9

12. Delerive P, De Bosscher K, Besnard S, et al. PPARα negatively regulates the vascular wall inflammatory gene response by negative cross-talk with transcription factors NF-κB and AP-1. J Biol Chem 1999; 274:32048–54

13. Delerive P, Martin F, Chinetti G, et al. PPAR activators inhibit thrombin-induced endothelin-1 production in human vascular endothelial cells by inhibiting the AP-1 signalling pathways. Circ Res 1999; 85:394–402

14. Jiang C, Ting AT, Seed B. PPAR-gamma agonists inhibit production of monocyte inflammatory cytokines. Nature (Lond) 1998; 391:82–6

15. Ricote M, Li AC, Willson TM, et al. The peroxisome proliferator-activated receptor-gamma is a negative regulator of macrophage activation. Nature (Lond) 1998; 391:79–82

16. Sakai M, Matsushima-Hibiya Y, Nishizawa M, et al. Suppression of rat gluthatione transferase P expression by peroxisome proliferators:interaction between Jun and peroxisome proliferator-activated receptor α. Cancer Res 1995; 53:5370–6

17. Staels B, Koenig W, Habib A, et al. Activation of human aortic smooth-muscle cells is inhibited by PPARalpha but not by PPARgamma activators. Nature (Lond) 1998; 393:790–3

18. Zhou YC, Waxman DJ. Cross-talk between janus kinase-signal transducer and activator of transcription (JAK-STAT) and peroxisome proliferator-activated receptor-alpha (PPARα) signalling pathways. Growth hormone inhibition of PPARα transcriptional activity mediated by STAT5b. J Biol Chem 1999; 274:2672–81

19. Delerive P, Gervois P, Fruchart JC, et al. Induction of IkappaBalpha expression as a mechanism contributing to the anti-inflammatory activities of peroxisome proliferator-activated receptor-alpha activators. J Biol Chem 2000; 275:36703–7

20. Gervois P, Kleemann R, Pilon A, et al. Global suppression of IL-6–induced acute phase response gene expression after in vivo chronic treatment with the peroxisome proliferator-activated receptor α activator fenofibrate. J Biol Chem 2004; 279:16154–60

21. Lemberger T, Staels B, Saladin R, et al. Regulation of the peroxisome proliferator-activated receptor alpha gene by glucocorticoids. J Biol Chem 1994; 269:24527–30

22. Steineger HH, Sorensen HN, Tugwood JD, et al. Dexamethasone and insulin demonstrate marked and opposite regulation of the steady-state mRNA level of the peroxisomal proliferator-activated receptor (PPAR) in hepatic cells. Hormonal modulation of fatty acid-induced transcription. Eur J Biochem 1994; 225:967–74

23. Wang MY, Unger RH. Novel form of lipolysis induced by leptin. J Biol Chem 1999; 274:17541–4

24. Zhou YT, Wang ZW, Higa M, et al. Reversing adipocyte differentiation: implications for treatment of obesity. Proc Natl Acad Sci USA 1999; 96:2391–5

25. Kersten S, Seydoux J, Peters JM, et al. Peroxisome proliferator-activated receptor alpha mediates the adaptive response to fasting. J Clin Invest 1999; 103:1489–98

26. Lemberger T, Saladin R, Vazquez M, et al. Expression of the peroxisome proliferator-activated receptor alpha gene is stimulated by stress and follows a diurnal rhythm. J Biol Chem 1996; 271:1764–9

27. Palmer CN, Hsu MH, Griffin KJ, et al. Peroxisome proliferator activated receptor-alpha expression in human liver. Mol Pharmacol 1998; 53:14–22

28. Gervois P, Pineda Torra I, Chinetti G, et al. A truncated human PPARα splice variant with dominant negative activity. Mol Endocrinol 1999; 13:1535–49

29. Zhu Y, Qi C, Korenberg JR, et al. Structural organization of mouse peroxisome proliferator-activated receptor gamma (mPPAR gamma) gene: alternative promoter use and different splicing yield two mPPAR gamma isoforms. Proc Natl Acad Sci USA 1995; 92:7921–5

30. Fajas L, Auboeuf D, Raspe E, et al. The organization, promoter analysis, and expression of the human PPARgamma gene. J Biol Chem 1997; 272:18779–89

31. Werman A, Hollenberg A, Solanes G, et al. Ligand-independent activation domain in the N terminus of peroxisome proliferator-activated receptor gamma (PPARgamma). Differential activity of PPARgamma1 and -2 isoforms and influence of insulin. J Biol Chem 1997; 272:20230–5

32. Wu Z, Bucher NL, Farmer SR. Induction of peroxisome proliferator-activated receptor gamma during the conversion of 3T3 fibroblasts into adipocytes is mediated by C/EBPbeta, C/EBPdelta, and glucocorticoids. Mol Cell Biol 1996; 16:4128–36

33. Juge-Aubry CE, Hammar E, Siegrist-Kaiser C, et al. Regulation of the transcriptional activity of the peroxisome proliferator-activated receptor alpha by phosphorylation of a ligand-independent transactivating domain. J Biol Chem 1999; 274:10505–10

34. Shao D, Rangwala SM, Bailey ST, et al. Interdomain communication regulating ligand binding by PPARgamma. Nature (Lond) 1998; 396:377–80

35. Shalev A, Siegrist-Kaiser CA, Yen PM, et al. The peroxisome proliferator-activated receptor alpha is a phosphoprotein: regulation by insulin. Endocrinology 1996; 137:4499–502

36. Adams M, Reginato MJ, Shao D, et al. Transcriptional activation by peroxisome proliferator-activated receptor gamma is inhibited by phosphorylation at a consensus mitogen-activated protein kinase site. J Biol Chem 1997; 272:5128–32

37. Hu E, Kim JB, Sarraf P, et al. Inhibition of adipogenesis through MAP kinase-mediated phosphorylation of PPARgamma. Science 1996; 274:2100–3

38. Camp HS, Tafuri SR, Leff T. c-Jun N-terminal kinase phosphorylates peroxisome proliferator-activated receptor-γ1 and negatively regulates its transcriptional activity. Endocrinology 1999; 140:392–7

39. Hauser S, Adelmant G, Sarraf P, et al. Degradation of the peroxisome proliferator-activated receptor gamma is linked to ligand-dependent activation. J Biol Chem 2000; 275:18527–33

40. Blanquart C, Barbier O, Fruchart JC, et al. Peroxisome proliferator-activated receptor alpha (PPARalpha) turnover by the ubiquitin-proteasome system controls the ligand-induced expression level of its target genes. J Biol Chem 2002; 277:37254–9

41. Hirotani M, Tsukamoto T, Bourdeaux J, et al. Stabilization of peroxisome proliferator-activated receptor alpha by the ligand. Biochem Biophys Res Commun 2001; 288:106–10

42. Willson TM, Wahli W. Peroxisome proliferator-activated receptor agonists. Curr Opin Chem Biol 1997; 1:235–41

43. Nagy L, Tontonoz P, Alvarez JG, et al. Oxidized LDL regulates macrophage gene expression through ligand activation of PPARγ. Cell 1998; 93:229–40

44. Xu HE, Lambert MH, Montana VG, et al. Molecular recognition of fatty acids by peroxisome proliferator-activated receptors. Mol Cell 1999; 3:397–403

45. Berger J, Leibowitz MD, Doebber TW, et al. Novel peroxisome proliferator-activated receptor (PPAR) gamma and PPARdelta ligands produce distinct biological effects. J Biol Chem 1999; 274:6718–25

46. Oliver WR, Shenk JL, Snaith MR, et al. A selective peroxisome proliferator-activated receptor delta agonist promotes reverse cholesterol transport. Proc Natl Acad Sci USA 2001; 98:5306–11

47. Hashimoto T, Fujita T, Usuda N, et al. Peroxisomal and mitochondrial fatty acid beta-oxidation in mice nullizygous for both peroxisome proliferator-activated receptor alpha and peroxisomal fatty acyl-CoA oxidase. Genotype correlation with fatty liver phenotype. J Biol Chem 1999; 274:19228–36

48. Qi C, Zhu Y, Pan J, et al. Absence of spontaneous peroxisome proliferation in enoyl-CoA Hydratase/L-3–hydroxyacyl-CoA dehydrogenase-deficient mouse liver. Further support for the role of fatty acyl-CoA oxidase in PPAR alpha ligand metabolism. J Biol Chem 1999; 274:15775–80

49. Aoyama T, Peters JM, Iritani N, et al. Altered constitutive expression of fatty acid-metabolizing enzymes in mice lacking the peroxisome proliferator-activated receptor alpha (PPARalpha). J Biol Chem 1997; 273:5678–84

50. Martin G, Schoonjans K, Lefebvre AM, et al. Coordinate regulation of the expression of the fatty acid transport protein and acyl-CoA synthetase genes by PPARalpha and PPARgamma activators. J Biol Chem 1997; 272:28210–17

51. Motojima K, Passilly P, Peters JM, et al. Expression of putative fatty acid transporter genes are regulated by peroxisome proliferator-activated receptor alpha and gamma activators in a tissue- and inducer-specific manner. J Biol Chem 1998; 273:16710–14

52. Mascaro C, Acosta E, Ortiz JA, et al. Control of human muscle-type carnitine palmitoyltransferase I gene transcription by peroxisome proliferator-activated receptor. J Biol Chem 1998; 273:8560–73

53. Brandt JM, Djouadi F, Kelly DP. Fatty acids activate transcription of the muscle carnitine palmitoyltransferase I gene in cardiac myocytes via the peroxisome proliferator-activated receptor alpha. J Biol Chem 1998; 273:23786–92

54. Yu GS, Lu YC, Gulick T. Co-regulation of tissue-specific alternative human carnitine palmitoyltransferase Ibeta gene promoters by fatty acid enzyme substrate. J Biol Chem 1998; 273:32901–9

55. Djouadi F, Weinheimer CJ, Saffitz JE, et al. A gender-related defect in lipid metabolism and glucose

homeostasis in peroxisome proliferator-activated receptor alpha-deficient mice. J Clin Invest 1998; 102:1083–91

56. Leone TC, Weinheimer CJ, Kelly DP. A critical role for the peroxisome proliferator-activated receptor alpha (PPARalpha) in the cellular fasting response: The PPARalpha-null mouse as a model of fatty acid oxidation disorders. Proc Natl Acad Sci USA 1999; 96:7473–8

57. Kelly LJ, Vicario PP, Thompson GM, et al. Peroxisome proliferator-activated receptors gamma and alpha mediate in vivo regulation of uncoupling protein (UCP-1, UCP-2, UCP-3) gene expression. Endocrinology 1998; 139:4920–7

58. Brun S, Carmona MC, Mampel T, et al. Activators of peroxisome proliferator-activated receptor-alpha induce the expression of the uncoupling protein-3 gene in skeletal muscle: a potential mechanism for the lipid intake-dependent activation of uncoupling protein-3 gene expression at birth. Diabetes 1999; 48:1217–22

59. Tsuboyama-Kasaoka N, Takahashi M, Kim H, et al. Up-regulation of liver uncoupling protein-2 mRNA by either fish oil feeding or fibrate administration in mice. Biochem Biophys Res Commun 1999; 257: 879–85

60. Hertz R, Bishara-Shieban J, Bar-Tana J. Mode of action of peroxisome proliferators as hypolipidemic drugs. Suppression of apolipoprotein C-III. J Biol Chem 1995; 270:13470–5

61. Staels B, Vu-Dac N, Kosykh V, et al. Fibrates down-regulate apolipoprotein C-III expression independent of induction of peroxisomal acyl co-enzyme A oxidase. J Clin Invest 1995; 95:705–12

62. Schoonjans K, Peinado-Onsurbe J, Lefebvre AM, et al. PPARalpha and PPARgamma activators direct a distinct tissue-specific transcriptional response via a PPRE in the lipoprotein lipase gene. EMBO J 1996; 15:5336–48

63. Peters JM, Hennuyer N, Staels B, et al. Alterations in lipoprotein metabolism in peroxisome proliferator-activated receptor alpha-deficient mice. J Biol Chem 1997; 272:27307–12

64. Vu-Dac N, Chopin-Delannoy S, Gervois P, et al. The nuclear receptors peroxisome proliferator-activated receptorα and Rev-erbα mediate the species-specific regulation of apolipoprotein A-I expression by fibrates. J Biol Chem 1998; 273:25713–20

65. Raspe E, Duez H, Mansen A, et al. Identification of Rev-erbalpha as a physiological repressor of apoC-III gene transcription. J Lipid Res 2002; 43:2172–9

66. Packard CJ. Overview of fenofibrate. Eur Heart J 1998; 19 (Suppl A):A62–5

67. Pennacchio LA, Olivier M, Hubacek JA, et al. An apolipoprotein influencing triglycerides in humans and mice revealed by comparative sequencing. Science 2001; 294:169–73

68. Tugwood JD, Aldridge TC, Lambe KG, et al. Peroxisome proliferator-activated receptor-alpha and

the pleiotropic responses to peroxisome proliferators. Arch Toxicol Suppl 1998; 20:377–86

69. Vu-Dac N, Gervois P, Jakel H, et al. Apolipoprotein A5, a crucial determinant of plasma triglyceride levels, is highly responsive to peroxisome proliferator activated receptor alpha. J Biol Chem 2003; 278:17982–5

70. Miller GJ, Miller NE. Plasma-high-density-lipoprotein concentration and development of ischaemic heart-disease. Lancet 1975; 1:16–19

71. Balfour JA, McTavish D, Heel RC. Fenofibrate. A review of its pharmacodynamic and pharmacokinetic properties and therapeutic use in dyslipidaemia. Drugs 1990; 40:260–90

72. Bard JM, Parra HJ, Camare R, et al. A multicenter comparison of the effects of simvastatin and fenofi-brate therapy in severe primary hypercholes-terolemia, with particular emphasis on lipoproteins defined by their apolipoprotein composition. Metabolism 1992; 41:498–503

73. Malmendier CL, Delcroix C. Effects of fenofibrate on high and low density lipoprotein metabolism in heterozygous familial hypercholesterolemia. Arteriosclerosis 1985; 55:161–9

74. Berthou L, Duverger N, Emmanuel F, et al. Opposite regulation of human versus mouse apolipoprotein A-I by fibrates in human apolipoprotein A-I transgenic mice. J Clin Invest 1996; 97:2408–16

75. Vu-Dac N, Schoonjans K, Laine B, et al. Negative regulation of the human apolipoprotein A-I promoter by fibrates can be attenuated by the inter-action of the peroxisome proliferator-activated recep-tor with its response element. J Biol Chem 1994; 269:31012–18

76. Vu-Dac N, Schoonjans K, Kosykh V, et al. Fibrates increase human apolipoprotein A-II expression through activation of the peroxisome proliferator-activated receptor. J Clin Invest 1995; 96:741–50

77. Acton S, Rigotti A, Landschulz KT, et al. Identi-fication of scavenger receptor SR-BI as a high density lipoprotein receptor. Science 1996; 271:518–20

78. Calvo D, Gomez-Coronado D, Lasuncion MA, et al. CLA-1 is an 85–kD plasma membrane glycoprotein that acts as a high-affinity receptor for both native (HDL, LDL, and VLDL) and modified (OxLDL and AcLDL) lipoproteins. Arterioscler Thromb Vasc Biol 1997; 17:2341–9

79. Chinetti G, Griglio S, Antonucci M, et al. Activation of proliferator-activated receptors alpha and gamma induces apoptosis of human monocyte-derived macrophages. J Biol Chem 1998; 273:25573–80

80. Chinetti G, Gbaguidi GF, Griglio S, et al. CLA-1/SR-BI is expressed in atherosclerotic lesion macrophages and regulated by activators of peroxisome prolifera-tor-activated receptors. Circulation 2000; 101: 2411–17

81. Chinetti G, Lestavel S, Bocher V, et al. PPAR-alpha and PPAR-gamma activators induce cholesterol removal from human macrophage foam cells through

stimulation of the ABCA1 pathway. Nature Med 2001; 7:53–8

82. Chawla A, Boisvert WA, Lee CH, et al. A PPAR gamma-LXR-ABCA1 pathway in macrophages is involved in cholesterol efflux and atherogenesis. Mol Cell 2001; 7:161–71

83. Tobin KA, Steineger HH, Alberti S, et al. Cross-talk between fatty acid and cholesterol metabolism mediated by liver X receptor-alpha. Mol Endocrinol 2000; 14:741–52

84. Staels B, Peinado-Onsurbe J, Auwerx J. Down-regulation of hepatic lipase gene expression and activity by fenofibrate. Biochim Biophys Acta 1992; 1123:227–30

85. Staels B, van Tol A, Skretting G, et al. Lecithin:cholesterol acyltransferase gene expression is regulated in a tissue-selective manner by fibrates. J Lipid Res 1992; 33:727–35

86. Bouly M, Masson D, Gross B, et al. Induction of the phospholipid transfer protein gene accounts for the high density lipoprotein enlargement in mice treated with fenofibrate. J Biol Chem 2001; 276:25841–7

87. Lee Y, Yu X, Gonzales F, et al. PPAR alpha is necessary for the lipopenic action of hyperleptinemia on white adipose and liver tissue. Proc Natl Acad Sci USA 2002; 99:11848–53

88. Guerre-Millo M, Gervois P, Raspe E, et al. Peroxisome proliferator-activated receptor alpha activators improve insulin sensitivity and reduce adiposity. J Biol Chem 2000; 275:16638–42

89. Mancini FP, Lanni A, Sabatino L, et al. Fenofibrate prevents and reduces body weight gain and adiposity in diet-induced obese rats. FEBS Lett 2001; 491:154–8

90. Ye JM, Iglesias PJ, Watson DG, et al. Peroxisome proliferator-activated receptor (PPAR)-alpha activation lowers muscle lipids and improves insulin sensitivity in high fat-fed rats: comparison with PPAR-gamma activation. Diabetes 2001; 50:411–17

91. Ip E, Farrell GC, Robertson G, et al. Central role of PPARalpha-dependent hepatic lipid turnover in dietary steatohepatitis in mice. Hepatology 2003; 38:123–32

92. Chou CJ, Haluzik M, Gregory C, et al. WY14,643, a peroxisome proliferator-activated receptor alpha (PPARalpha) agonist, improves hepatic and muscle steatosis and reverses insulin resistance in lipoatrophic A-ZIP/F-1 mice. J Biol Chem 2002; 277: 24484–9

93. He TC, Chan TA, Vogelstein B, et al. PPARdelta is an APC-regulated target of nonsteroidal anti-inflammatory drugs. Cell 1999; 99:335–45

94. Lim H, Dey SK. PPARdelta functions as a prostacyclin receptor in blastocyst implantation. Trends Endocrinol Metab 2000; 11:137–42

95. Tan NS, Michalik L, Noy N, et al. Critical roles of PPAR beta/delta in keratinocyte response to inflammation. Genes Dev 2001; 15:3263–77

96. Wang YX, Lee CH, Tiep S, et al. Peroxisome proliferator-activated receptor delta activates fat metabolism to prevent obesity. Cell 2003; 113:159–70

97. Tanaka T, Yamamoto J, Iwasaki S, et al. Activation of peroxisome proliferator-activated receptor delta induces fatty acid beta-oxidation in skeletal muscle and attenuates metabolic syndrome. Proc Natl Acad Sci USA 2003; 100:15924–9

98. Dressel U, Allen TL, Pippal JB, et al. The peroxisome proliferator-activated receptor beta/delta agonist, GW501516, regulates the expression of genes involved in lipid catabolism and energy uncoupling in skeletal muscle cells. Mol Endocrinol 2003; 17:2477–93

99. Gilde AJ, van der Lee KA, Willemsen PH, et al. Peroxisome proliferator-activated receptor (PPAR) alpha and PPARbeta/delta, but not PPARgamma, modulate the expression of genes involved in cardiac lipid metabolism. Circ Res 2003; 92:518–24

100. Muoio DM, MacLean PS, Lang DB, et al. Fatty acid homeostasis and induction of lipid regulatory genes in skeletal muscles of peroxisome proliferator-activated receptor (PPAR) alpha knock-out mice. Evidence for compensatory regulation by PPAR delta. J Biol Chem 2002; 277:26089–97

101. Luquet S, Lopez-Soriano J, Holst D, et al. Peroxisome proliferator-activated receptor delta controls muscle development and oxidative capability. FASEB J 2003; 17:2299–301

102. Holst D, Luquet S, Kristiansen K, et al. Roles of peroxisome proliferator activated receptors delta and gamma in myoblast transdifferentiation. Exp Cell Res 2003; 288:168–76

103. Vosper H, Patel L, Graham TL, et al. The peroxisome proliferator-activated receptor delta promotes lipid accumulation in human macrophages. J Biol Chem 2001; 276:44258–65

104. Chawla A, Lee CH, Barak Y, et al. PPARdelta is a very low-density lipoprotein sensor in macrophages. Proc Natl Acad Sci USA 2003; 100:1268–73

105. Sood V, Colleran K, Burge MR. Thiazolidinediones: a comparative review of approved uses. Diabetes Technol Ther 2000; 2:429–40

106. Sfeir Z, Ibrahimi A, Amri E, et al. Regulation of FAT/CD36 gene expression: further evidence in support of a role of the protein in fatty acid binding/transport. Prost Leuk Ess Fatty Acids 1997; 57:17–21

107. Tontonoz P, Hu E, Graves RA, et al. mPPAR gamma 2: tissue-specific regulator of an adipocyte enhancer. Genes Dev 1994; 8:1224–34

108. Tontonoz P, Hu E, Devine J, et al. PPAR gamma 2 regulates adipose expression of the phosphoenolpyruvate carboxykinase gene. Mol Cell Biol 1995; 15:351–7

109. Schoonjans K, Watanabe M, Suzuki H, et al. Induction of the acyl-coenzyme A synthetase gene by fibrates and fatty acids is mediated by a peroxisome proliferator response element in the C promoter. J Biol Chem 1995; 270:19269–76

110. Schoonjans K, Staels B, Grimaldi P, et al. Acyl-CoA synthetase mRNA expression is controlled by fibric-

acid derivatives, feeding and liver proliferation. Eur J Biochem 1993; 216:615–22

111. Guan Y, Zhang Y, Davis L, et al. Expression of peroxisome proliferator-activated receptors in urinary tract of rabbits and humans. Am J Physiol 1997; 273:F1013–22

112. De Vos P, Lefebvre AM, Miller SG, et al. Thiazolidinediones repress ob gene expression in rodents via activation of peroxisome proliferator-activated receptor gamma. J Clin Invest 1996; 98:1004–9

113. Yamauchi T, Kamon J, Waki H, et al. The fat-derived hormone adiponectin reverses insulin resistance associated with both lipoatrophy and obesity. Nature Med 2001; 7:941–6

114. Maeda N, Takahashi M, Funahashi T, et al. PPARgamma ligands increase expression and plasma concentrations of adiponectin, an adipose-derived protein. Diabetes 2001; 50:2094–9

115. Berg AH, Combs TP, Du X, et al. The adipocyte-secreted protein Acrp30 enhances hepatic insulin action. Nature Med 2001; 7:947–53

116. Iwaki M, Matsuda M, Maeda N, et al. Induction of adiponectin, a fat-derived antidiabetic and antiatherogenic factor, by nuclear receptors. Diabetes 2003; 52:1655–63

117. Stevenson RW, Hutson NJ, Krupp MN, et al. Actions of novel antidiabetic agent englitazone in hyperglycemic hyperinsulinemic ob/ob mice. Diabetes 1990; 39:1218–27

118. Sohda T, Mizuno K, Momose Y, et al. Studies on antidiabetic agents. 11. Novel thiazolidinedione derivatives as potent hypoglycemic and hypolipidemic agents. J Med Chem 1992; 35:2617–26

119. Kemnitz JW, Elson DF, Roecker EB, et al. Pioglitazone increases insulin sensitivity, reduces blood glucose, insulin, and lipid levels, and lowers blood pressure, in obese, insulin- resistant rhesus monkeys. Diabetes 1994; 43:204–11

120. Young PW, Cawthorne MA, Coyle PJ, et al. Repeat treatment of obese mice with BRL 49653, a new potent insulin sensitizer, enhances insulin action in white adipocytes. Association with increased insulin binding and cell-surface GLUT4 as measured by photoaffinity labeling. Diabetes 1995; 44:1087–92

121. Lohray BB, Bhushan V, Rao BP, et al. Novel euglycemic and hypolipidemic agents. 1. J Med Chem 1998; 41:1619–30

122. Reddy KA, Lohray BB, Bhushan V, et al. Novel antidiabetic and hypolipidemic agents. 5. Hydroxyl versus benzyloxy containing chroman derivatives. J Med Chem 1999; 42:3265–78

123. Lefebvre AM, Peinado-Onsurbe J, Leitersdorf I, et al. Regulation of lipoprotein metabolism by thiazolidinediones occurs through a distinct but complementary mechanism relative to fibrates. Arterioscler Thromb Vasc Biol 1997; 17:1756–64

124. Herzig S, Hedrick S, Morantte I, et al. CREB controls hepatic lipid metabolism through nuclear hormone receptor PPAR-gamma. Nature (Lond) 2003; 426:190–3

125. Watkins SM, Reifsnyder PR, Pan HJ, et al. Lipid metabolome-wide effects of the PPARgamma agonist rosiglitazone. J Lipid Res 2002; 43:1809–17

126. Bedoucha M, Atzpodien E, Boelsterli UA. Diabetic KKAy mice exhibit increased hepatic PPARgamma1 gene expression and develop hepatic steatosis upon chronic treatment with antidiabetic thiazolidinediones. J Hepatol 2001; 35:17–23

127. Gavrilova O, Haluzik M, Matsusue K, et al. Liver peroxisome proliferator-activated receptor gamma contributes to hepatic steatosis, triglyceride clearance, and regulation of body fat mass. J Biol Chem 2003; 278:34268–76

128. He W, Barak Y, Hevener A, et al. Adipose-specific peroxisome proliferator-activated receptor gamma knockout causes insulin resistance in fat and liver but not in muscle. Proc Natl Acad Sci USA 2003; 100:15712–17

129. Savage DB, Tan GD, Acerini CL, et al. Human metabolic syndrome resulting from dominant-negative mutations in the nuclear receptor peroxisome proliferator-activated receptor-gamma. Diabetes 2003; 52:910–17

130. Mayerson AB, Hundal RS, Dufour S, et al. The effects of rosiglitazone on insulin sensitivity, lipolysis, and hepatic and skeletal muscle triglyceride content in patients with type 2 diabetes. Diabetes 2002; 51:797–802

131. Carey DG, Cowin GJ, Galloway GJ, et al. Effect of rosiglitazone on insulin sensitivity and body composition in type 2 diabetic patients. Obes Res 2002; 10:1008–15

132. Bajaj M, Suraamornkul S, Pratipanawatr T, et al. Pioglitazone reduces hepatic fat content and augments splanchnic glucose uptake in patients with type 2 diabetes. Diabetes 2003; 52:1364–70

133. Neuschwander-Tetri BA, Brunt EM, Wehmeier KR, et al. Improved nonalcoholic steatohepatitis after 48 weeks of treatment with the PPAR-gamma ligand rosiglitazone. Hepatology 2003; 38:1008–17

134. Neuschwander-Tetri BA, Brunt EM, Wehmeier KR, et al. Interim results of a pilot study demonstrating the early effects of the PPAR-gamma ligand rosiglitazone on insulin sensitivity, aminotransferases, hepatic steatosis and body weight in patients with non-alcoholic steatohepatitis. J Hepatol 2003; 38:434–40

135. Kaplan F, Al-Majali K, Betteridge DJ. PPARS, insulin resistance and type 2 diabetes. J Cardiovasc Risk 2001; 8:211–17

136. Minamikawa J, Tanaka S, Yamauchi M, et al. Potent inhibitory effect of troglitazone on carotid arterial wall thickness in type 2 diabetes. J Clin Endocrinol Metab 1998; 83:1818–20

137. Kipnes MS, Krosnick A, Rendell MS, et al. Pioglitazone hydrochloride in combination with sulfonylurea therapy improves glycemic control in patients with type 2 diabetes mellitus: a randomized,

placebo-controlled study. Am J Med 2001; 111:10–17

138. Gegick CG, Altheimer MD. Comparison of effects of thiazolidinediones on cardiovascular risk factors: observations from a clinical practice. Endocr Pract 2001; 7:162–9

139. Sidhu JS, Kaposzta Z, Markus HS, et al. Effect of rosiglitazone on common carotid intima-media thick-ness progression in coronary artery disease patients without diabetes mellitus. Arterioscler Thromb Vasc Biol 2004; 24:930–4

140. Smith U. Pioglitazone: mechanism of action. Internal J Clin Pract Suppl 2001; 13–18

141. Gale EA. Lessons from the glitazones: a story of drug development. Lancet 2001; 357:1870–5

Adipocytes and their secretory products 14

J.B. Prins

BACKGROUND

History of adipokines

As the prevalence of obesity is at near-epidemic proportions in many societies scientific and medical attention has focused on the fat cell. Traditionally regarded as a cell providing energy storage and insulation, the adipocyte is now recognized to be a complex and metabolically active cell with a prominent endocrine function.[1,2] The adipocyte is highly responsive to central and local signals and nutritional status, and produces a number of proteins and molecules which have autocrine, paracrine and endocrine effects. These molecules are collectively known as adipokines.

The existence of adipokines has been postulated for decades,[3] and then the discovery of leptin in 1994[4] set in train a remarkable era of research and discovery that has completely changed our understanding of, and approach to, adipose cells and adipose tissue. This research effort shows no signs of abating, encouraged by both an intense scientific interest in a completely 'new' endocrine organ – adipose tissue – and by the need for treatments for obesity and its related metabolic disorders.

For both the researcher in the field and for interested onlookers, this era of discovery has been exciting and impressive in its pace. From the initial discovery of each adipokine to the stage of establishing a reasonable understanding of its role, regulation and effects has sometimes taken only months. Whilst we still lack an overall understanding of the adipokine system and network, significant patterns are now emerging regarding the secretory aspects of adipose tissue.

Adipokines and the metabolic syndrome

A major reason for the intense research interest in adipokines is their likely role as mediators of the metabolic syndrome.[5–7] It is now clear that dysregulation of adipokine production occurs in obesity, and that the altered adipokine milieu underpins, at a biochemical level, the insulin resistance and cardiovascular and metabolic abnormalities that characterize the syndrome. The question still remains as to which occurs first – the adipokine dysregulation or the obesity? The observation that abnormalities in adipokine production seen in obesity can be largely reversed with weight loss argues that obesity may be the primary problem. However recent data indicating roles for adipokines in appetite and metabolic rate regulation suggest that inherited 'abnormalities' in adipokine production (which may be evolutionarily advantageous) may be the fundamental defect, only expressed in settings of positive energy balance. It is remarkable that most identified adipokines appear to have some relationship with the metabolic syndrome. It is as yet unclear whether this is indeed the case, or whether it is a bias produced by experimental approaches based on metabolic syndrome or obesity models.

Adipokine regulation: evolutionary and genetic aspects

Whilst much adipokine research is centred on obesity models, from an evolutionary point of view, many adipokines are starvation molecules.[8,9] Indeed, the levels of obesity seen today (and represented by some animal models) have a very short history and are unlikely to have significantly impacted on the genome. For example, leptin was touted as an obesity hormone immediately after its discovery. As further research was undertaken it has become apparent that its major role is to signal that sufficient energy stores exist to allow reproduction.[8,9] It is now no surprise to researchers that the regulation and function of leptin are impaired in obese states, and similar patterns of regulation are recognized much more quickly in the newly discovered adipokines.

The corollary to this is that the fundamental function of many adipokines is to maximize weight gain. For millennia this was an essential system for survival and those with the most 'active' adipokine system survived best in situations of low food availability. In our current situation of excess food availability in many societies, this metabolic efficiency has driven the obesity epidemic. The discovery of adipokines has afforded some insight into the mediators of this 'thrifty genotype'.

We still understand little about the diversity of body weight, and why some individuals remain lean in situations of energy excess and vice versa. Very lean individuals remain little studied, but will reveal insights into energy homeostasis and adipokine regulation. Twin and other studies demonstrate clearly a substantial inheritability of body weight and metabolic dysfunction,[10–13] but in very few individuals can this be explained on the basis of single-gene defects. The single-gene defects leading to obesity or the metabolic syndrome are often of adipokine genes, and have provided superb insight into adipokine physiology.[14]

Adipokines and medical therapy

The strong relationship between adipokine dysregulation and metabolic dysfunction provides clearly identified targets and opportunities for therapeutic intervention. These opportunities have attracted scientists and pharmaceutical companies to the research area with a resultant rapid advance in understanding. To date, however, strategies to block the action or reduce expression of over-produced adipokines have had little impact on metabolic dysfunction in man,[15] despite, in some instances, promising results in murine models. Such results have re-affirmed the complexity of metabolic regulation, and have also led to the identification of important differences between man and other species and recognition of the need for good experimental models.

ADIPOKINES

Adipocyte secretory products include hormones, cytokines, growth factors and fats, leading to the adoption of the 'umbrella' term – adipokine. In this chapter, adipokines are grouped based on their putative major function, but it is apparent that most adipokines have multiple roles. In many instances, the major function is controversial or unclear, and may also change according to the body weight of the subject. For example, in starvation, leptin has a metabolic role, signalling to the hypothalamus that energy stores are low and thus stimulating appetite and suppressing ovulation. In the setting of obesity, these functions of leptin are superfluous, and prominent functions now include deleterious effects on the vasculature and glucose homeostasis.

'Metabolic' adipokines

Leptin

The discovery of leptin,[4] first postulated decades before, began the current era of intense research into adipose tissue as an endocrine organ. It is still regarded as the prototypical adipokine whose secretion is normal at normal body weight but is abnormal in situations of either decreased[16] or increased fat stores.[1]

Leptin is secreted almost exclusively by adipocytes and acts via a family of plasma membrane receptors.[17,18] The functional long form of the receptor (Ob-Rb) is expressed in several sites in the hypothalamus and brainstem[19] and signals via the STAT-3 pathway to alter expression of a number of genes involved in energy homeostasis.[20,21] Leptin receptors are also expressed in many peripheral tissues[22-33] and leptin appears to have actions in adipose tissue, skeletal muscle and the pancreas. Regulation of energy balance appears to be through both central mechanisms[34] (appetite and metabolic rate) and peripheral mechanisms (activation of 5'-AMP-activated protein kinase (AMPK) expression in muscle and liver).[35] In addition to regulation of energy balance, leptin has important roles in fertility (outlined above)[36-39] and immune function as the immunosuppression seen in starvation or nutrient deprivation appears due to leptin deficiency.[40,41]

Circulating concentrations of leptin are proportional to fat mass, but the fact that the high leptin levels in obesity do not suppress appetite indicates that leptin resistance may be a fundamental pathology in obesity.[32,33] This resistance is in part due to impaired transport of leptin into the cerebrospinal fluid, and in part due to reduced activation at the target tissue level.

The importance of normal leptin levels is elegantly demonstrated by the rare individuals with leptin deficiency and their response to leptin replacement therapy, with virtual normalization of extreme metabolic dysfunction.[14,42,43] In contrast, trials of leptin supplementation in obese humans have shown considerably less promise.[44]

Adiponectin

Adiponectin (AdipQ, Acrp30, apMl) is secreted exclusively by adipocytes and, in contrast to leptin, circulating levels are inversely proportional to fat mass.[45,46] Serum levels are very high (3–30 nM) and, like leptin, are 2–3-fold higher in females than in males.[6] Adiponectin has roles in glucose and lipid homeostasis[5–7,47,48] and as an anti-atherogenic protein.[7]

Adiponectin is a prototypical adipokine involved in the 'cross-talk' between insulin target tissues.[49] This cross-talk is demonstrated by the FIRKO mouse, which lacks adipose tissue insulin receptors, has low adiponectin levels and is insulin resistant in muscle and liver.[50] Adiponectin has a major role to enhance hepatic insulin sensitivity, and the fall in adiponectin levels with weight gain appears responsible for associated hepatic insulin resistance and non-suppression of hepatic glucose output. With weight loss, the rise in adiponectin levels correlates strongly with the return of insulin sensitivity.[6]

Adiponectin expression is increased by PPAR-γ agonists such as thiazolidinediones and this function may be central to their efficacy as insulin sensitizers[5,51,52] Additionally, the decreased adiponectin seen in obesity may mediate the enhanced adipocyte TNF-α production, postulated to underpin the insulin resistance.[5]

In mice, recombinant adiponectin decreases hepatic gluconeogenesis by reducing expression of phosphoenolpyruvate carboxykinase (PEPCK). Adiponectin also reduces lipid accumulation in non-adipose tissues via activation of AMPK.[6] Adiponectin actions are mediated by the receptors AdipoR1 and AdipoR2.[53] These findings indicate substantial promise for adiponectin as a therapeutic agent in patients with the metabolic syndrome.

Free fatty acids

Free, or non-esterified, fatty acids are a mechanism for energy transport and redistribution.[54] They are derived from diet, hepatic synthesis and lipolysis, dependent on nutritional status and acute energy balance. Because lipolysis is a major source of free fatty acids (FFAs) (especially in obesity), these molecules are regarded as adipokines. The major regulators of FFA concentration are catecholamines (favouring lipolysis) and insulin (favouring lipogenesis, which is essentially triglyceride re-esterification). Obesity is a state of high catecholamine levels and insulin resistance and the net effect of these abnormalities, plus ongoing positive energy balance, leads to increase FFA concentrations in the circulation.

Increased FFA concentrations lead to further metabolic dysfunction through effects to decrease insulin production[55,56] and to impair insulin action[57] leading to reduced insulin-stimulated glucose uptake. It is clear that all FFA are not alike, with some providing metabolic benefit. This benefit, particularly with respect to insulin sensitivity, may be due to alterations in plasma membrane fluidity or may be due to particular FFA (or metabolites) activating members of the PPAR family of transcription factors.[58,59]

Steroid hormones

Adipocytes have an important role in steroid hormone metabolism, and there has been much recent emphasis on this role in the development of the metabolic syndrome.

Adipocytes express the enzyme 11β-hydroxysteroid dehydrogenase (11β-HSD) which converts circulating inactive cortisone to the active hormone cortisol, thus regulating adipose tissue (and perhaps systemic) corticosteroid concentrations.[60] Adipose tissue corticosteroid produced by this reaction could then promote pre-adipocyte replication and differentiation, thus promoting obesity, and contribute to insulin resistance. Observations in support of this theory are that 11β-HSD activity is greater in omental adipose tissue and dysregulated in obesity.[60,61] Compelling supporting data come from transgenic studies in which mice overexpressing 11β-HSD demonstrate features of the metabolic syndrome[62] whilst the 11β-HSD knockout mouse is relatively protected from metabolic dysfunction.[63] Further evidence defining the importance of the 11β-HSD system will come from clinical trials of the 11β-HSD inhibitors under development by many groups.

Adipocytes also have an important role in sex-steroid metabolism. Androgens are converted to oestrogens in fat by a cytochrome P450-dependent aromatase. This reaction is the major source of oestrogens in men and post-menopausal women, and a significant contributor in pre-menopausal women. Additionally, adipose tissue 17β-hydroxysteroid oxidoreductase converts oestrone to oestradiol and androstenedione (from the adrenal) to testosterone. In obesity there is increased net sex steroid interconversion which may contribute to the metabolic syndrome and to regulation of adipose tissue distribution.[1]

'Vascular' adipokines

The relationship between the microvasculature within adipose tissue and adipose cell growth and activity has been an active area of research for some time. This relates to the observation that (sometimes enormous) change in fat mass must be accompanied by a similar change in vasculature.[64] It is unclear which comes first. In settings of positive energy balance, an obvious sequence of events is that the need for lipid storage drives increase in size and number of adipocytes, which in turn signals growth in the vasculature.[65] This possibility is supported by the identification of pro-vascularization adipokines. The alternative possibility is that neo-vascularization occurs first, with the microvasculature then signalling adipogenesis.[66] This is supported by observations that anti-angiogenic drugs can cause weight loss[66] and that adipose-tissue-derived microvascular endothelial cells produce factors that promote human pre-adipocyte replication.[67]

Adipokines that promote vascular growth

Monobutyrin is a pro-angiogenic lipid that may promote expansion of the microvasculature during adipose tissue growth.[68] Angiopoietin-1 is produced by adipocytes and endothelial cells and expression is altered in settings of adipose tissue growth and regression.[69] A number of groups have presented evidence that vascular endothelial growth factor (VEGF) is an adipokine involved in neo-vascularization, and that the relationship may be reciprocal.[70] This importance of the relationship is confirmed by the demonstration that blocking VEGF receptors inhibits adipose tissue development in vivo.[71]

Hormones of the renin–angiotensin–aldosterone system

Adipose tissue synthesizes all components of the renin–angiotensin–aldosterone system (RAAS) and expresses angiotensin II receptors.[72] Adipose tissue angiotensinogen production is increased by overnutrition and insulin, suggesting that overactivity of the RAAS may be a link between obesity and hypertension.[73] Angiotensin II increases lipogenesis[74] in human adipocytes and promotes pre-adipocyte differentiation,[72] suggesting a role for the RAAS in regulation of body weight. The RAAS has also been implicated in the development of myocardial dysfunction and hence may have a role in the development of the cardiomyopathy commonly seen in obesity and diabetes.[75]

Plasminogin activator inhibitor-1

Plasminogin activator inhibitor-1 (PAI-1) is a major anti-fibrinolytic protein produced by liver and fat. Circulating levels of PAI-1 are increased in obesity and PAI-1 production is greater in omental than subcutaneous adipose tissue,[76] suggesting a link between adipose tissue PAI-1 production and the cardiovascular disease component of the metabolic syndrome.[7] PAI-1 appears to be involved in the pathogenesis of cardiovascular disease as levels are increased in association with myocardial infarction and venous thrombosis.[1] PAI-1 production by adipocytes is increased by insulin, glucose and corticosteroids and decreased by thiazolidinediones.[77–79] It is also possible that statin therapy lowers PAI-1.[7] Increased PAI-1 levels also predict type 2 diabetes and are a core feature of the insulin resistance syndrome.

'Immune' adipokines

Adipsin (complement factor D) was one of the first recognized[80] adipokines and is now but one of a large group of 'immune' or 'inflammatory' compounds recognized to be produced by fat.[81] Many of these adipokines have purported metabolic function in addition to their immune role as most cause insulin resistance in vitro or, when overexpressed, in vivo. Debate continues as to their true role in adipose tissue, and this debate has been accelerated by the identification of C-reactive protein (CRP) as a risk factor for cardiovascular disease.[6] It has been recently proposed that 'immune' adipokines may contribute to the elevated CRP seen in obesity and the metabolic syndrome. This family of adipokines has increased production in obesity, with return toward normal levels with weight loss.[6] In health, it appears that adipose tissue is a significant contributor to circulating levels of most of these compounds. All are also produced by immune tissues and levels seen in inflammation far exceed those seen in (even morbid) obesity.

Tumour necrosis factor alpha

Tumour necrosis factor alpha (TNF-α) is produced by lymphoid cells, skeletal muscle and fat cells, and is a postulated 'link' between obesity and type 2 diabetes.[82–86] This postulate is based on observations that TNF-α knockout mice are relatively protected from obesity-related diabetes,[87] and anti-TNF-α strategies have been shown to ameliorate diabetes in obese animals.[84]

Adipose tissue and circulating TNF-α levels are increased in obese animals and humans, and these levels tend to normalize with weight loss.[88] In several studies, change in insulin sensitivity parallels the change in TNF-α level. TNF-α disrupts insulin signalling at a number of levels, including the insulin receptor, IRS-1 and GLUT 4.[85,89–95] Despite these findings, few data have been published showing TNF-α-induced inhibition of glucose uptake in insulin-responsive tissues. Of importance, effective anti-TNF-α strategies have no effect on glucose homeostasis in humans with type 2 diabetes.[96,97]

TNF-α has also been proposed to have a role in the regulation of adipose tissue mass. It impairs human pre-adipocyte differentiation in vitro,[98] and induces apoptosis of human pre-adipocytes and adipocytes in vitro.[99] It also induces lipolysis,[100,101] so TNF-α may have a net role in reducing adipose tissue mass. This would certainly be logical in an evolutionary sense, as it would serve to mobilize energy in settings of inflammation.

Overall, despite the wealth of data about TNF-α as a key adipokine, currently available evidence does not strongly support a role for TNF-α as underpinning the metabolic syndrome in man.

Interleukin 6

Interleukin-6 (IL-6) is a potent anti-inflammatory cytokine which also has endocrine actions.[2,102] These include postulated roles in glucose and lipid metabolism.[5] Like TNF-α, circulating IL-6 levels and production by adipose tissue are increased in obesity and fall with weight loss.[103] In health, adipose tissue is a major source of circulating IL-6. IL-6 production is greater in omental than subcutaneous fat, and this may be relevant to the metabolic syndrome.[104] IL-6 has a postulated role in the development of vascular disease in obesity.[7] IL-6 knockout mice have altered appetite and energy expenditure and IL-6 is produced in the hypothalamus.[105] These findings suggest a broader role for IL-6 than TNF-α in energy metabolism.

Complement pathway components

Complement factors B, C3 and D (adipsin) are produced by adipose tissue.[81] Adipsin was the first adipokine identified[80] and a potential metabolic role was suggested by the observation that adipsin levels were decreased in murine obese models.[106] Subsequent human studies demonstrated the opposite – that adipsin expression is increased in obesity and with feeding and reduced in cachexia, lipodystrophy and fasting.[107]

In recent years it has been postulated that the metabolic role for factors B, C3 and adipsin as adipokines is through the formation of acyla-tion-stimulating protein (ASP).[108] ASP level increases post-prandially and is involved in the stimulus and storage of triglycerides.[109] ASP knockout animals are lean and have high post-prandial FFA levels and increased metabolic rate,[110] but humans with adipsin deficiency have no obvious metabolic derangement and are normal weight.[111]

RELATIONSHIP OF ADIPOKINES TO THE METABOLIC SYNDROME

Overall, the relationship of adipokines to the metabolic syndrome remains one of correlation, rather than cause–effect. It is becoming clear that murine models of obesity do not truly reflect the obese human state. For example, the ob/ob mouse allowed facilitated identification of leptin and provided enormous amounts of data and impetus to obesity research. However, the leptin-deficient mouse differs significantly from the leptin-deficient humans described to date, the former displaying decreased metabolic rate and skeletal and muscle abnormalities not prominent in the humans.[42] Also, transgenic studies provide valuable clues and suggestions as to the roles of adipokines, but do not necessarily provide key data of relevance to the 'average' obese man or woman. This is exemplified by the TNF-α studies, which demonstrate efficacy of anti-TNF-α strategies in mice with the metabolic syndrome, whilst identical strategies in man are ineffective.

The fundamental issue is that prolonged overfeeding induces obesity which, in evolutionary terms, is an abnormal state. Strategies utilized by adipose tissue in settings of starvation are ill developed in obesity and hence are dysregulated. This concept is exemplified by leptin and adiponectin. In starvation, leptin levels are low, signalling to the hypothalamus to both increase feeding behavior and suppress ovulation – strategies of clear survival advantage. Similarly, adiponectin levels are high, maximizing insulin sensitivity to promote energy storage and utilization. In obesity, these actions of leptin and adiponectin are not needed for survival, so appropriate regulatory mechanisms are not in place.

It seems likely that obesity drives abnormal adipokine production and this, in turn, contributes to the many facets of the metabolic syndrome. It is unclear whether inherited perturbations in adipokine production might underlie the metabolic syndrome. In some ways it is surprising that numerous large-scale genetics studies have failed to show clear evidence for adipokine sequence variations as potential causes of the metabolic syndrome. On the other hand, this could be expected in view of the fact that the metabolic syndrome is so common, and is quite a subtle disorder, taking many decades to develop in most instances. It seems certain that the metabolic syndrome is a multi-gene disorder.[112] Future large-scale genetic studies with extensive phenotyping and genotyping may indeed unravel and identify contributory mutations.

A further layer of complexity is the inter-relationship between many of the adipokines. If alteration in the production or action of one adipokine was the primary event (which seems unlikely), this could lead to abnormalities of expression or function in many of the others. It may therefore be unrealistic to expect that therapeutic modulation of a single adipokine would be efficacious in the metabolic syndrome.

REGULATION OF KEY ADIPOKINE PRODUCTION

A number of regulators of adipokine production have been identified. This section will concentrate on acute regulation, as opposed to defining the relationship between fat mass and adipokine production, which is detailed in the sections above. Adipokine production is regulated acutely by both nutritional status and a number of drugs, as well as by other adipokines.

Leptin

Feeding has an obvious effect to reduce appetite and this may in part be due to stimulation of leptin expression.[1] In contrast, food deprivation in the mouse and man is associated with an acute fall in leptin expression.[5,113,114] These observations are consistent with the appetite-suppressive effects of the adipokine. Leptin expression is reduced by thiazolinedione (TZDs) and β-agonists and increased by insulin and glucocorticoids.[5,115] These observations are consistent with the appetite-suppressive effects of the adipokine. Weight loss induced by lifestyle intervention induces a fall in leptin,[116] but this may simply reflect the reduction in fat mass. Insulin is a potent acute regulator of leptin expression and may mediate the post-prandial changes seen.[21] It is not clear whether the hyperinsulinaemia seen in obesity or the metabolic syndrome underlies the relationship between leptin levels and fat mass.

Adiponectin

Adiponectin expression is reduced in fasting and restored by refeeding.[5,114] This may be due to an effect of the stomach-derived peptide, ghrelin, to suppress adiponectin expression.[117] TZDs have been shown by many groups to increase adiponectin expression and this may be a significant contributor to their efficacy as insulin sensitizers.[51,52] Interestingly, this effect may be depot-specific, with a greater adiponectin response in omental, compared to subcutaneous, adipose tissue.[52] Of further therapeutic interest, adiponectin expression is increased by blockade of the RAS with either angiotensin-converting enzyme inhibitor or angiotensin II receptor blockade.[118] Of interest, exercise does not alter adiponectin expression despite significant promotion of insulin sensitivity.[116,119] In contrast to leptin, adiponectin expression is decreased by insulin and glucocorticoids,[5] perhaps explaining the decrease in adiponectin levels seen in obese, insulin-resistant subjects.

POTENTIAL FOR ADIPOKINE-BASED MEDICAL THERAPIES

As outlined above, the relationship between metabolic dysfunction and altered adipokine levels is now well established. The opportunity is thus provided for therapeutic interventions aimed at normalizing adipokine levels and hence improving metabolic dysfunction. At a superficial level, strategies to increase leptin in obesity with a view to suppressing appetite or increasing adiponectin levels to improve insulin sensitivity would seem likely to be successful. However, the complexities of the regulatory systems mean that such simplistic strategies are not always efficacious. On a more positive note, such therapeutic attempts have increased our understanding of the metabolic roles of adipokines.

Another important consideration is that the underlying reason for adipokine dysregulation may in itself make therapy ineffective. An example is seen with insulin therapy in type 2 diabetes, where progressively larger doses of insulin are needed to overcome the insulin resistance – the basic initial abnormality.

Leptin therapy has been trialled in obesity with disappointing results. The leptin 'resistance' of obesity necessitates high dosage, and this in turn leads to increased insulin resistance with little reduction in appetite or weight. Current strategies are aimed at developing receptor-specific leptin analogues in an effort to improve the efficacy/adverse effect ratio.

Adiponectin has obvious therapeutic potential with the theoretical attraction of being a 'replacement' therapy rather than a supplementation to supra-physiological concentrations. If effective, adiponectin therapy could induce insulin sensitivity, improve lipids and decrease vascular inflammation. Such strategies are effective in rodent models with evident significant side-effects. A potential concern is that significant improvement in insulin sensitivity may induce weight gain, but this is not apparent in animal studies published to date.

Strategies to reduce circulating levels of immune adipokines are also theoretically attractive. Anti-TNF-α therapeutics are effective in rheumatoid arthritis and Crohn's disease in man, and in murine models have efficacy in type 2 diabetes. In human trials, however, similar agents do not alter insulin sensitivity or weight. The reason for this species specificity of effect is not clear. Strategies to reduce levels of IL-6 or PAI-1 may also be of benefit in reducing insulin resistance and vascular disease. The potential problem with such interventions is the risk of compromising the immune response, with consequent increased risk of infection, autoimmunity and malignancy.

As outlined above, corticosteroids are implicated in many aspects of the metabolic syndrome. Many companies have inhibitors of 11β-HSD in development with the promise of reducing adipose tissue and possibly systemic corticosteroid levels. The advantage of this strategy over, for example, corticosteroid receptor blockers is that the stress response is unlikely to be significantly compromised.

The development of effective therapeutic interventions based on the adipokine system is completely reliant on a sound and detailed understanding of the (patho)-physiology of the system in sickness and in health. At the current rate of research progress, such understanding will be rapidly obtained, and it is hoped that effective therapies will result in the near future.

References

1. Ahima RS, Flier J. Adipose tissue as an endocrine organ. Trends Endocrinol Metab 2000; 11:327–9
2. Mohamed-Ali V, Pinkney J, Coppack AW. Adipose tissue as an endocrine and paracrine organ. Int J Obesity 1998; 22:1145–58
3. Coleman DL. Effects of parabiosis of obese with diabetes and normal mice. Diabetologia 1973; 9:294–8
4. Zhang Y, Proenca R, Maffei M, et al. Positional cloning of the mouse obese gene and its human homologue. Nature 1994; 372:425–32
5. Fasshauer M, Paschke R. Regulation of adipocytokines and insulin resistance. Diabetologia 2003
6. Rajala M, Scherer P. Minireview: The adipocyte – at the crossroads of energy homeostasis, inflammation, and athersclerosis. Endocrinology 2003; 144:3765–73

7. Lyon C, Law R, Hsueh WA. Minireview: Adiposity, inflammation and atherogenesis. Endocrinology 2003; 144:2195–200

8. Ahima RS, Prabakaran D, Mantzoros C, et al. Role of leptin in the neuroendocrine response to fasting. Nature 1996; 382:250–2

9. Flier JS. What's in a name? In search of leptin's physiological role. J Clin Endocrinol Metab 1998; 83:1407–13

10. Borjesson M. The aetiology of obesety in children. A study of 101 twin pairs. Acta Paediatr Scand 1976; 65:279–87

11. Bouchard C, Tremblay A, Depr,s J-P, et al. Overfeeding in identical twins: 5–tear postoverfeeding results. Metabolism 1996; 45:1042–50

12. Carey D, Campbell L, Chisholm D, et al. Genetic influences on central abdominal fat: a twin study. Int J Obesity (Suppl) 1994; 18 (Supp 2):116

13. Mauriege P, Depres J-P, Marcotte M, et al. Adipose tissue lipolysis after long-term overfeeding in identical twins. Int J Obesity 1992; 16:219–25

14. O'Rahilly S, Farooqi IS, Yeo GSH, et al. Minireview: human obesity—lessons from monogenic disorders. Endocrinology 2003; 144:3757–64

15. Lee DW, Leinung MC, Rozhavskaya-Arena M, et al. Leptin and the treatment of obesity: its current status. Eur J Pharmacol 2002; 440:129–39

16. Oral E, Simha V, Ruiz E, et al. Leptin-replacement therapy for lipodystrophy. N Engl J Med 2002; 346:570–2

17. Tartaglia LA. The leptin receptor. J Biol Chem 1997; 272:6093–6

18. Tartaglia LA, Dembski M, Weng X, et al. Identification and expression cloning of a leptin receptor, OB-R. Cell 1995; 83:1263–71

19. Lynn RB, Cao G-Y, Considine RV, et al. Autoradiographic localization of leptin binding in the choroid plexus of {Iob/ob} and {Idb/db} mice. Biochem Biophys Res Commun 1996; 219:884–9

20. White DW, Kuropatwinski KK, Devos R, et al. Leptin receptor (OB-R) signalling. J Biol Chem 1997; 272:4065–71

21. Zigman JM, Elmquist JK. Minireview: From anorexia to obesity—the yin and yang of body weight control. Endocrinology 2003; 144:3749–56

22. Wang Y, Kuropatwinski KKK, White DW, et al. Leptin receptor action in hepatic cells. J Biol Chem 1997; 272:16216–23

23. Serradeil-Le Gal C, Raufaste D, Brossard G, et al. Characterization and localization of leptin receptors in the kidney. FEBS Lett 1997; 404:185–91

24. Hoggard N, Mercer JG, Rayner DV, et al. Localization of leptin receptor mRNA splice variants in murine peripheral tissues by RT-PCR and {in situ} hybridization. Biochem Biophys Res Commun 1997; 232:383–7

25. Cao G-Y, Considine RV, Lynn RB. Leptin receptors in the adrenal medulla of the rat. Am J Physiol 1997; 273:E448–52

26. Walder K, Filippis A, Clark S, et al. Leptin inhibits insulin binding in isolated rat adipocytes. J Endocrinol 1997; 155:R5–7

27. Karlsson C, Lindell K, Svensson E, et al. Expression of functional leptin receptors in the human ovary. J Clin Endocrinol Metab 1997; 82:4144–8

28. Lostao MP, Urdaneta E, Martinez-Ans¢ E, et al. Presence of leptin receptors in rat small intestine and leptin effect on sugar absorption. FEBS Lett 1998; 423:302–6

29. Wang M-Y, Zhou YT, Newgard CB, et al. A novel leptin receptor isoform in rat. FEBS Lett 1996; 392:87–90

30. Kieffer TJ, Heller RS, Habener JF. Leptin receptors expressed on pancreatic á-cells. Biochem Biophys Res Commun 1996; 224:522–7

31. Emilsson V, Liu Y-L, Cawthorne MS, et al. Expression of the functional leptin receptor mRNA in pancreatic islets and direct inhibitory action of leptin on insulin secretion. Diabetes 1997; 46:313–16

32. El-Haschimi K, Pierroz D, Hileman S, et al. Two defects contribute to hypothalamic leptin resistance in mice with diet-induced obesity. J Clin Invest 2000; 105:1827–32

33. Bjírb'k C, Elmquist JK, Frantz JD, et al. Identification of SOCS-3 as a potential mediator of central leptin resistance. Mol Cell 1998; 1:619–25

34. White DW, Tartaglia LA. Leptin and OB-R: body weight regulation by a cytokine receptor. Cytokine Growth Fact Rev 1997; 7:303–9

35. Minokoshi Y, Kim YB, Peroni OD, et al. Leptin stimulates fatty-acid oxidation by activating AMP-activated protein kinase. Nature 2002; 415:268–9

36. Barash IA, Cheung CC, Weigle DS, et al. Leptin is a metabolic signal to the reproductive system. Endocrinology 1996; 137:3144–7

37. Mounzih K, Lu R, Chehab FF. Leptin treatment rescues the sterility of genetically obese {lob/ob} males. Endocrinology 1997; 138:1190–3

38. Hamilton BS. A new role for a fat actor. Nature Med 1996; 2:272–3

39. Chehab FF, Lim ME, Lu R. Correction of the sterility defect in homozygous obese female mice by treatment with the human recombinant leptin. Nature Genet 1996; 12:318–20

40. Farooqi IS, Matarese G, Lord GM, et al. Beneficial effects of leptin on obesity, T cell hyporesponsiveness, and neuroendocrine/metabolic dysfunction of human congenital leptin deficiency. J Clin Invest 2002; 110:1093–103

41. Lord GM, Matarese G, Howard JK, et al. Leptin modulates the T-cell immune response and reverses starvation-induced immunosuppression. Nature 1998; 394:897–901

42. Montague CT, Farooqi IS, Whitehead JP, et al. Congenital leptin deficiency is associated with severe early-onset obesity in humans. Nature 1997; 387:903–8

43. Farooqi I, Jebb SA, Langmack G, et al. Effects of

recombinant leptin therapy in a child with congenital leptin deficiency. N Engl J Med 1999; 341:879–84

44. Heymsfield S, Greenberg A, Fujioka K, et al. Recombinant leptin for weight loss in obese and lean adults: a randomized, controlled, dose-escalation trial. JAMA 2000; 283:1567–8

45. Hu E, Liang P, Spiegelman BM. AdipoQ is a novel adipose-specific gene dysregulated in obesity. J Biol Chem 1996; 271:10697–703

46. Arita Y, Kihara S, Ouchi N, et al. Paradoxical decrease on an adipose-specific protein, adiponectin, in obesity. Biochem Biophys Res Commun 1999; 257:79–83

47. Combs T, Berg A, Obici S, et al. Endogenous glucose production is inhibited by the adipose-derived protein Acrp30. J Clin Invest 2001; 108:1875–81

48. Berg A, Combs T, Scherer P. ACRP30/adiponectin: an adipokine regulating glucose and lipid metabolism. Trends Endocrinol Metab 2002; 13:84–9

49. Berg A, Combs T, Du X, et al. The adipocyte-secreted protein Acrp30 enhances hepatic insulin action. Nature Med 2001; 7:947–53

50. Bluher M, Michael M, Peroni O, et al. Adipose tissue selective insulin receptor knockout protects against obesity and obesity-related glucose intolerance. Develop Cell 2002; 3:25–38

51. Hirose H, Kawai T, Yamamoto Y, et al. Effects of pioglitazone on metabolic parameters, body fat distribution, and serum adiponectin levels in Japanese male patients with type 2 diabetes*1. Metabolism 2002; 51:314–17

52. Motoshima H, Wu X, Sinha MK, et al. Differential regulation of adiponectin secretion from cultured human omental and subcutaneous adipocytes: effects of insulin and rosiglitazone. J Clin Endocrinol Metab 2002; 87:5662–7

53. Yamauchi T, Kamon J, Ito Y, et al. Cloning of adiponectin receptors that mediate antidiabetic metabolic effects. Nature 2003; 423:762–9

54. Kraegan E, Cooney GJ. The role of free fatty acids in muscle insulin resistance. In: Marshall S, Home P, Rizza R, eds. The Diabetes Annual 12. Amsterdam: Elsevier, 1999: 141–60

55. Bollheimer LC, Skelly RH, Chester MW, et al. Chronic exposure to free fatty acid reduces pancreatic β cell insulin content by increasing basal insulin secretion that is not compensated for by a corresponding increase in proinsulin biosynthesis translation. J Clin Invest 1998; 101:1094–101

56. Dobbins RL, Chester MW, Stevenson BE, et al. A fatty acid-dependent step is critically important for both glucose- and non-glucose stimulated insulin secretion. J Clin Invest 1998; 101:2370–6

57. Storlein LH, Kriketos AD, Calvert GD, et al. Fatty acids, triglycerides and syndromes of insulin resistance. Prost Leuk Ess Fatty Acids 1997; 57:379–85

58. Kliewer SA, Sundseth SS, Jones SA, et al. Fatty acids and eicosanoids regulate gene expression through direct interactions with peroxisome proliferator-activated receptors α and γ. Proc Natl Acad Sci USA 1997; 94:4318–23

59. Forman BM, Chen J, Evans RM. Hypolipidemic drugs, polyunsaturated fatty acids, and eicosanoids are ligands for peroxisome proliferator-activated receptors α and γ. Proc Natl Acad Sci USA 1997; 94:4312–17

60. Stewart P, Boulton A, Kumar S, et al. Cortisol metabolism in human obesity: impaired cortisone to cortisol conversion in subjects with central adiposity. J Clin Endocrinol Metab 1999; 84:1022–7

61. Bujalska I, Kumar S, Stewart PM. Does central obesity reflect 'Cushing's disease of the omentum'? Lancet 1997; 349:1210–13

62. Masuzaki H, Paterson J, Shinyama H, et al. A transgenic model of visceral obesity and the metabolic syndrome. Science 2001; 294:2166–70

63. Kotelevtsev Y, Holmes MC, Burchell A, et al. 11beta-Hydroxysteroid dehydrogenase type 1 knockout mice show attenuated glucocorticoid-inducible responses and resist hyperglycemia on obesity or stress. Proc Natl Acad Sci USA 1997; 94:14924–9

64. Ailhaud G, Grimaldi P, Negrel J. Cellular and molecular aspects of adipose tissue development. Ann Rev Nutr 1992; 12:207–33

65. Prins JB, O'Rahilly S. Regulation of adipose cell number in man. Clin Sci 1997; 92:3–11

66. Rupnick MA, Panigrahy D, Zhang C-Y, et al. From the cover: adipose tissue mass can be regulated through the vasculature. Proc Natl Acad Sci USA 2002; 99:10730–5

67. Hutley L, Herington A, Shurety W, et al. Human adipose tissue endothelial cells promote preadipocyte proliferation. Am J Physiol Endocrinol Metab 2001; 281:E1037–44

68. Wilkison W, Spiegelman B. Biosynthesis of the vasoactive lipid monobutyrin. Central role of diacylglycerol. J Biol Chem 1993; 268:2844–9

69. Dallabrida SM, Zurakowski D, Shih S-C, et al. Adipose tissue growth and regression are regulated by angiopoietin-1. Biochem Biophys Res Commun 2003; 311:563–71

70. Fukumura D, Ushiyama A, Duda DG, et al. Paracrine regulation of angiogenesis and adipocyte differentiation during in vivo adipogenesis. Circ Res 2003; 93:88–97

71. Shibuya M. VEGF-receptor inhibitors for anti-angiogenesis. Folia Pharmacol Jap 2003; 122:498–503

72. Karlsson C, Lindell K, Ottosson M, et al. Human adipose tissue expresses angiotensinogen and enzymes required for its conversion to angiotensin II. J Clin Endocrinol Metab 1998; 83:3925–9

73. Frederich RC, Kahn B, Peach M, et al. Tissue-specific nutritional regulation of angiotensinogen in adipose tissue. Hypertension 1992; 19:339–44

74. Jones BH, Standridge MK, Moustaid N. Angiotensin II increases lipogenesis in 3T3-L1 and human adipose cells. Endocrinology 1997; 138:1512–19

75. Malik F, Lavie C, Mehra M, et al. Renin–angiotensin system: genes to bedside. Am Heart J 1998; 136:562–3

76. Shimomura I, Funahashi T, Takahashi M, et al. Enhanced expression of PAI-1 in visceral fat: possible contributor to vascular disease in obesity. Nature Med 1994; 2:800–3

77. Morange P-E, Aubert J, Pieretti F, et al. Glucocorticoids and insulin promote plasminogen activator inhibitor 1 production by human adipose tissue. Diabetes 1999; 48:890–5

78. Marx N, Bourcier T, Sukhova G, et al. PPARγ activation in human endothelial cells increases plasminogen activator inhibitor type-1 expression. Thromb Vasc Biol 1999; 19:546–51

79. He G, Bruun JM, Lihn AS, et al. Stimulation of PAI-1 and adipokines by glucose in human adipose tissue in vitro. Biochem Biophys Res Commun 2003; 310:878–83

80. Flier JS, Cook KS, Usher P, et al. Severely impaired adipsin expression in genetic and acquired obesity. Science 1987; 237:405–8

81. Choy LN, Rosen BS, Spiegelman BM. Adipsin and an endogenous pathway of complement from adipose cells. J Biol Chem 1992; 267:12736–41

82. Hotamisligil GS, Arner P, Caro JF, et al. Increased adipose tissue expression of tumor necrosis factor-α in human obesity and insulin resistance. J Clin Invest 1995; 95:2409–15

83. Hotamisligil GS, Peraldi P, Spiegelman BM. The molecular link between obesity and diabetes. Curr Opin Endocrinol Diabetes 1996; 3:16–23

84. Hotamisligil GS, Shargill NS, Spiegelman BM. Adipose expression of tumor necrosis factor-α: direct role in obesity-linked insulin resistance. Science 1993; 259:87–91

85. Hotamisligil GS, Spiegelman BM. Tumor necrosis factor alpha: a key component of the obesity-diabetes link. Diabetes 1994; 43:1271–8

86. Jequier E. A metabolic perspective on the interaction between obesity and diabetes. Curr Opin Endocrinol Diabetes 1996; 3:10–15

87. Uysal KT, Wiesbrock SM, Marino MW, et al. Protection from obesity-induced insulin resistance in mice lacking TNF-α function. Nature 1997; 389:610–14

88. Ledgerwood EC, Prins JB. TNF alpha. In: Marshall SM, Home PD, Rizza R, eds. Diabetes Annual 12, 1st edn. Oxford: Elsevier, 1998

89. Hotamisligil GS. Molecular mechanisms of insulin resistance and the role of the adipocyte. Int J Obesity 2000; 24(Suppl 4):S23–7

90. Liu LS, Spelleken M, R'hrig K, et al. Tumor necrosis factor α acutely inhibits insulin signaling in human adipocytes. Diabetes 1998; 47:515–22

91. Peraldi P, Hotamisligil GS, Buurman WA, et al. Tumor necrosis factor (TNF)-α inhibits insulin signaling through stimulation of the p55 TNF receptor and activation of sphingomyelinase. J Biol Chem 1996; 271:13018–22

92. Hube F, Hauner H. The two tumor necrosis factor receptors mediate opposite effects on differentiation and glucose metabolism in human adipocytes in primary culture. Endocrinology 2000; 141:2582–8

93. Stephens JM, Lee J, Pilch PF. Tumor necrosis factor-α-induced insulin resistance in 3T3–L1 adipocytes is accompanied by a loss of insulin receptor substrate-1 and GLUT4 expression without a loss of insulin-receptor-mediated signal transduction. J Biol Chem 1997; 272:971–6

94. Kanety H, Feinstein R, Papa MZ, et al. Tumor necrosis factor α-induced phosphorylation of insulin receptor substrate-1 (IRS-1). J Biol Chem 1995; 270:23780–4

95. Hotamisligil GS, Peraldi P, Budavari A, et al. IRS-1–mediated inhibition of insulin receptor tyrosine kinase activity in TNF-α- and obesity-induced insulin resistance. Science 1996; 271:665–8

96. Scheen AJ, Castillo MJ, Paquot N, et al. Neutralization of TNFα in obese insulin-resistant human subjects: no effect on insulin sensitivity. Diabetes (Suppl) 1996; 45:286A

97. Ofei F, Hurel S, Newkirk J, et al. Effects of engineered human anti-TNFα antibody (CDP571) on insulin sensitivity and glycemic control in patients with NIDDM. Diabetes 1996; 45:881–5

98. Petruschke TH, Hauner H. Tumor necrosis factor-α prevents the differentiation of human adipocyte precurser cells and causes delipidation of newly developed fat cells. J Clin Endocrinol Metab 1993; 76:742–7

99. Prins JB, Niesler CU, Winterford CM, et al. Tumor necrosis factor-α induces apoptosis of human adipose cells. Diabetes 1997; 46:1939–44

100. Hauner H, Petruschke T, Russ M, et al. Effects of tumour necrosis factor alpha (TNFα) on glucose transport and lipid metabolism of newly-differentiated human fat cells in culture. Diabetologia 1995; 38:764–71

101. Van der Poll T, Romijn JA, Endert E, et al. Tumor necrosis factor mimics the metabolic response to acute infection in healthy humans. Am J Physiol 1991; 261:E457–65

102. Jones TH. Interleukin-6 an endocrine cytokine. Clin Endocrinol 1994; 40:703–13

103. Bastard J-P, Jardel C, Bruckert E, et al. Elevated levels of interleukin 6 are reduced in serum and subcutaneous adipose tissue of obese women after weight loss. J Clin Endocrinol Metab 2000; 85:3338–42

104. Fried SK, Bunkin DA, Greenberg AS. Omental and subcutaneous adipose tissue depots of obese subjects release interleukin-6: depot difference and regulation by glucocorticoid. J Clin Endocrinol Metab 1998; 83:847–50

105. Wallenius V, Wallenius K, Ahrén B, et al. Interleukin-6–deficient mice develop mature-onset obesity. Nature Med 2002; 8:75–9

106. Rosen BS, Cook KS, Yaglom J, et al. Adipsin and complement factor D activity: an immune-related defect in obesity. Science 1989; 244:1483–7

107. Napolitano A, Lowell BB, Damm D, et al.

Concentration of adipsin in blood and rates of adipsin secretion by adipose tissue in humans with normal, elevated and diminished adipose tissue mass. Int J Obesity 1994; 18:213–18

108. Sniderman AD, Cianflone K. The adipsin-ASP pathway and regulation of adipocyte function. Ann Med 1994; 26:389–93

109. Baldo A, Sniderman AD, St-Luce S, et al. The adipsin-acylation stimulating protein system and regulation of intracellular triglyceride synthesis. J Clin Invest 1993; 92:1543–7

110. Murray I, Havel P, Sniderman AD, et al. Reduced body weight, adipose tissue, and leptin levels despite increased energy intake in female mice lacking acyla-tion-stimulating protein. Endocrinology 2000; 141:1041–9

111. Biesma D, Hannema A, van Velzen-Blad H, et al. A family with complement factor D deficiency. J Clin Invest 2001; 108:233–40

112. Tang W, Miller MB, Rich SS, et al. Linkage analysis of a composite factor for the multiple metabolic syndrome: The National Heart, Lung, and Blood Institute Family Heart Study. Diabetes 2003; 52:2840–7

113. Zhang Y, Matheny M, Zolotukhin S, et al. Regulation of adiponectin and leptin gene expression in white and brown adipose tissues: influence of

[beta]3–adrenergic agonists, retinoic acid, leptin and fasting. Biochim Biophys Acta (BBA) Mol Cell Biol Lipids 2002; 1584:115–22

114. Gui Y, Silha JV, Mishra S, et al. Changes in adipokine expression during food deprivation in the mouse and the relationship to fasting-induced insulin resistance. Can J Physiol Pharmacol 2003; 81:979–85

115. Zhang B, Graziano MP, Doebber TW, et al. Down-regulation of the expression of the {1obese} gene by and antidiabetic thiazolidinedione in Zucker diabetic fatty rats and {1db/db} mice. J Biol Chem 1996; 271:9455–9

116. Monzillo LU, Hamdy O, Horton ES, et al. Effect of lifestyle modification on adipokine levels in obese subjects with insulin resistance. Obes Res 2003; 11:1048–54

117. Ott V, Fasshauer M, Dalski A, et al. Direct peripheral effects of ghrelin include suppression of adiponectin expression. Horm Metab Res 2002; 34:640–5

118. Furuhashi M, Ura N, Higashiura K, et al. Blockade of the renin–angiotensin system increases adiponectin concentrations in patients with essential hyperten-sion. Hypertension 2003; 42:76–81

119. Hulver MW, Zheng D, Tanner CJ, et al. Adiponectin is not altered with exercise training despite enhanced insulin action. Am J Physiol Endocrinol Metab 2002; 283:E861–5

Regulation of adipocyte triglyceride storage

15

F. Karpe and G.D. Tan

ADIPOCYTE TRIGLYCERIDE STORAGE AND CARDIOVASCULAR RISK FACTORS

A major function of adipose tissue is to store energy for later use. In this respect, adipose tissue is the most specialized and efficient organ for energy storage. In fact, adipose tissue is the ultimate repository of dietary fat. In obesity, i.e. a condition of long-term energy excess, adipose tissue might store triglycerides worth months of whole-body energy expenditure. Obesity is a high-risk syndrome for cardiovascular disease and some of the underlying risk factors can be traced back to inefficient storage of fatty acids in adipose tissue.[1] It is also recognized that differentiated adipocytes from various adipose tissue stores have functional differences in terms of fatty acid handling. This chapter will describe the principal pathways for storage and release of fatty acids in adipocytes and how they are regulated. The clinical relevance for the respective pathways and how this might relate to cardiovascular risk factors will also be highlighted.

BACKGROUND TO ADIPOCYTE FAT STORAGE AND FAT RELEASE

Adipogenesis is regulated by two major transcriptional factors: peroxisomal proliferator activated receptor gamma (PPAR-γ) and the sterol regulatory element binding protein 1 (SREBP-1).[2–4] PPAR-γ appears to regulate a set of genes for triglyceride storage, whereas SREBP-1 is often seen as the ultimate transcriptional signal for the lipogenic pathway induced by insulin signalling. The CCAAT/enhancer-binding protein (C/EBP) also plays a role in the early differentiation of adipocytes.[2–4]

Triglycerides are stored in a large lipid droplet within the adipocyte. Adipocyte triglyceride synthesis is under acute and long-term transcriptional regulation by insulin. The acute regulation may involve cAMP activated dependent protein kinase regulation of glycerol-3 phosphate acyl-transferase (GPAT). Elevated intracellular concentrations of cAMP inactivate GPAT. The acute regulation of diacylglycerol acyl-transferase (DGAT) is, however, largely unknown.[5]

Mobilization of fatty acids from the adipocyte triglyceride stores is mediated by hormone-sensitive lipase (HSL). A recently discovered additional triglyceride hydrolase might also be of importance in the mobilization of intracellular triglycerides.[6] Recent characterization of the processes of lipid mobilization has shown that the abundant adipocyte protein perilipin A covers the lipid droplet, which on the one hand appears to function as a barrier and on the other as a facilitating protein for HSL action. Regulation of lipolysis by HSL has recently been outlined by Holm et al.[7] HSL is regulated by the reversible phosphorylation of serine residues. This event marks the end of several lipolytic signals culminating in the modulation of the intracellular cAMP concentration. Most lipolytic signals derive from a range of G-protein-coupled receptors, which are outlined later in this chapter. The dominant lipolytic stimulus is likely to be the signalling of catecholamines through β-adrenoreceptors. Upon stimulation, adenylyl cyclase activity increases and this generates cAMP from ATP. Subsequent phosphorylation of the HSL sites Ser_{659} and Ser_{660} by cAMP-dependent protein kinase A appears to activate HSL. However, HSL activation alone is not enough for effective lipolysis to occur; HSL needs to be in physical contact with its substrate, the triglyceride droplet. Crucially, phosphorylated HSL translocates from the cytoplasm to the lipid droplet.[8] Here, the protein envelope of the lipid droplet, perilipin A, plays a role. Like HSL, perilipin A is phosphorylated by the lipolytic signal, and it is thought that perilipin A phosphorylation facilitates HSL's access to its substrate. In contrast, the unphosphorylated perilipin A protects the lipid droplet from lipolysis by HSL. The physiological role of perilipin A has been investigated by the targeted disruption of the perilipin A gene (*PLIN*) in mice. These mice were healthy and exhibited resistance to diet-induced obesity. They were leaner than control mice and had reduced adipocyte triglyceride stores with small and dispersed intracellular lipid droplets. Physiologically, they showed constitutively activated lipolysis.[9,10] These data clearly highlight the important role of perilipin A in lipid droplet formation and the control of lipolysis.

Insulin provides the powerful inhibitory control of fat mobilization from adipocytes. This is mediated through a signal chain involving the insulin receptor, via PI_3-kinase forming PIP_3, which in turn activates PKB/Akt. PKB then phosphorylates and activates cAMP-phosphodiesterase 3B (PDE3B). PDE3B hydrolyses cAMP to AMP, thereby reducing cAMP concentrations.[7] The cellular cAMP concentration is therefore an integrator of the regulation of fat mobilization.

STORAGE

Transport of fatty acids

Most of the fat stored in adipocytes derives from triglyceride-rich lipoproteins such as chylomicrons and very low density lipoproteins (VLDLs). The triglycerides contained in these lipoproteins are hydrolysed at the vascular endothelium by lipoprotein lipase. The fatty acids produced are transported along the prevailing concentration gradient. In the fed state, when the generation of fatty acids by adipocytes is low, fatty acids flow through the endothelium to the adipocyte. In contrast, in the fasted state, the gradient is in the opposite direction and a majority of the fatty acids produced by the hydrolysis of VLDL are unlikely to enter the adipocyte, and instead enter the systemic circulation.

The mechanism by which fatty acids are transported across the adipocyte plasma membrane is controversial. There are two distinct pathways, which may co-exist, although it is unclear which is dominant. Fatty acids are translocated across membranes either by transporter proteins or by non-protein-mediated mechanisms. A number of fatty acid transport proteins have been identified. In adipocytes, FATP-1 and FAT/CD36 are the two major proteins with this function. The activation of FATP-1 by insulin has recently been described in adipocytes.[11] Insulin mediates translocation of FATP-1 to the plasma membrane within minutes of insulin exposure, to facilitate the uptake of long-chain fatty acids. Alternatively, there is a distinct possibility that a major proportion of fatty acid uptake is non-protein-mediated.[12,13] This movement can be described by a simple flip-flop mechanism by which fatty acids bind with high affinity to the phospholipids in the plasma membrane, traverse the membrane and are esterified in the cell.

Both these mechanisms are passive and dependent on the concentration gradient of fatty acids from the endothelium to the adipocytes. Interference with these mechanisms is therefore unlikely to provide promising targets for the alteration of adipocyte fatty acid uptake.

Lipogenesis and triglyceride synthesis

Adipocyte lipogenesis can be divided into triglyceride synthesis and de novo lipogenesis.

Data in humans indicate that de novo lipogenesis is a minor pathway in adipose tissue. Under most metabolic conditions, it is assumed that de novo lipogenesis is minimal. However, under extreme conditions such as hypercaloric carbohydrate feeding, it may occur. De novo lipogenesis may also take place in the liver, but the quantitative contribution is likely to be small. It has therefore been assumed that other tissues such as adipose tissue might contribute. The very last step in de novo lipogenesis, stearoyl-CoA desaturase, is enhanced by the PPAR-γ agonist rosiglitazone in humans.[14] Although lipogenesis might not be particularly active, some of the enzymes and regulatory properties of the pathways involved appear to have significant effects on adipocyte function. Essentially, all steps of lipogenesis and triglyceride synthesis are positively regulated by SREBP-1c. SREBP-1c is localized to the endoplasmic reticulum (ER). The protein undergoes a sequence of protein cleavages to release a final peptide fragment that translocates to the nucleus to act as a transcriptional activator. A cofactor of SREBP-1c, the membrane-spanning SREBP cleavage activating peptide (SCAP) is sensitive to the membrane lipid/cholesterol content. The SCAP molecule has seven membrane-spanning domains, which convey sterol sensing. When activated, presumably by a certain cholesterol density in the membrane or a low abundance of polyunsaturated acyl chains in the phospholipid structures, SCAP promotes the activity of a site-1 protease. This allows, in turn, for a site-2 protease that cleaves off the final signalling peptide derived from the SREBP-1c protein. The cleaved peptide leaves the ER to enter the nucleus and binds to a sterol-regulated element (SRE). A large number of genes involved in fatty acid synthesis are induced by activation of SREBP-1c. Fatty acid synthase (FAS), acetyl CoA carboxylase (ACC), stearoyl CoA desaturase (SCD-1) and GPAT have SREs and they will co-ordinately promote synthesis of triglycerides.

The SCD-1 step is normally seen as the final step in de novo lipogenesis. It converts palmitic acid to monounsaturated palmitoleic acid. The conversion appears to have major significance in biological terms. Hypothetically, this can be explained by the biological effect of the biophysical state of the fatty acid: palmitic acid is crystalline, whereas palmitoleic acid is liquid at 37°C. Therefore, overincorporation of palmitic acid into phospholipids in a biological membrane might substantially alter function. The activation of SCD-1 by SREBP-1c might therefore be seen as an important feedback loop to control membrane function. In this context it has also been proposed that the actual cholesterol content of the adipocyte might serve as an internal signal for triglyceride storage.[15]

In mice with targeted disruption of the SCD-1 gene, the storage of triglycerides in adipose tissue is reduced. The mice are lean and do not accumulate adipose tissue when fed a high-fat diet. Fat oxidation is increased and the animals are insulin sensitive, suggesting that the SCD-1 gene disruption alters the fuel utilization.[16]

The final committed step in triglyceride synthesis in the adipocyte is DGAT. This pathway is dealt with in detail in Chapter 3.

Insulin signalling co-ordinates adipocyte lipogenesis. A review of the molecular events of insulin signalling has recently been published.[17] It has been proposed that a prolonged or intensified signal would enhance the overall action of insulin[18] and in turn adipocyte lipogenesis. In general terms, this can be achieved by insulin sensitizers such as thiazolidinediones, but their molecular mechanism of action is still unclear. Another option is to interfere with the insulin signalling pathway directly, i.e. with one of the sequential steps regulating the intracellular phosphorylation status. For this reason protein phosphatase inhibitors can be seen as insulin sensitizers and potentially promote adipocyte fat storage. The particular step that has been targeted so far is the protein tyrosine phosphatase 1B (PTP1B), for which there is abundant in vitro evidence of functional effects by using PTP1B inhibitors.[18] However, the action of this system in terms of adipocyte triglyceride storage is unclear. As a proof of concept, ablation of PTP1B activity creates a lean phenotype in mice,[19] which would be incompatible with enhanced adipocyte triglyceride storage due to a maintained high state of insulin signalling. These mice have increased insulin sensitivity, which is particularly enhanced in skeletal muscle. This paradox is explained by an increased energy expenditure, whose relationship to the PTP1B has not been fully explored.

Thiazolidinediones are known to be insulin sensitizers and ligands to PPAR-γ, which is a transcription factor enhancing several lipogenic enzymes. PPAR-γ is highly expressed in adipocytes, but it is unclear whether the effects on lipogenesis or fatty acid metabolism in adipose tissue are related to the insulin sensitization. Thiazolidinediones appear to reduce the concentration of non-esterified fatty acids in rodents,[20,21] but this effect is much less marked in humans.[22–25] It was recently proposed that thiazolidinediones induce glycerol kinase activity in adipocytes and that this would be the mechanistic background to lowering of plasma NEFA concentrations as well as retention of triglycerides within adipocytes.[26] However, this does not seem to hold true for humans, in whom induction of glycerol kinase is absent in response to rosiglitazone.[27]

METABOLISM OF FATTY ACIDS IN HUMAN ADIPOCYTES

Human adipose tissue and adipocytes have a very low oxidative capacity. This is a key feature of white adipose tissue in humans: it stores fat but does not metabolize it. In contrast, brown adipose tissue has high oxidative capacity and the uncoupling process gives rise to non-shivering thermogenesis. Neonates may have some brown adipose tissue, but the feature of non-shivering thermogenesis is lost early during development.

The activation of brown adipose tissue has been studied in detail in hibernating animals and in rodents. There is a strong central regulation through sympathetic activation signalling through β-adrenoreceptors. The atypical β3-adrenoreceptor has attracted partic-

ular attention as it seems specific for this tissue in mammals. It has therefore been suggested that agonists for this receptor might play a role in enhancing uncoupling in brown adipose tissue.[28] The role of the receptor in human adipose tissue is still controversial. The receptor is also found in human white adipose tissue and it has therefore been speculated that such agonists might stimulate non-shivering thermogenesis in humans. Alternatively, it might simply be involved in the regulation of lipolysis, in particular the differential regulation between subcutaneous and visceral adipose tissue.[29] One line of evidence to suggest a function of the β3-adrenoreceptor in humans has been the phenotype of a common genetic variant, which sometimes shows an association with obesity; but the results from a large number of association studies are conflicting,[30,31] One of the problems in employing β3-adrenoreceptor agonists has been the lack of specific compounds; activation of β2- and β1-adrenoreceptors might be an underlying cause for unwanted cardiovascular side-effects.

The expression of uncoupling protein-1 (UCP-1) is crucial for the mitochondrial uncoupling process; it cannot be replaced by other uncoupling proteins such as UCP-2 or UCP-3.[32] As more and more factors that determine adipocyte differentiation become known, it has been speculated that white adipose tissue adipocyte characteristics might not be static; could it be possible to interfere with the process and actually turn white adipocytes into brown adipocytes that burn fat?[33,34] Theoretically, this would be a very attractive approach to dispose of excess energy and therefore serve as a potential anti-obesity treatment. The expression of PPAR-γ cofactor-1α (PGC-1α) in brown adipose tissue is linked to UCP-1 expression. Tiraby and colleagues recently tested whether transient overexpression of PGC-1α in adipocytes affected UCP-1 expression.[35] Indeed, the mRNA content of UCP-1 increased, suggesting that a transcriptional program linked to energy dissipation had been turned on. Similar effects were seen in mice after transgenic induction of the PGC-1α like product, PGC-1β.[36] The latter observation is, however, made in a species that already harbours brown adipocytes and is therefore less conclusive. There are two other examples of UCP-1 induction in mouse adipose tissue by enhancing upstream regulatory factors. First, adipose tissue-specific induction of PPAR-δ appears to induce UCP-1 and physiological studies also demonstrated increased uncoupling.[37] These mice gained less weight when provoked with a high-fat diet compared with the wild type. Second, the translational inhibitor 4E-BP1, which is a protein that is highly phosphorylated in response to insulin signalling and thereby releases a polypeptide (eIF4E) that is involved in translation initiation, appears to constitutively depress PGC-1 expression and thereby UCP-1.[38] Mice with a disruption of the 4E-BP1 gene show a lean and fat-burning phenotype.

In summary, these data demonstrate the distinct possibility of converting the characteristics of adipocytes from white adipose tissue to those from brown adipose tissue. If this could be therapeutically exploited it might open new ways for pharmacological treatment of obesity and its related cardiovascular complications. PPAR-δ agonists are promising agents in this respect.

LIPOLYSIS

Adrenoreceptor function in adipocytes

Catecholamine-induced lipolysis is probably the major trigger for fat mobilization. In human white adipose tissue adipocytes, the adrenergic response is balanced by the lipolytic response from β2-adrenoreceptors and the anti-lipolytic response of α2-adrenoreceptors. The relative role of β3-adrenoreceptors is controversial.[39] The receptor distribution varies depending on adipose tissue location and this is likely to be an important underlying factor determining the characteristics of the different adipose tissue depots.[39] Buttock fat appears to be resistant to lipolytic stimulus, whereas adipocytes from visceral fat stores are very sensitive. The upper body subcutaneous adipose tissue is more responsive than the

lower body store. The endogenous ligands for the adrenoreceptors (adrenaline (epinephrine) and noradrenaline (norepinephrine)) have different relative agonist actions to the β2- and α2-adrenoreceptors, respectively. These catecholamines reach the tissue by different routes. There is evidence for innervation of adipose tissue,[40] which would invoke noradrenaline release upon sympathetic activation. In contrast adrenaline is released from the adrenal medulla and reaches the tissue by the blood stream. Noradrenaline has higher agonist specificity for β2-adrenoreceptors than adrenaline, but is a weaker α2-adrenoreceptor agonist. In isolated cellular systems, noradrenaline therefore gives rise to a higher lipolytic stimulus than adrenaline.[41]

The effects resulting from sympathetic activation of adipose tissue are complex. The delivery of the products of lipolysis, non-esterified fatty acids, from adipose tissue is enhanced by a simultaneous increase in blood flow. Food intake is followed by insulin secretion that inhibits HSL action, whilst the post-meal sympathetic activation enhances the blood flow.[42] Obviously, the inhibitory lipolytic signal of insulin is stronger than that of the insulinaemia-induced lipolytic stimulus by sympathetic activation. However, there might be tissue-specific differences whereby certain adipose tissue depots, perhaps in particular visceral fat stores, are particularly sensitive to sympathetic activation and insensitive to the anti-lipolytic action of insulin. It has been speculated that the readiness to respond to sympathetic activation is maintained by pulsatile signals to the tissue in the resting state,[43–45] which has recently been confirmed in humans.

In exercise there is a need for lipid mobilization. In physical exercise, lipolysis is partly promoted by β2-adrenoreceptor activation in adipocytes.

There is substantial genetic heterogeneity in the β2-adrenoreceptor gene and this has implications for responsiveness to the lipolytic signals. Three common haplotypes have been described for the β2-adrenoreceptor gene.[46] Recent in vitro data show that there is a 500-fold difference in terbutaline sensitivity between the extreme variants.[47] This finding is likely to have substantial pharmacogenomic impact, either when the dyslipidaemic effects of β-adrenoreceptor blockers are evaluated or when novel therapeutic approaches are tested in this system.

Atrial natriuretic peptide

Natriuretic peptides have emerged as new and potent lipolytic factors.[48–50] Atrial natriuretic peptide (ANP) is released from the atrium whereas the brain natriuretic peptide (BNP) is primarily released from the cardiac ventricle, although it was first identified in the brain. The stimulus for release is stretching of the cardiomyocytes. ANP and BNP bind to either of two G-protein-coupled receptors on adipocytes, the A-type primarily expressed by adipocytes and the more ubiquitously expressed B-type, both of which activate guanylate cyclase giving rise to increased concentrations of cGMP. A third receptor, the C-type, lacks the intracellular domain of the receptor structure and has therefore been suggested to take part in catabolizing ANP and BNP. Almost all other lipolytic responses in adipocytes signal through cAMP, and thus the signalling of ANP by cGMP is unique in this respect. It gives rise to HSL and perilipin phosphorylation through the cGMP-dependent protein kinase I.[51]

The plasma concentrations of these peptides are in the range which is found to stimulate lipolysis from adipocytes in vitro. Physical activity leads to stimulation of sympathetic activation and in turn lipolysis. However, there is a paradoxically low proportion of this lipolytic stimulus that can be blocked by β-adrenoreceptor blockade. It is likely that ANP released as a result of the increased performance of the heart plays a role. Systemic administration of β-adrenoreceptor blockers increases the plasma concentrations of ANP. This is likely to depend on the negative chronotropic effect of these drugs and the increased end-diastolic filling pressure of the atrium. It is tempting to speculate that this might lead to increased lipolysis and partly explain the dysmetabolic effects of β-adrenoreceptor blockers. It is therapeutically interesting to interfere with the ANP system from a metabolic point of view, but there is still a lack of potent non-peptide antagonists.

Adenosine receptors

Adenosine produced by the adipocyte exerts a negative feedback in response to lipolytic stimuli.[52,53] It was later discovered that adenosine acts via an inhibitory G-protein-coupled receptor, reducing the adenylate cyclase activity and, in turn, lowering cAMP concentrations.[54] Adipocytes express two types of adenosine receptors, A1 and A2. The A1 receptor is found in mature adipocytes and conveys the classic inhibition of cAMP, whereas A2 is found in pre-adipocytes and is stimulatory.[55] Overexpression of A1 in mice protects them against obesity-related insulin resistance.[56] The development of A1 agonists is, however, hampered by the wide tissue distribution of the receptor, leading to potential side-effects on heart rate or kidney function. In adipocytes A1 appears to be tonically activated at physiological nanomolar concentrations. There is a substantial receptor reserve[57] and it has been postulated that this receptor reserve can be used therapeutically.[58] The rapid downregulation of the A1 receptor is another caveat in the development of long-term anti-lipolytic drugs.

Nicotinic acid receptor

Specific binding of nicotinic acid to adipose tissue was demonstrated 40 years ago.[59] The binding of nicotinic acid to a putative G-protein-coupled receptor has been demonstrated in membranes prepared from adipocytes.[60] More recently, Tunaru and colleagues[61] and Wise and colleagues[62] used genomic approaches to screen for genes encoding orphan G-protein-coupled receptors with a tissue distribution resembling that of nicotinic acid binding, i.e. adipose tissue, spleen and macrophages. Both groups recognized that the new receptor had already been cloned as PUMA-G in macrophages (protein upregulated in macrophages by interferon-γ)[63] and as HM74[64] in monocytes, respectively. In addition, Wise et al cloned a gene with a 96% predicted amino acid sequence similarity to HM74 (HM74A),[62] whose gene product appears to be the high-affinity receptor for nicotinic acid. Receptor activation by nicotinic acid showed binding to the G-protein-coupled receptor subunit GTPγS with subsequent cellular response.[62] Mice made deficient of the receptor were viable without any obviously abnormal phenotype, but failed to suppress lipolysis after nicotinic acid administration.[61]

Although nicotinic acid has proved to be a very useful lipid-modifying agent, its use has always been hampered by side-effects that patients have found difficult to tolerate. The nicotinic-acid-specific flush is uncomfortable and if new molecules signalling through this receptor pathway could be developed that would be seen as a major step forward in the management of hypertriglyceridaemias. The endogenous ligand of the nicotinic acid receptor is unknown, but the cloning of this receptor is likely to pave the way for anti-lipolytic drugs that can be used either as hypolipidaemic drugs or possibly as anti-diabetic drugs.

ADIPOCYTE CORTISOL METABOLISM

Hypercortisolism has profound effects on adipose tissue distribution and adipocyte function. Systemic exposure to cortisol produces a specific pattern of adipose tissue depletion in limbs, whilst trunk and visceral adipose tissue expands. The clinical similarity of the adipose tissue distribution in Cushing's syndrome and in the male-pattern fat distribution is enigmatic, in the sense that the hypothalamo–pituitary axis is not obviously disturbed in the latter condition. The paradox could be explained by local adipose tissue generation of cortisol which increases with increasing obesity. Cortisol generated locally would be functionally antagonistic to insulin. The local cortisol generation affects the adipocytes but has little effect on systemic cortisol concentrations. The enzyme responsible for the conversion of biologically inert cortisone to cortisol in adipose tissue is the 11β-hydroxysteroid dehydrogenase type 1 (11β-HSD1). The role of 11β-HSD has recently been reviewed.[65,66] Inhibitors of 11β-HSD1 might be a particularly interesting target to alter adipocyte function in the metabolic syndrome.[67]

ACKNOWLEDGEMENTS

F Karpe is a Senior Wellcome Trust Clinical Research Fellow and G Tan is a Medical Research Council Training Fellow.

References

1. Sniderman AD, Cianflone K, Arner P, et al. The adipocyte, fatty acid trapping and atherogenesis. Arterioscler Thromb Vasc Biol 1998; 18:147–51
2. Rangwala SM, Lazar MA. Transcriptional control of adipogenesis. Annu Rev Nutr 2000; 20:535–59
3. Tong Q, Hotamisligil GS. Molecular mechanisms of adipocyte differentiation. Rev Endocr Metab Disord 2001; 2:349–55
4. Camp HS, Ren D, Leff T. Adipogenesis and fat-cell function in obesity and diabetes. Trends Mol Med 2002; 8:442–7
5. Coleman RA, Lewin TM, Muoio DM. Physiological and nutritional regulation of enzymes of triacylglycerol synthesis. Annu Rev Nutr 2000; 20:77–103
6. Zimmerman R, Strauss JG, Haemmerle G, et al. Fat mobilization in adipose tissue is promoted by adipose triglyceride lipase. Science 2004; 306:1383–6
7. Holm C, Osterlund T, Laurell H, et al. Molecular mechanisms regulating hormone-sensitive lipase and lipolysis. Annu Rev Nutr 2000; 20:365–93
8. Clifford GM, Londos C, Kraemer FB, et al. Translocation of hormone-sensitive lipase and perilipin upon lipolytic stimulation of rat adipocytes. J Biol Chem 2000; 275:5011–15
9. Martinez-Botas J, Anderson JB, Tessier D, et al. Absence of perilipin results in leanness and reverses obesity in Lepr(db/db) mice. Nat Genet 2000; 26:474–9
10. Tansey JT, Sztalryd C, Gruia-Gray J, et al. Perilipin ablation results in a lean mouse with aberrant

adipocyte lipolysis, enhanced leptin production, and resistance to diet-induced obesity. Proc Natl Acad Sci USA 2001; 98:6494–9

11. Stahl A, Evans JG, Pattel S, et al. Insulin causes fatty acid transport protein translocation and enhanced fatty acid uptake in adipocytes. Dev Cell 2002; 2:477–88

12. Kamp F, Guo W, Souto R, et al. Rapid flip-flop of oleic acid across the plasma membrane of adipocytes. J Biol Chem 2003; 278:7988–95

13. Scow RO, Blanchette-Mackie EJ. Why fatty acids flow in cell membranes. Prog Lipid Res 1985; 24:197–241

14. Riserus U, Tan GD, Fielding BA, et al. Rosiglitazone increases indexes of stearoyl-CoA desaturase activity in humans: link to insulin sensitization and the role of dominant-negative mutation in Peroxisome Proliferator-Activated Receptor-γ. Diabetes 2005; 54:1379–84

15. Dugail I, Le Lay S, Varret M, et al. New insights into how adipocytes sense their triglyceride stores. Is cholesterol a signal? Horm Metab Res 2003; 35:204–10

16. Ntambi JM, Miyazaki M, Stoehr JP, et al. Loss of stearoyl-CoA desaturase-1 function protects mice against adiposity. Proc Natl Acad Sci USA 2002; 99:11482–6

17. Saltiel AR, Pessin JE. Insulin signaling pathways in time and space. Trends Cell Biol 2002; 12:65–71

18. Xie L, Lee SY, Andersen JN, et al. Cellular effects of small molecule PTP1B inhibitors on insulin signaling. Biochemistry 2003; 42:12792–804

19. Klaman LD, Boss O, Peroni OD, et al. Increased energy expenditure, decreased adiposity, and tissue-specific insulin sensitivity in protein-tyrosine phosphatase 1B-deficient mice. Mol Cell Biol 2000; 20:5479–89

20. Zhou YT, Grayburn P, Karim A, et al. Lipotoxic heart disease in obese rats: implications for human obesity. Proc Natl Acad Sci USA 2000; 97:1784–9

21. Finegood DT, McArthur MD, Kojwang D, et al. Beta-cell mass dynamics in Zucker diabetic fatty rats. Rosiglitazone prevents the rise in net cell death. Diabetes 2001; 50:1021–9

22. Maggs DG, Buchanan TA, Burant CF, et al. Metabolic effects of troglitazone monotherapy in type 2 diabetes mellitus. A randomized, double-blind, placebo-controlled trial. Ann Intern Med 1998; 128:176–85

23. Mayerson AB, Hundal RS, Dufour S, et al. The effects of rosiglitazone on insulin sensitivity, lipolysis, and hepatic and skeletal muscle triglyceride content in patients with type 2 diabetes. Diabetes 2002; 51:797–802

24. Hällsten K, Virtanen KA, Lönnqvist F, et al. Rosiglitazone but not metformin enhances insulin- and exercise-stimulated skeletal muscle glucose uptake in patients with newly diagnosed type 2 diabetes. Diabetes 2002; 51:3479–85

25. Tan GD, Fielding BA, Currie JM, et al. Nitric oxide and beta-adrenergic stimulation are majhor regulators of preprandial and postprandial subcutaneous adipose tissue blood flow in humans. Circulation 2004; 109:47–52

26. Guan HP, Li Y, Jensen MV, et al. A futile metabolic cycle activated in adipocytes by antidiabetic agents. Nat Med 2002; 8:1122–8

27. Tan GD, Debard C, Tiraby C, et al. A 'futile cycle' induced by thiazolidinediones in human adipose tissue? Nat Med 2003; 9:811–12

28. Arch JR. beta(3)-Adrenoceptor agonists: potential, pitfalls and progress. Eur J Pharmacol 2002; 440:99–107

29. Lönnqvist F, Thome A, Nilsell K, et al. A pathogenic role of visceral fat beta 3-adrenoceptors in obesity. J Clin Invest 1995; 95:1109–16

30. Fujisawa T, Ikegami H, Kawaguchi Y, et al. Meta-analysis of the association of Trp64Arg polymorphism of beta 3-adrenergic receptor gene with body mass index. J Clin Endocrinol Metab 1998; 83:2441–4

31. Allison DB, Heo M, Faith MS, et al. Meta-analysis of the association of the Trp64Arg polymorphism in the beta3 adrenergic receptor with body mass index. Int J Obes Relat Metab Disord 1998; 22:559–66

32. Nedergaard J, Golozoubova V, Matthias A, et al. UCP1: the only protein able to mediate adaptive non-shivering thermogenesis and metabolic inefficiency. Biochim Biophys Acta 2001; 1504:82–106

33. Chen HC, Farese RV, Jr. Turning WAT into BAT gets rid of fat. Nat Med 2001; 7:1102–3

34. Walczak R, Tontonoz P. Setting fat on fire. Nat Med 2003; 9:1348–9

35. Tiraby C, Tavernier G, Lefort C, et al. Acquirement of brown fat cell features by human white adipocytes. J Biol Chem 2003; 278:33370–6

36. Kamei Y, Ohizumi H, Fujitani Y, et al. PPARgamma coactivator 1beta/ERR ligand 1 is an ERR protein ligand, whose expression induces a high-energy expenditure and antagonizes obesity. Proc Natl Acad Sci USA 2003; 100:12378–83

37. Wang YX, Lee CH, Tiep S, et al. Peroxisome-proliferator-activated receptor delta activates fat metabolism to prevent obesity. Cell 2003; 113:159–70

38. Tsukiyama-Kohara K, Poulin F, Kohara M, et al. Adipose tissue reduction in mice lacking the translational inhibitor 4E-BP1. Nat Med 2001; 7:1128–32

39. Lafontan M, Berlan M. Do regional differences in adipocyte biology provide new pathophysiological insights? Trends Pharmacol Sci 2003; 24:276–83

40. Dodt C, Lönnroth P, Wellhoner JP, et al. Sympathetic control of white adipose tissue in lean and obese humans. Acta Physiol Scand 2003; 177:351–7

41. Carpene C, Bousquet-Melou A, Galitzky J, et al. Lipolytic effects of beta 1-, beta 2-, and beta 3-adrenergic agonists in white adipose tissue of mammals. Ann NY Acad Sci 1998; 839:186–9

42. Ardilouze JL, Fielding BA, Currie JM, et al. Nitric oxide and beta-adrenergic stimulation are major regulators of preprandial and postprandial subcutaneous adipose tissue blood flow in humans. Circulation 2004; 109:47–52

43. Hucking K, Hamilton-Wessler M, Ellmerer M, et al. Burst-like control of lipolysis by the sympathetic nervous system in vivo. J Clin Invest 2003; 111:257–64

44. Getty L, Panteleon AE, Mittelman SD, et al. Rapid oscillations in omental lipolysis are independent of changing insulin levels in vivo. J Clin Invest 2000; 106:421–30

45. Karpe F, Fielding BA, Coppack SW, et al. Oscillations of fatty acid and glycerol release from human subcutaneous adipose tissue in vivo. Diabetes 2005; 54:1297–303

46. Drysdale CM, McGraw DW, Stack CB, et al. Complex promoter and coding region beta 2-adrenergic receptor haplotypes alter receptor expression and predict in vivo responsiveness. Proc Natl Acad Sci USA 2000; 97:10483–8

47. Eriksson P, Dahlman I, Ryden M, et al. Relationship between beta-2 adrenoceptor gene haplotypes and adipocyte lipolysis in women. Int J Obes Relat Metab Disord 2004; 28:185–90

48. Sengenes C, Berlan M, De Glisczinski I, et al. Natriuretic peptides: a new lipolytic pathway in human adipocytes. FASEB J 2000; 14:1345–51

49. Moro C, Galitzky J, Sengenes C, et al. Functional and pharmacological characterization of the natriuretic peptide-dependent lipolytic pathway in human fat cells. J Pharmacol Exp Ther 2004; 308:984–92

50. Dessi-Fulgheri P, Sarzani R, Rappelli A. Role of the natriuretic peptide system in lipogenesis/lipolysis. Nutr Metab Cardiovasc Dis 2003; 13:244–9

51. Sengenes C, Bouloumie A, Hauner H, et al. Involvement of a cGMP-dependent pathway in the natriuretic peptide-mediated hormone-sensitive lipase phosphorylation in human adipocytes. J Biol Chem 2003; 278:48617–26

52. Ho R, Russell TR, Asakawa T, et al. Cellular levels of feedback regulator of adenylate cyclase and the effect of epinephrine and insulin. Proc Natl Acad Sci USA 1975; 72:4739–43

53. Ho RJ, Sutherland EW. Action of feedback regulator on adenylate cyclase. Proc Natl Acad Sci USA 1975; 72:1773–7

54. Londos C, Cooper DM, Schlegel W, et al. Adenosine analogs inhibit adipocyte adenylate cyclase by a GTP-dependent process: basis for actions of adenosine and methylxanthines on cyclic AMP production and lipolysis. Proc Natl Acad Sci USA 1978; 75:5362–6

55. Borglum JD, Vassaux G, Richelsen B, et al. Changes in adenosine A1- and A2-receptor expression during adipose cell differentiation. Mol Cell Endocrinol 1996; 117:17–25

56. Dong Q, Ginsberg HN, Erlanger BF. Overexpression of the A1 adenosine receptor in adipose tissue protects mice from obesity-related insulin resistance. Diabetes Obes Metab 2001; 3:360–6

57. Liang HX, Belardinelli L, Ozeck MJ, et al. Tonic activity of the rat adipocyte A1-adenosine receptor. Br J Pharmacol 2002; 135:1457–66

58. Dhalla AK, Shryock JC, Shreeniwas R, et al. Pharmacology and therapeutic applications of A1 adenosine receptor ligands. Curr Top Med Chem 2003; 3:369–85

59. Carlson LA, Hanngren Å. Initial distribution in mice of 3H-labelled nicotinic acid studied with autoradiography. Life Sci 1964; 3:867–71

60. Lorenzen A, Stannek C, Lang H, et al. Characterization of a G protein-coupled receptor for nicotinic acid. Mol Pharmacol 2001; 59:349–57

61. Tunaru S, Kero J, Schaub A, et al. PUMA-G and HM74 are receptors for nicotinic acid and mediate its antilipolytic effect. Nat Med 2003; 9:352–5

62. Wise A, Foord SM, Fraser NJ, et al. Molecular identification of high and low affinity receptors for nicotinic acid. J Biol Chem 2003; 278:9869–74

63. Schaub A, Futterer A, Pfeffer K. PUMA-G, an IFN-gamma-inducible gene in macrophages is a novel member of the seven transmembrane spanning receptor superfamily. Eur J Immunol 2001; 31:3714–25

64. Nomura H, Nielsen BW, Matsushima K. Molecular cloning of cDNAs encoding a LD78 receptor and putative leukocyte chemotactic peptide receptors. Int Immunol 1993; 5:1239–49

65. Seckl JR, Walker BR. Minireview: 11beta-hydroxysteroid dehydrogenase type 1 – a tissue-specific amplifier of glucocorticoid action. Endocrinology 2001; 142:1371–6

66. Stulnig TM, Waldhäusl W. 11beta-Hydroxysteroid dehydrogenase type 1 in obesity and type 2 diabetes. Diabetologia 2004; 47:1–11

67. Walker BR, Seckl JR. 11beta-Hydroxysteroid dehydrogenase type 1 as a novel therapeutic target in metabolic and neurodegenerative disease. Expert Opin Ther Targets 2003; 6:771–83

16

Role of innate immunity in atherosclerosis: immune recognition, immune activation and the atherosclerostic process

J-M. Fernández-Real

Humans live in close association with vast numbers of microorganisms that are present on the external and internal surfaces of our body. The ability to mount a prominent inflammatory response to pathogens confers a continuous advantage in our fight against pathogens. All metazoan organisms have evolved complex immune defence systems, used to repel invasive microbes that would parasitize or kill them. Innate immunity is the most universal and the most rapidly acting and most organisms survive through the action of this mechanism alone. After any trauma or infection, organisms mount a homeostatic response to injury which is called an acute-phase response, a highly complex process. In the acute phase, the response is protective because it counteracts the effects of injury and improves survival. Long-term exposure to stressful stimuli (mucositis, aging, increased fat intake, periodontitis, etc.), however, may result in disease (atherosclerosis) rather than repair.

There exist two arms of innate immunity: the sensing arm (those mechanisms involved in the continuous sensing and perception of infection) and the effector arm, the sophisticated processes aimed at eradication of infection and tissue repair. Each of these arms may be subdivided into humoral and cellular processes which are tightly co-ordinated in the inflammatory process.[1]

In this chapter we will evaluate each part of the innate immune defence in relation to the atherosclerotic process.

AFFERENT ARM OF INNATE IMMUNITY AND ATHEROSCLEROSIS (Figure 1)

Cellular sensing

The chronic inflammatory process of atherosclerosis is triggered and sustained by unknown factors. Among the candidate triggers are oxidized or enzymatically modified low-density lipoproteins, heat shock proteins and infectious pathogens. Interestingly, in recent years it has become clear that all these triggers and

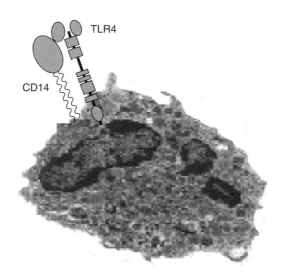

Figure 1 Afferent arm of innate immunity and atherosclerosis. *Cellular* components simultaneously involved in innate immune sensing and the atherosclerotic process

ligands could be recognized and sensed by the same cell and the same receptor.

Macrophages play a primary role in host defence against infection, utilizing a range of receptors to recognize microbes by opsonic as well as direct interactions. The term 'pathogen-associated molecular patterns' (PAMPs) was coined to describe those microbial principles that triggered an innate immune response.[2] PAMPs were said to act via 'pattern recognition receptors' (PRR),[2] i.e. those sensors that could recognize a pattern on a microbe. Binding of targets via PRR results in phagocytosis and killing. Macrophages express a broad repertoire of PRR (e.g. scavenger and lectin-like). In this sense, the amount of lipid retained in macrophages during the atherosclerotic process depends on the unregulated uptake of oxidized lipoproteins by scavenger receptors, counterbalanced by degradation and cholesterol efflux. This scavenger receptor also plays a major role in microbial uptake in the absence of opsonins.

The principal signalling receptors of the innate immune system – through which the greater part of the host awareness of infection is processed – are the toll-like receptor (TLR) family of transmembrane molecules. The best understood TLR, both in terms of ligand binding and signal transduction, is the lipopolysaccharide (LPS) receptor, TLR4.

Toll-like receptor-4

An involvement of toll-like receptor-4 (TLR4) in the pathogenesis of atherosclerosis has been recently emphasized. Expression of TLR4 is clearly detected by immunohistochemistry in macrophages of lipid-rich, human atherosclerotic plaques and in lesions of atherosclerosis-susceptible mice deficient for apolipoprotein E.[3] This expression (evaluated by immunohistochemistry and semiquantitative polymerase chain reaction) was paralleled with inflammatory activation in the lesions as assessed by nuclear translocation of NF-κB.[4] Fibrous plaques and normal arteries show almost no TLR4 expression.[3] Basal TLR4 messenger RNA expression of human monocyte-derived macrophages is markedly upregulated upon in-vitro loading by oxidized LDL.

TLR ligation transmits transmembrane signals that activate NF-κB and mitogen-activated protein kinase (MAPK) pathways, inducing expression of a wide variety of genes such as those encoding proteins involved in leukocyte recruitment, production of reactive oxygen species and phagocytosis. Activation of TLR will also elicit the production of cytokines that potentiate local inflammation.

In the last few years, retrospective and prospective studies of markers of inflammation in humans have shown that a range of different infectious agents may be associated with accelerated atherosclerosis. Very recently, a direct link between microbial infection and lipid accumulation in macrophages has also been demonstrated.[5] A family of transcriptional regulators in macrophages (named liver X receptors, LXR) can modulate LPS-induced TLR4 pathways, and selected TLRs can inhibit LXR function by cross-talk.[5,6] Given that LXR promotes synthesis of ABCA1 and other transporters, which reduce intracellular levels of cholesterol, these observations could aid in the prevention of atherosclerosis.

A polymorphism in the TLR4 gene affects the inflammatory response to lipopolysaccharide (LPS), with impact on the risk of Gram-negative infections and septic shock.[7] Two co-segregating mutations in the gene region coding for the extracellular domain of TLR4, characterized by a substitution at amino acid position 299 (glycine for aspartate) and another at position 399 (isoleucine for threonine), are relatively common. A study reported an association of this *TLR4* polymorphism with atherogenesis.[8] These variants, Asp299Gly and Thr399Ile, lead to a blunted immunological response to inhaled LPS[9] and to lower levels of pro-inflammatory cytokines, acute-phase reactants, fibrinogen, systemic interleukin-6 and soluble adhesion molecules.[8] Last, and most strikingly, they appear to be associated with reduced extent and progression of carotid atherosclerosis as quantified by B-mode ultrasound.[8]

The TLR4 gene polymorphism has also been evaluated in a study in 655 men with angiographically documented coronary atherosclerosis, who participated in a prospective cholesterol-lowering trial. These patients were randomly assigned to either pravastatin or placebo for 2 years, for evaluation of the effect on coronary artery disease. There were no significant differences between genetically defined sub-groups with respect to baseline risk factors, treatment or in-trial changes of lipid, lipoprotein or angiographic measurements. Genotype was not associated with progression of atherosclerosis. In the pravastatin group, 299Gly carriers had a lower risk of cardiovascular events during follow-up than non-carriers (2.0% versus 11.5%, p = 0.045). Among non-carriers, pravastatin reduced the risk of cardiovascular events from 18.1% to 11.5% (p = 0.03), whereas among 299Gly carriers this risk was strikingly reduced from 29.6% to 2.0% (p = 0.0002, p = 0.025 for interaction).[10] These results suggested that the TLR4 Asp299Gly polymorphism was associated with the risk of cardiovascular events and also modified the efficacy of statins in preventing cardiovascular events.[10]

In another study, however, no association of the *TLR4* polymorphism with individual parameters of sub-clinical inflammation or with parameters of the metabolic syndrome (a situation with a well-described increased pro-inflammatory response) was found.[11] Subjects with one or two alleles causing the 299Gly TLR4 did not differ from carriers of TLR4 Asp homozygotes with regard to hypertension, obesity, waist circumference or HDL-cholesterol levels. Differences were also not observed for systemic levels of IL-6, IL-6 receptor, C reactive protein or fibrinogen. Of all parameters analysed, only the prevalence of hypertension showed a trend (p = 0.07), leaving the possibility of a mild protective effect of the Gly299 TLR4 allele.[11]

Heat shock protein 60 (hsp60) is a putative endogenous ligand of the TLR4 complex.[12] Since hsp60 is an important player in chronic inflammatory conditions, the TLR4 polymorphism may regulate through hsp60 the subclinical inflammation underlying the pathogenesis of arteriosclerosis. In fact, in a femoral artery cuff model in the atherosclerotic ApoE3 (Leiden) transgenic mouse, TLR4 activation by LPS stimulated plaque formation and subsequent outward arterial remodelling. With the use of the same model in wild-type mice, neointima formation and outward remodelling occurred. In TLR4-deficient mice, however, no outward arterial remodelling was observed independent of neointima formation. Carotid artery ligation in wild-type mice resulted in outward remodelling without neointima formation in the contralateral artery. This was associated with an increase in TLR4 expression and Hsp60 mRNA levels. In contrast, outward remodelling was not observed after carotid ligation in TLR4-deficient mice. These findings provided genetic evidence that TLR4 is involved in outward arterial remodelling.[13] TLR4-deficient mice also sustained smaller infarctions and exhibit less inflammation after myocardial ischaemia-reperfusion injury.[14]

CD14 receptor

The CD14 receptor, as TLR4, is in the crossroads between infection and the immune system. Several molecules bind lipopolysaccharide (LPS) and subsequently activate the resting monocyte/macrophages, playing an important role in the internalization and detoxification of LPS. However, CD14 is the main LPS receptor that can activate monocytes in conjunction with serum LPS-binding protein and TLR4 at low (<10 ng/ml) clinically significant concentrations of LPS. CD14 interacts with different components of Gram-negative and -positive bacteria and fungi, defining CD14 as a central PRR in innate immunity. Other agonists, notably the heat shock protein HSP70, also activate monocytes by binding to CD14.[15]

CD14 is a membrane glycoprotein (with a glycosyl-phosphatidyl inositol (GPI) anchor) which is present on the surface of different myeloid cells and at very low numbers on B-lymphocytes, basophils and gingival fibroblasts. The CD14 protein has no transmembrane or cytoplasmic domain. CD14 is a constituent of a multi-ligand PRR complex, in which TLRs show a major impact on CD14 signalling in macrophages.

Two European groups reported a relationship between promoter polymorphism in the CD14 gene and increased risk of atherosclerosis. One group found that T>C at position –260 was associated with increased risk of myocardial infarction, and the other reported C>T was more frequent in myocardial infarction survivors than controls.[16,17]

Two Japanese groups confirmed the occurrence of the C (–260) nucleotide change and an associated predisposition to increased risk of coronary artery disease.[18,19] The polymorphism was apparently associated with an enhanced risk for myocardial infarction (MI), particularly in patients who did not otherwise have any significant risk profile for atherosclerosis.

More recently, this functional polymorphism in the promoter region of the CD14 gene was studied to determine its impact on common carotid artery (CCA) intima-media thickness (IMT) and any interactions with environmental inflammatory stimuli. The *CC* genotype was associated with increased CCA IMT. The age- and sex-adjusted odds ratio for IMT above the 75th percentile was 1.63 (95% CI, 1.19 to 2.24; $p = 0.002$) and 1.70 (95% CI, 1.18 to 2.44; $p = 0.004$) after additional adjustment for conventional risk factors. This gene effect was found only in current smokers and ex-smokers. Multivariate analysis in this group ($n = 503$) increased the odds ratio to 2.02 (95% CI, 1.23 to 3.34; $p = 0.006$). No significant interactions were found in non-smokers. This study suggested that CD14 may modulate the inflammatory effects of smoking in atherogenesis.[20]

These observations are interesting because bacterial LPS, a potent mediator of inflammation, has been identified as an active component of cigarette smoke,[21] and smokers have elevated plasma levels of LPS.[22] Circulating levels of LPS, in turn, have been shown to independently predict incident atherosclerosis measured by carotid ultrasound,[22] but the ability of LPS to promote atherogenesis appears to be dependent on the degree of inflammatory response it provokes.[23]

Because the polymorphism is associated with an upregulation of CD14 receptors on monocytes, these observations corroborate the growing evidence that chronic infections of, e.g. *Chlamydia pneumonia*, *Helicobacter pylori*, Epstein Barr virus, etc., or other inflammatory triggers (smoking) may be important risk factors for the development of atherosclerosis and consequently of MI.

Humoral sensing (Figure 2)

Pentraxins

The pentraxin family, named, for its electron micrographic appearance, from the Greek *penta* (five) and *ragos* (berries),[24] comprises C-reactive protein (CRP) and serum amyloid P (SAP) component in man, and is highly conserved in evolution, with homologous proteins throughout the vertebrates and even in the phylogenetically distant arthropod, *Limulus polyphemus*, and the horseshoe crab.[25] SAP, named for its universal presence in amyloid deposits, is a constitutive, non-acute-phase plasma glycoprotein in man and all other species studied, except the mouse, in which it is the major acute-phase protein.

Human CRP is a calcium-dependent ligand-binding protein, which binds with highest affinity to phosphocholine residues. Extrinsic ligands include many glycan, phospholipid and other components of micro-organisms, such as capsular and somatic components of bacteria, fungi and parasites, as well as plant products. Autologous ligands include native and modified plasma lipoproteins, damaged cell membranes, a number of different phospholipids and related compounds, small nuclear ribonucleoprotein particles and apoptotic cells (reviewed in references 26 and 27).

When human CRP is ligand-bound, it is recognized by C1q and potently activates the classical complement pathway, engaging C3, the main adhesion molecule of the complement system, and the terminal membrane attack complex, C5–C9. Bound CRP may also provide secondary binding sites for factor H, and thereby regulate alternative pathway amplification and C5 convertases.[26]

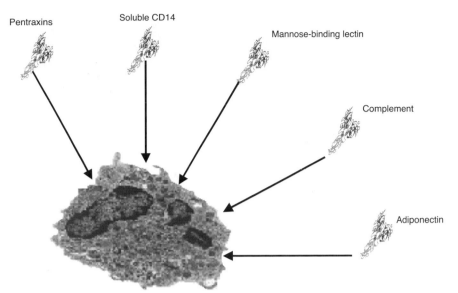

Figure 2 Afferent arm of innate immunity and atherosclerosis. *Humoral* components simultaneously involved in innate immune sensing and the atherosclerotic process

The first suggestion of a possible relationship of CRP to atherosclerosis came when it was demonstrated that aggregated, but not native, non-aggregated, CRP selectively bound just LDL and some VLDL from whole serum. Native CRP also binds to oxidized LDL. There is robust immunohistochemical evidence of CRP deposition within all acute myocardial infarcts, co-localized with activated complement components.[28] Thus, CRP could contribute to complement activation and inflammation in the plaques.[27]

Endothelial dysfunction, a marker of atherosclerosis related to coronary events, is associated in epidemiological studies with markers of systemic inflammation, including CRP production. It is well demonstrated that circulating CRP concentration in apparently healthy people predicts future cardiovascular events.[29–32] Finally, there exists an epidemiological association between higher peak CRP values and poor prognosis of ischaemic heart disease.[27]

In recent years, a number of new pentraxins have been discovered, including pentraxin 3 (PTX3), neuronal pentraxin 1 and neuronal pentraxin 2. These molecules are known as long pentraxins and are approximately twice the size of the prototypic pentraxins CRP and SAP. PTX3 was the first long pentraxin to be discovered and its expression is induced in response to inflammatory stimuli, including tumour necrosis factor-alpha (TNF-α), interleukin (IL)-1β and LPS. PTX3 is produced by a range of cell types, including monocytes/macrophages, endothelial cells and fibroblasts, but is not produced by hepatocytes, which are a major source of CRP. Like CRP, PTX3 is able to bind the C1q complement component and it has been proposed that PTX3 may play the same function in the periphery as CRP does in the circulation.

Strong PTX3 staining has been found in macrophages and endothelial cells in advanced atherosclerotic lesions and in smooth muscle cells.[33] In contrast, sections from non-atherosclerotic internal mammary arteries did not express PTX3. Increased serum PTX3 has been also detected in the blood of patients with acute MI.[34]

Soluble CD14

CD14 also exists as a soluble form (sCD14) found in normal human serum. sCD14 is apparently derived both from secretion of CD14 and from enzymatically cleaved GPI-anchored tissue

CD14. Soluble CD14 has been shown to enhance the endotoxin-neutralization capacity of plasma.[35–37] In fact, plasma lipoproteins promote the release of bacterial LPS from the monocyte cell surface and sCD14 is involved in this process. Neutralization of LPS by reconstituted lipoprotein particles is accelerated more than 30-fold by addition of sCD14.[38,39]

Circulating sCD14 concentration has been found to be associated with several cardiovascular risk factors such as waist diameter, blood pressure, insulin resistance, plasma triglycerides and serum uric acid concentration.[40] This observation is important in the sense that LPS, one of the most potent biological response modifiers currently recognized, circulates in normal humans attached to triglyceride-rich lipoproteins.[41,42] LPS is extraordinarily ubiquitous in nature, being present in food and water, and in normal indoor environments as a constituent of house dust.[43] Endogenous LPS is continually produced within the gut by the death of Gram-negative bacteria and is absorbed into intestinal capillaries. Low-grade portal venous LPS has been claimed to be the status quo in humans.[44] Decreased efficiency in neutralizing LPS-induced responses was hypothesized to lead to a chronic pro-inflammatory response and insulin resistance.[40] This was further supported by the finding of negative correlations betweeen serum sCD14 and circulating concentrations of soluble TNF-α receptors in healthy subjects.[40] sCD14 concentration has also been described to be linked to aortic stiffness.[45]

Mannose-binding lectin

Mannose-binding lectin (MBL) is a circulating immune factor responsible for opsonization of pathogens by binding mannose moieties on their surface and directly activating complement via the lectin pathway before antibody formation. Common variations in the MBL gene are responsible for an opsonic deficiency that affects 5% to 7% of Caucasian subjects. Deficiencies in MBL can be caused by three single nucleotide polymorphisms within exon 1 of the MBL gene on chromosome 10: allele B at codon 54 (G54D), allele C at codon 57 (G57E) and allele D at codon 52 (R52C), with the most common codon at these loci designated allele A. This effect is substantially modulated by at least four promoter polymorphisms, including the H/L and X/Y systems, which show reductions of MBL of up to 85% among individuals homozygous for the LX ('low') promoters.[46] The structural variations have typically been labelled 'O' alleles, in contrast to the most common 'A' allele. The presence of a heterozygous genotype (AO) results in an approximate 8-fold reduction in MBL levels, but there is considerable overlap in the distribution of MBL levels in those with AA and AO genotypes. These structural variations leading to decreased circulating MBL concentration were associated with increased risk of certain infectious conditions[47,48] and, interestingly, were also predictive of coronary artery disease (CAD) in a recent study in American Indians of different ethnicity living in three different locations.[49] This was particularly remarkable in this population given the marked presence of other CAD risk factors such as type 2 diabetes, hypertension and albuminuria. A significant association between persistent infection with *Chlamydia pneumoniae* and CAD has also been reported, but only in the context of OO or AO structural MBL genotypes.[50] An early report of an association between MBL genotypes and CAD from Norway indicated that the prevalence of homozygous structural (but not heterozygous) genotypes predicting low levels of MBL was increased among those with prior coronary artery bypass procedures compared with normal blood donors.[51] MBL variants were also associated with a slightly higher mean area of plaque detected in the carotid artery in whites at high risk for CAD.[52] In another study of US physicians, no relationship was noted between MBL levels and self-reported peripheral arterial disease.[53]

Complement

Complement is a term referring to a collection of plasma proteins, specific cellular receptors and cell surface regulatory molecules. Complement represents an important innate immune defence system to discriminate 'self' from 'non-self'. Invading pathogens are normally attacked by alternative and MBL pathways (triggered by the surface composition of the invader) and also by the classical pathway (triggered by specific antibodies targeted towards the intruder or directly as, for example, in the case of several viruses and bacteria). Chemotaxis of phagocytic cells, opsonization and lysis of the microbe then mostly lead to limitation of the attack and control of the infection. This type of humoral innate host defence plays a crucial role and is executed on viruses, bacteria, fungi and parasites.[54]

Activation of the complement system to completion results in the formation of C5b-9 terminal complexes. These complexes have been observed in human atherosclerotic lesions by immunohistochemistry. Endothelial cell damage leads to complement activation and endothelial cells overlying atherosclerotic lesions have been observed to contain C3 and C5b-9 antigens. Cardiac myocytes stain for complement proteins (C3, C4 and C5b-9) following MI. Infarct size and extent of inflammatory cell infiltrates are diminished by decomplementation prior to experimentally induced myocardial ischaemia. Following MI and ulceration of atherosclerotic lesions in human patients there is an increase in circulating complement activation products and a decrease in the level of native C1 through C4 proteins.[55]

Macrophage complement receptors, C3b receptor (CR1) and C3bi receptor, were also expressed in the atherosclerotic lesions when the complement system was activated.[56]

Thus, complement plays an important role in immune recognition, immune response, in atherogenesis and its sequelae.

Adiponectin

Adiponectin (also called Acrp30 or adipoQ in mice) is a 244-amino-acid protein synthesized and secreted exclusively by the adipose tissue.[57,58] It is a close homologue of the complement protein C1q, which is involved in the recognition of microbial surfaces.

In vitro, adiponectin inhibited monocyte adhesion to endothelial cells, decreased lipid accumulation in human monocyte-derived macrophages and diminished scavenger receptor expression in these cells.[59,60] In cultured human endothelial cells, adiponectin down-regulated expression of intracellular adhesion molecules.[60] It shows anti-inflammatory properties as suggested by the suppressive effect of adiponectin on phagocytic activity and lipopolysaccharide-induced TNF-α production in cultured macrophages.[61] Adiponectin has been shown to inhibit TNF-α induction of nuclear factor κB through activation of the cAMP–protein kinase A pathway.[61] Adiponectin also seems to stimulate the production of nitric oxide in vascular endothelial cells in in vitro studies.[62]

Decreased adiponectin was originally described in patients with coronary artery disease.[63,64] The incidence of cardiovascular death was found to be higher in renal failure patients with low plasma adiponectin compared with those with higher plasma adiponectin levels.[65] Adiponectin has also been found to be associated with vascular function in addition to its well-known positive effects on insulin action. Shimabukuro et al evaluated forearm blood flow (FBF) using plethysmography in 76 Japanese subjects without a history of cardiovascular disease or diabetes mellitus.[66] They found positive associations between FBF and adiponectin. Ouchi et al also reported a significant and positive association between adiponectin and endothelium-dependent vasodilation among hypertensive patients.[67]

Increased nitroglycerin-induced vasodilation of forearm conduit vessels has also been observed in those apparently healthy subjects with the highest circulating adiponectin concentration.[68] However, when established cardiovascular risk factors were present, such as impaired fasting glucose, glucose intolerance or type 2 diabetes, no significant associations between endothelial or vascular dysfunction and adiponectin were found. It could be that, once hypoadiponectinaemia develops, homeostatic mechanisms are lost.[68]

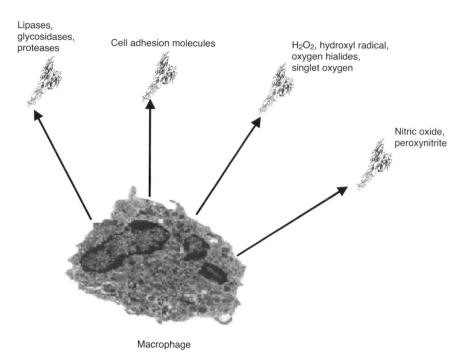

Lipases,
glycosidases,
proteases

Cell adhesion molecules

H₂O₂, hydroxyl radical,
oxygen hialides,
singlet oxygen

Nitric oxide,
peroxynitrite

Macrophage

Figure 3 Efferent arm of innate immunity and atherosclerosis. *Cellular* components simultaneously involved in innate immune action and the atherosclerotic process

Adiponectin null-mice formed 2-fold more neointima in response to external vascular cuff injury than wild-type mice.[69] In fact, in wild-type mice, adiponectin infiltrated rapidly into the subendothelial space of the vascular wall when the endothelial barrier of the arterial wall was injured by balloon angioplasty.[70] Adenovirus-mediated supplement of adiponectin improved the intimal thickening in adiponectin null-mice to the wild-type level.[71] In these studies, the protective effect of adiponectin seemed to be a direct consequence of adiponectin action on the vascular wall and/or macrophages rather than an indirect consequence of alteration of conventional atherosclerotic risk factors in vivo.[69,71]

EFFERENT ARM OF INNATE IMMUNITY AND ATHEROSCLEROSIS

From a historical point of view, the cellular effector arm was the first to be characterized and the best understood in this context.

Cellular response (Figure 3)

It is not enough for the host to sense microbes. It must kill microbes as well. In vertebrates, innate immunity is largely dependent upon myeloid cells: professional immunocytes that engulf and destroy pathogens.[1] Myeloid cells include mononuclear phagocytes and polymorphonuclear phagocytes. The mononuclear phagocytes are the macrophages, derived from blood monocytes. A higher peripheral white blood cell count has been associated with insulin resistance and with atherosclerosis.[72] Peripheral white blood cell count correlated significantly with insulin-mediated glucose disposal during a euglycaemic clamp.[72] In subsequent studies, it was demonstrated that neutrophil and lymphocyte count correlated positively with several components of the insulin resistance syndrome, and that plasma insulin concentration was specifically associated with the number of lymphocytes and monocytes.[73]

Macrophages are distributed throughout the body of the host, in some cases (e.g. heart, brain, lung and liver) lying within the parenchyma of major organs. Macrophages are not a uniform population of cells; rather they are morphologically diverse, encompassing the spindle-shaped tissue histiocyte, the flattened Küpffer cell of the hepatic sinusoids and the stellate microglial cell of the central nervous system.[1]

Should an infectious inoculum be introduced by any route, a macrophage will rarely be far away from the invasive organism. This function seems directly involved in development of atherosclerosis. The accumulation of cholesterol-rich lipoproteins in the arterial wall results in recruitment of blood monocytes and their differentiation into lipid-laden foam cells, which drive the disease process of atherosclerosis. The most convincing evidence that atherosclerosis is an inflammatory process, and not merely a process of depositions of lipids in the arterial wall, is the continous presence and accumulation of monocyte-derived macrophages and T lymphocytes in fatty streaks and advanced atherosclerotic lesions.

Monocyte migration is integral to the development of atherosclerosis. Early in the process of atherosclerosis, circulating monocytes adhere to the endothelial layer of the vessel wall, migrate into the vascular interstitium and phagocytize oxidized low density lipoprotein cholesterol. This process results in the formation of lipid-laden foam cells, which accumulate within the arterial wall to form fatty streaks. Ultimately, these early lesions evolve into advanced atherosclerotic plaques that contain necrotic lipid cores surrounded by a proteoglycan matrix and covered by a fibrous cap and thickened intima. This structure defines an organized atherosclerotic plaque.[74]

According to a recent review, a number of approaches have been used to cripple macrophage activity in genetically prone mouse models of atherosclerosis, all of which attenuated the atherosclerotic process.[74] These include mouse models deficient for expression of:

- Macrophage chemoattractive protein-1 (MCP-1), which stimulates macrophage movement into the vessel wall;

- Chemokine receptor-2, a macrophage receptor that binds MCP-1;
- Macrophage colony stimulating factor, which enhances conversion of monocytes to macrophages;
- Macrophage osteopontin, which may prevent macrophage apoptosis, similar to its effects on endothelial cell survival.

These observations underscore the prominent role of the macrophage in the pathogenesis of atherosclerosis.

The cellular response results in the production of lipases, glycosidases, proteases, antimicrobial peptides, cell adhesion molecules, H_2O_2, hydroxyl radicals, oxygen hialides, singlet oxygen, nitric oxide (NO), peroxynitrite and others. These substances are simultaneously involved in the fight against infection and in the atherosclerotic process. For instance, the NO system appears to play a major role.[75] NO is an important messenger molecule that plays a critical role in a wide variety of physiological functions, including immune modulation, vascular relaxation, neuronal transmission and cytotoxicity. There are at least three isotypes of NO synthase (NOS): endothelial cell NOS (eNOS), the neuronal type NOS (nNOS) and the so-called inducible NOS (iNOS). iNOS is implicated in host defence and is synthesized de novo in response to a variety of inflammatory stimuli. Studies in humans indicate that NO production is decreased during hypertension.[76] A polymorphism within the promoter of the iNOS candidate gene, NOS2A, revealed both increased allele sharing among sibpairs and positive association of NOS2A to essential hypertension.[77] These facts are linked to another major cardiovascular risk factor, insulin resistance, because insulin stimulation of glucose uptake in skeletal muscles and adipose tissues in vivo seem to be NO dependent.[78] Moreover, iNOS has recently been shown to be crucial for the development of insulin resistance.[79] NO also antagonizes the effects of angiotensin II on vascular tone and growth and also downregulates the synthesis of angiotensin-converting enzyme and angiotensin II type 1 (AT-1) receptors.[80] Angiotensin

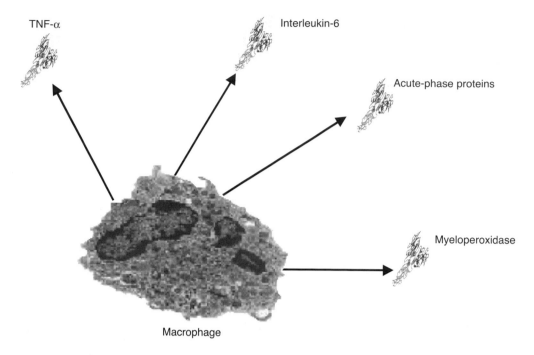

Figure 4   Efferent arm of innate immunity and atherosclerosis. *Humoral* components simultaneously involved in innate immune action and the atherosclerotic process

II is important in stimulating the production of reactive oxygen species and the activation of ancient inflammatory mechanisms through its AT1 receptor.[81]

Humoral response (Figure 4)

The humoral response of the innate immune system results in the production of different cytokines (the major cytokines are TNF-α and IL-6), acute phase reactants, lysozyme, lactoferrin and myeloperoxidase, among others, aimed at tissue repair.

Tumour necrosis factor-alpha and interleukin-6

The available information on the effects of TNF-α and IL-6 in experimental models and the transversal and prospective observations in humans suggest that they are involved in the

pathophysiology of hypertension, abdominal obesity, dyslipidaemia and disorders of glucose metabolism.[82]

The liver is the target of these systemic inflammatory mediators. Among the most important aspects of this response is the reprioritization of hepatic protein synthesis with the increased production of a number of plasma proteins (positive acute-phase proteins) and reduced production of a number of normal export proteins (negative acute-phase proteins). Although the concentrations of multiple components of the acute-phase response increase together, not all of them increase uniformly in all patients. These variations indicate that the components of the acute-phase response are individually regulated, and this may be caused in part by differences in the pattern of production of specific cytokines. These facts would explain increased susceptibility to increased inflammatory activity among healthy volunteers with genetically increased rates of some cytokines (reviewed in reference 82).

Given that abnormalities in immune system function and inflammatory mediators have been found to be associated with several classical cardiovascular risk factors such as hypertension, dyslipidaemia, obesity, insulin resistance and others like endothelial dysfunction and clotting activation, cardiovascular disease seems to be the endpoint, common to metabolic and inflammatory pathways.

Human atherosclerotic lesions have been found to contain TNF-α mRNA. The accumulation of cholesteryl esters in macrophages exposed to LDL is associated with increased synthesis and release of TNF-α. The associations of TNF-α gene polymorphism and MI have been investigated in several studies.[83–87] The *TNFA2* allele, linked to increased transcription rate of the cytokine, was associated with parental history of MI.[83] The odds ratio for myocardial infarction tended to be higher (albeit not significantly) in *TNF2* homozygotes in Brazil.[84] These authors also described a tendency toward increased risk of MI conferred by obesity. In another study, the *TNF2* allele was associated with increased plasma homocysteine levels, a known potentiator of lipid-related oxidation.[85] *TNF2* homozygotes (*n* = 10) also tended to have more fibrous lesions and calcification in their coronary arteries in an autopsy series.[86] An association between –308 TNF-α gene polymorphism and ischaemic heart disease has been recently described, mainly attributed to women with type 2 diabetes.[87]

IL-6 has also been speculated to play a key role in the development of coronary artery disease through a number of metabolic, endothelial and procoagulant mechanisms (reviewed in references 88 and 89). Damage to the vessel wall causes endothelial cell disruption, resulting in exposure of the underlying vascular smooth muscle cells. Endothelial and smooth muscle cells produce IL-6 and IL-6 gene transcripts are expressed in human atherosclerotic lesions. Prospective studies of apparently healthy and high-risk individuals indicate that increased IL-6 levels predict cardiovascular events.[82] IL-6 has been demonstrated to be a strong independent marker of increased mortality in unstable CAD and identifies patients who benefit most from a strategy of early invasive management.

Myeloperoxidase

Myeloperoxidase (MPO), an enzyme principally associated with host defence mechanisms, has also been associated with CRP levels and cardiovascular risk.[90] MPO seems to modulate vascular signalling and vasodilatory function of nitric oxide, linking fight against infection with metabolic events.[91] Importantly, circulating myeloperoxidase levels, in contrast to troponin T, creatine kinase MB isoform and CRP levels, identified patients at risk for cardiac events in the absence of myocardial necrosis, highlighting its potential usefulness for risk stratification among patients who present with chest pain.[92]

CONCLUSIONS

The ability to mount a prominent inflammatory response to pathogens confers an advantage in innate immune defence. Several factors seem to be implicated in the recognition of microbial surfaces, external and endogenous ligands and in their elimination. These pathways are simultaneously involved in atherosclerosis and in metabolic pathways.[82] Thus, different metabolic pathways might have evolved in parallel with several mechanisms involved in our fight against infection.

All the associations described between innate immune components and atherosclerosis might be interpreted as a body's response to chronic tissue injury (the response-to-injury hypothesis), cardiovascular disease being a byproduct of the inflammatory cascade triggered by physical, environmental and infectious agents. Although it seems unlikely that one specific agent causes atherosclerosis, the infectious burden and environmental exposure related to bacterial products (smoking, LPS) are increasingly claimed to be involved in the triggering and development of atherosclerosis.[93]

Research on factors involved in innate immunity and the inflammatory cascade will probably help to characterize individuals prone to cardiovascular disease, and to develop new therapeutic targets aimed at preventing this important cause of death.

References

1. Beutler B. Innate immunity: an overview. Mol Immunol 2004; 40:845–59
2. Janeway CA Jr, Medzhitov R. Innate immune recognition. Ann Rev Immunol 2002; 20:197–216
3. Xu XH, Shah PK, Faure E, et al. Toll-like receptor-4 is expressed by macrophages in murine and human lipid-rich atherosclerotic plaques and upregulated by oxidized LDL. Circulation 2001;104:3103–8
4. Edfeldt K, Swedenborg J, Hansson GK, et al. Expression of toll-like receptors in human atherosclerotic lesions: a possible pathway for plaque activation. Circulation 2002; 105:1158–61
5. Castrillo A, Joseph SB, Vaidya SA, et al. Crosstalk between LXR and Toll-like receptor signaling mediates bacterial and viral antagonism of cholesterol metabolism. Mol Cell 2003; 12:805–16
6. Joseph SB, Castrillo A, Laffitte BA, et al. Reciprocal regulation of inflammation and lipid metabolism by liver X receptors. Nat Med 2003; 9:213–19
7. Agnese DM, Calvano JE, Hahm SJ, et al. Human toll-like receptor 4 mutations but not CD14 polymorphisms are associated with an increased risk of gram-negative infections. J Infect Dis 2002; 186:1522–5
8. Kiechl S, Lorenz E, Reindl M, et al. Toll-like receptor 4 polymorphisms and atherogenesis. N Engl J Med 2002; 347:185–92
9. Arbour NC, Lorenz E, Schutte BC, et al. TLR4 mutations are associated with endotoxin hyporesponsiveness in humans. Nat Genet 2000; 25:187–91
10. Boekholdt SM, Agema WR, Peters RJ, et al. Variants of toll-like receptor 4 modify the efficacy of statin therapy and the risk of cardiovascular events. Circulation 2003; 107:2416–21
11. Illig T, Bongardt F, Schopfer A, et al. The endotoxin receptor TLR4 polymorphism is not associated with diabetes or components of the metabolic syndrome. Diabetes 2003; 52:2861–4
12. Ohashi K, Burkart V, Flohe S, et al. Cutting edge: heat shock protein 60 is a putative endogenous ligand of the toll-like receptor-4 complex. J Immunol 2000; 164:558–61
13. Hollestelle SC, De Vries MR, Van Keulen JK, et al. Toll-like receptor 4 is involved in outward arterial remodeling. Circulation 2004; 109:393–8
14. Oyama J, Blais C Jr, Liu X, et al. Reduced myocardial ischemia-reperfusion injury in toll-like receptor 4-deficient mice. Circulation 2004;109:784–9
15. Asea A, Kraeft SK, Kurt-Jones EA, et al. HSP70 stimulates cytokine production through a CD14-dependent pathway, demonstrating its dual role as a chaperone and cytokine. Nat Med 2000; 6:435–42
16. Unkelbach K, Gardemann A, Kostrzewa M, et al. A new promoter polymorphism in the gene of lipopolysaccharide receptor CD14 is associated with expired myocardial infarction in patients with low atherosclerotic risk profile. Arterioscler Thromb Vasc Biol 1999; 19:932–8
17. Hubacek JA, Rothe G, Pit'ha J, et al. C (-260)- T polymorphism in the promoter of the CD14 monocyte receptor gene as a risk factor for myocardial infarction. Circulation 1999; 99:3218–20
18. Ito D, Murata M, Tanahashi N, et al. Polymorphism in the promoter of lipopolysaccharide receptor CD14 and ischemic cerebrovascular disease. Stroke 2000; 31:2661–4
19. Shimada K, Watanabe Y, Mokuno H, et al. Common polymorphism in the promoter of the CD14 monocyte receptor gene is associated with acute myocardial infarction in Japanese men. Am J Cardiol 2000; 86:682–4
20. Risley P, Jerrard-Dunne P, Sitzer M, et al. Carotid Atherosclerosis Progression Study. Promoter polymorphism in the endotoxin receptor (CD14) is associated with increased carotid atherosclerosis only in smokers: the Carotid Atherosclerosis Progression Study (CAPS). Stroke 2003; 34:600–4
21. Hasday JD, Bascom R, Costa JJ, et al. Bacterial endotoxin is an active component of cigarette smoke. Chest 1999; 115:829–35
22. Wiedermann CJ, Kiechl S, Dunzendorfer S, et al. Association of endotoxemia with carotid atherosclerosis and cardiovascular disease: prospective results from the Bruneck study. J Am Coll Cardiol 1999; 34:1975–81
23. Wiedermann CJ, Kiechl S, Schratzberger P, et al. The role of immune activation in endotoxin-induced atherogenesis. J Endotoxin Res 2001; 7:322–6
24. Osmand AP, Friedenson B, Gewurz H, et al. Characterisation of C-reactive protein and the complement subcomponent Clt as homologous proteins displaying cyclic pentameric symmetry (pentraxins). Proc Natl Acad Sci USA 1977; 74:739–43
25. Robey FA, Liu T-Y. Limulin: a C-reactive protein from Limulus polyphemus. J Biol Chem 1981; 256:969–75

26. Ablij H, Meinders A. C-reactive protein: history and revival. Eur J Intern Med 2002; 13:412–22

27. Pepys MB, Hirschfield GM. C-reactive protein: a critical update. J Clin Invest 2003; 111:1805–12

28. Lagrand WK, Niessen HW, Wolbink GJ, et al. C reactive protein colocalizes with complement in human hearts during acute myocardial infarction. Circulation 1997; 95:97–103

29. Ridker PM, Buring JE, Shih J, et al. Prospective study of C-reactive protein and the risk of future cardiovascular events among apparently healthy women. Circulation 1998; 98:731–3

30. Kuller LH, Tracy RP, Shaten J, et al for the MRFIT Research Group. Relationship of C-reactive protein and coronary heart disease in the MRFIT nested case-control study. Am J Epidemiol 1996; 144:537–47

31. Harris TB, Ferrucci L, Tracy RP, et al. Associations of elevated interleukin-6 and C-reactive protein levels with mortality in the elderly. Am J Med 1999; 106:506–12

32. Ridker PM, Rifai N, Stampfer MJ, et al. Plasma concentration of interleukin-6 and the risk of future myocardial infarction among apparently healthy men. Circulation 2000; 101:1767–72

33. Rolph MS, Zimmer S, Bottazzi B, et al. Production of the long pentraxin PTX3 in advanced atherosclerotic plaques. Arterioscler Thromb Vasc Biol 2002; 22:e10-4

34. Peri G, Introna M, Corradi D, et al. PTX3, a prototypical long pentraxin, is an early indicator of acute myocardial infarction in humans. Circulation 2000; 102:636–41

35. Hiki N, Berger D, Dentener MA, et al. Changes in endotoxin-binding proteins during major elective surgery: important role for soluble CD14 in regulation of biological activity of systemic endotoxin. Clin Diagn Lab Immunol 1999; 6:844–50

36. Haziot A, Rong GW, Lin XY, et al. Recombinant soluble CD14 prevents mortality in mice treated with endotoxin (lipopolysaccharide). J Immunol 1995; 154:6529–32

37. Haziot A, Rong GW, Bazil V, et al. Recombinant soluble CD14 inhibits LPS-induced tumor necrosis factor-alpha production by cells in whole blood. J Immunol 1994; 152:5868–76

38. Wurfel MM, Hailman E, Wright SD. Soluble CD14 acts as a shuttle in the neutralization of lipopolysaccharide (LPS) by LPS-binding protein and reconstituted high density lipoprotein. J Exp Med 1995; 181:1743–54

39. Kitchens RL, Wolfbauer G, Albers JJ, et al. Plasma lipoproteins promote the release of bacterial lipopolysaccharide from the monocyte cell surface. J Biol Chem 1999; 274:34116–22

40. Fernandez-Real JM, Broch M, Richart C, et al. CD14 monocyte receptor, involved in the inflammatory cascade, and insulin sensitivity. J Clin Endocrinol Metab 2003; 88:1780–4

41. Harris HW, Grunfeld C, Feingold KR, et al. Human very low density lipoproteins and chylomicrons can protect against endotoxin-induced death in mice. J Clin Invest 1990; 86:696–702

42. Eggesbo JB, Lyberg T, Aspelin T, et al. Different binding of 125I-LPS to plasma proteins from persons with high or low HDL. Scand J Clin Lab Invest 1996; 56:533–43

43. Michel OJ, Kips J, Duchateau J, et al. Severity of asthma is related to endotoxin in house dust. Am J Respir Crit Care Med 1996; 154:1641–6

44. Jacob AI, Goldberg PK, Bloom N, et al. Endotoxin and bacteria in portal blood. Gastroenterology 1977; 72:1268–70

45. Amar J, Ruidavets JB, Bal Dit Sollier C, et al. Soluble CD14 and aortic stiffness in a population-based study. J Hypertens 2003; 21:1869–77

46. Madsen HO, Garred P, Thiel S, et al. Interplay between promoter and structural gene variants control basal serum level of mannan-binding protein. J Immunol 1995; 155:3013–20

47. Summerfield JA, Sumiya M, Levin M, et al. Association of mutations in mannose binding protein gene with childhood infection in consecutive hospital series. BMJ 1997; 314:1229–32

48. Koch A, Melbye M, Sorensen P, et al. Acute respiratory tract infections and mannose-binding lectin insufficiency during early childhood. JAMA 2001; 285:1316–21

49. Best LG, Davidson M, North KE, et al. Prospective analysis of mannose-binding lectin genotypes and coronary artery disease in American Indians: the Strong Heart Study. Circulation 2004; 109:471–5

50. Rugonfalvi-Kiss S, Endresz V, Madsen HO, et al. Association of *Chlamydia pneumoniae* with coronary artery disease and its progression is dependent on the modifying effect of mannose-binding lectin. Circulation 2002; 106:1071–6

51. Madsen HO, Videm V, Svejgaard A, et al. Association of mannose-binding-lectin deficiency with severe atherosclerosis. Lancet 1998; 352:959–60

52. Hegele RA, Ban MR, Anderson CM, et al. Infection-susceptibility alleles of mannose-binding lectin are associated with increased carotid plaque area. J Investig Med 2000; 48:198–202

53. Albert MA, Rifai N, Ridker PM. Plasma levels of cystatin-C and mannose binding protein are not associated with risk of developing systemic atherosclerosis. Vasc Med 2001; 6:145–9

54. Joiner KA. Complement evasion by bacteria and parasites. Annu Rev Microbiol 1988; 42:201–30

55. Seifert PS, Kazatchkine MD. The complement system in atherosclerosis. Atherosclerosis 1988; 73:91–104

56. Saito E, Fujioka T, Kanno H, et al. Complement receptors in atherosclerotic lesions. Artery 1992; 19:47–62

57. Maeda K, Okubo K, Shimomura I, et al. cDNA cloning and expression of a novel adipose specific collagen-like factor, apM1 (AdiPose Most abundant Gene transcript 1). Biochem Biophys Res Commun 1996; 221:286–9

58. Scherer PE, Williams S, Fogliano M, et al. A novel serum protein similar to C1q, produced exclusively in adipocytes. J Biol Chem 1995; 270:26746–9

59. Ouchi N, Kihara S, Arita Y, et al. Adipocyte-derived plasma protein, adiponectin, suppresses lipid accumulation and class A scavenger receptor expression in human monocyte-derived macrophages. Circulation 2001; 103:1057–63

60. Yokota T, Oritani K, Takahashi I, et al. Adiponectin, a new member of the family of soluble defense collagens, negatively regulates the growth of myelomonocytic progenitors and the functions of macrophages. Blood 2000; 96:1723–32

61. Ouchi N, Kihara S, Arita Y, et al. Adiponectin, an adipocyte-derived plasma protein, inhibits endothelial NF-kappaB signaling through a cAMP-dependent pathway. Circulation 2000; 102:1296–301

62. Chen H, Montagnani M, Funahashi T, et al. Adiponectin stimulates production of nitric oxide in vascular endothelial cells. J Biol Chem 2003; 278:45021–6

63. Hotta K, Funahashi T, Arita Y, et al. Plasma concentrations of a novel, adipose-specific protein, adiponectin, in type 2 diabetic patients. Arterioscler Thromb Vasc Biol 2000; 20:1595–9

64. Ouchi N, Kihara S, Arita Y, et al. Novel modulator for endothelial adhesion molecules: adipocyte-derived plasma protein adiponectin. Circulation 1999; 100:2473–6

65. Zoccali C, Mallamaci F, Tripepi G, et al. Adiponectin, metabolic risk factors, and cardiovascular events among patients with end-stage renal disease. J Am Soc Nephrol 2002; 13:134–41

66. Shimabukuro M, Higa N, Asahi T, et al. Hypoadiponectinemia is closely linked to endothelial dysfunction in man. J Clin Endocrinol Metab 2003; 88:3236–40

67. Ouchi N, Ohishi M, Kihara S, et al. Association of hypoadiponectinemia with impaired vasoreactivity. Hypertension 2003; 42:231–4

68. Fernandez-Real JM, Castro A, Vazquez G, et al. Adiponectin is associated with vascular function independent of insulin sensitivity. Diabetes Care 2004; 27:739–45

69. Kubota N, Terauchi Y, Yamauchi T, et al. Disruption of adiponectin causes insulin resistance and neointimal formation. J Biol Chem 2002; 277:25863–6

70. Okamoto Y, Arita Y, Nishida M, et al. An adipocyte-derived plasma protein, adiponectin, adheres to injured vascular walls. Horm Metab Res 2000; 32:47–50

71. Matsuda M, Shimomura I, Sata M, et al. Role of adiponectin in preventing vascular stenosis. The missing link of adipo-vascular axis. J Biol Chem 2002; 277:37487–91

72. Facchini F, Hollenbeck CB, Chen YN, et al. Demonstration of a relationship between white blood cell count, insulin resistance, and several risk factors for coronary heart disease in women. J Intern Med 1992; 232:267–72

73. Targher G, Seidell JC, Tonoli M, et al. The white blood cell count: its relationship to plasma insulin and other cardiovascular risk factors in healthy male individuals. J Intern Med 1996; 239:435–41

74. Hansson GK, Peter Libby P, Schönbeck U, et al. Innate and adaptive immunity in the pathogenesis of atherosclerosis. Circ Res 2002; 91:281–91

75. Manning RD Jr, Hu L, Tan DY, et al. Role of abnormal nitric oxide systems in salt-sensitive hypertension. Am J Hypertens 2001; 14(6 Pt 2):68S–73S

76. Leclercq B, Jaimes EA, Raij L. Nitric oxide synthase and hypertension. Curr Opin Nephrol Hypertens 2002; 11:185–9

77. Rutherford S, Johnson MP, Curtain RP, et al. Chromosome 17 and the inducible nitric oxide synthase gene in human essential hypertension. Hum Genet 2001; 109:408–15

78. Roy D, Perreault M, Marette A. Insulin stimulation of glucose uptake in skeletal muscles and adipose tissues in vivo is NO dependent. Am J Physiol 1998; 274(4 Pt 1):E692–9

79. Perreault M, Marette A. Targeted disruption of inducible nitric oxide synthase protects against obesity-linked insulin resistance in muscle. Nat Med 2001; 7:1138–43

80. Bataineh A, Raij L. Angiotensin II, nitric oxide, and end-organ damage in hypertension. Kidney Int (Suppl) 1998; 68:S14–19

81. Luft FC. Angiotensin, inflammation, hypertension, and cardiovascular disease. Curr Hypertens Rep 2001; 3:61–7

82. Fernández-Real JM, Ricart W. Insulin resistance and chronic cardiovascular inflammatory syndrome. Endocr Rev 2003; 24:278–301

83. Herrmann SM, Ricard S, Nicaud V, et al. Polymorphisms of the tumour necrosis factor-α gene, coronary heart disease and obesity. Eur J Clin Invest 1998; 28:59–66

84. Padovani JC, Pazin-Filho A, Simoes MV, et al. Gene polymorphisms in the TNF locus and the risk of myocardial infarction. Thromb Res 2000; 100:263–9

85. Wang XL, Oosterhof J. Tumour necrosis factor α $G^{-308} \rightarrow$ A polymorphism and risk for coronary artery disease. Clin Sci 2000; 98:435–7

86. Keso T, Perola M, Laippala P, et al. Polymorphisms within the tumor necrosis factor locus and prevalence of coronary artery disease in middle-aged men. Atherosclerosis 2001; 154:691–7

87. Vendrell J, Fernandez-Real JM, Gutierrez C, et al. A polymorphism in the promoter of the tumor necrosis factor-alpha gene (–308) is associated with coronary heart disease in type 2 diabetic patients. Atherosclerosis 2003; 167:257–64

88. Yudkin JS, Kumari M, Humphries SE, et al. Inflammation, obesity, stress and coronary heart disease: is interleukin-6 the link? Atherosclerosis 2000; 148:209–14

89. Woods A, Brull DJ, Humprhies SE, et al. Genetics of inflammation and risk of coronary artery disease: the

central role of interleukin 6. Eur Heart J 2000; 21:1574–83

90. Zhang R, Brennan ML, Fu X, et al. Association between myeloperoxidase levels and risk of coronary artery disease. JAMA 2001; 286:2136–42

91. Eiserich JP, Baldus S, Brennan ML, et al. Myeloperoxidase, a leukocyte-derived vascular NO oxidase. Science 2002; 296:2391–4

92. Brennan ML, Penn MS, Van Lente F, et al. Prognostic value of myeloperoxidase in patients with chest pain. N Engl J Med 2003; 349:1595–604

93. Espinola-Klein C, Rupprecht HJ, Blankenberg S, et al. Impact of infectious burden on extent and long-term prognosis of atherosclerosis. Circulation 2002; 105:15–21

Role of CD44 in atherogenesis and its potential role as a therapeutic target

17

E. Puré

INTRODUCTION

In spite of the significant progress being made in understanding the cellular and molecular basis of atherosclerosis, cardiovascular disease remains the leading cause of morbidity and mortality in the United States. Multiple risk factors for development of atherosclerosis have been identified, including elevated levels of LDL-cholesterol and reduced levels of HDL. In addition to the contribution of lipoprotein metabolism, the inflammatory response in the vessel wall has proven to be a major component of the development and progression of atherosclerotic lesions, as well as an important factor in the risk of acute thrombotic events.

Atherosclerotic lesions develop at anatomical sites characterized by variations in haemodynamic and mechanical forces that induce the local expression of chemokines, cytokines and endothelial cell adhesion molecules.[1] The infiltrating inflammatory cells secrete soluble mediators that perpetuate the inflammatory response underlying the progression of atherosclerotic lesions. Vascular cells also play a critical part in disease progression. Activated endothelial cells (ECs), in addition to mediating inflammatory cell recruitment, regulate the function of vascular smooth muscle cells (VSMCs). In normal vessels, VSMCs reside predominantly in the media in a quiescent, contractile state, maintained in part by products of ECs such as prostacyclin, nitric oxide and TGF-β. Atherosclerotic lesions are characterized by dedifferentiation of VSMCs to a synthetic state characterized by proliferation and migration into the neointima.[2] In addition, VSMC dedifferentiation is associated with downregulation of contractile proteins such as α-smooth muscle actin, and upregulation of adhesion molecules,[3] as well as matrix components and inflammatory mediators.[2] In addition to mediating leukocyte recruitment, cell adhesion molecules (CAMs) mediate signal transduction and thereby regulate the function of leukocytes as well as vascular cells, thus providing potential targets for novel therapeutics designed to selectively regulate the inflammatory response in atherosclerosis.

CD44 is a widely expressed CAM that serves as a principal receptor for the extracellular matrix glycosaminoglycan hyaluronan (HA). CD44 can mediate atherogenic processes including inflammatory cell recruitment and cellular activation.[4-6] Importantly, the proinflammatory low molecular weight forms of HA (LMW-HA) accumulate in atherosclerotic lesions.[7-9] This evidence led to investigation of the potential for CD44 to modulate atherogenesis. Using a genetic approach it was demonstrated that CD44-null mice had markedly reduced atherosclerosis compared with CD44 heterozygote and wild-type littermates.[10] Furthermore, it was shown that CD44 promotes atherosclerosis by mediating inflammatory cell recruitment and leukocyte and vascular cell activation.[10] In addition, CD44-deficient mice were found to be protected against ischaemic brain injury.[11] Thus, CD44 appears to be an important factor, and potential therapeutic

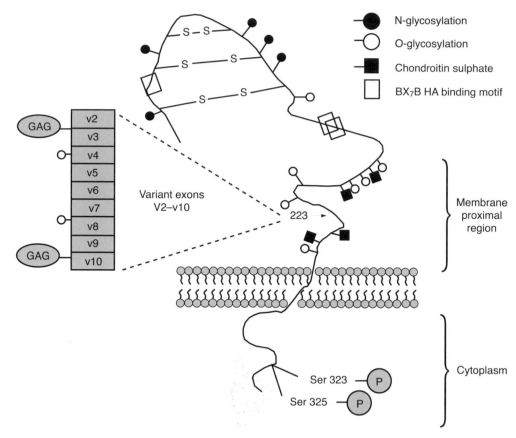

Figure 1   Schematic representation of CD44

target, in the two most devastating outcomes of cardiovascular disease, myocardial infarction and stroke. In this chapter, the mechanisms by which CD44 can contribute to atherogenesis at multiple levels and their potential as targets for therapeutic intervention in cardiovascular disease are discussed.

STRUCTURE, LIGANDS AND FUNCTION OF CD44 (Figure 1)

CD44 is a family of type I transmembrane glycoprotein products of a single gene generated by alternative RNA splicing. The gene for CD44 maps to chromosome 11 in humans and 2 in mice.[12] The CD44 gene consists of 20 exons. The most abundant isoform of CD44 (referred to as CD44s for 'standard') is encoded by 12 non-variant exons that encode for the extracellular domain, a transmembrane domain and an intracellular domain. The alternatively spliced isoforms are generated by inclusion of various numbers and combinations of one to 10 or 11 (depending on the species) variant exons that are inserted at a single site in the membrane-proximal region of the extracellular domain.[13,14] The predominant, and highly conserved, 72-amino-acid cytoplasmic domain can also be replaced by an alternatively spliced exon encoding a truncated form of the receptor.

CD44 is also subject to myriad post-translational modifications, including variations in the *N*- and *O*-linked carbohydrate structures and covalent modification with glycosaminoglycans, in a cell-type-specific fashion that also varies with activation and differentiation in some cell lineages. These modifications contribute to the large variation in the apparent molecular weight, pI and ligand binding function of CD44.

The first ~100 residues of the amino terminus of the extracellular domain constitute a structural 'link module' that contains one of the three potential HA binding motifs, $B(X_7)B$,[15] and defines the receptor as a member of the link module superfamily.[16] The N-terminus of the extracellular domain, including six cysteines that participate in intramoleclar disulphide bridging, and the transmembrane and intracellular domains are highly conserved (80–90% among species), while the membrane proximal region of the extracellular domain is less well conserved (~50%).

A soluble form of CD44 is found in plasma and other body fluids.[17,18] Although found in significant levels in normal plasma, immune activation and inflammation are often associated with increased plasma levels of soluble CD44. These findings suggest that release of CD44 correlates with enhanced local proteolytic activity and matrix remodelling and have generated interest in CD44 as a potential biomarker for inflammation. Recent evidence suggests that, in addition to the transmembrane and soluble forms, CD44 also exists as an integral component of extracellular matrix that may be an important reservoir of the soluble CD44 released into the fluid phase in inflammation.[19,20] Furthermore, cleavage of the extracellular domain leads to sequential proteolytic processing of the transmembrane domain and the release of the intracellular domain (by a presenilin-dependent gamma secretase), that translocates to the nucleus where it may regulate gene transcription, and the extracellular release of a so-called CD44β-peptide.[21,22] The function of the latter is unknown, but is reminiscent of the presenilin-dependent processing of β-amyloid precursor protein leading to the release of amyloid β peptide(s) implicated in Alzheimer's disease. Cleavage of CD44 may also be ligand induced

as cross-linking the receptor with anti-CD44 antibodies leads to release of soluble CD44.[23,24] Endogenous membrane metalloproteinases, including MT1-MMP and MT3-MMP, and disintegrins and metalloproteases (ADAM)[25] have been implicated in the shedding of CD44 based on pharmacological evidence.[24,26] Shedding of CD44 appears to be controlled at least in part by Ras and Rho GTPases (Cdc42 and Rac1), possibly through regulation of the actin cytoskeleton.[24,27] Finally, an alternatively spliced variant may generate a soluble form of CD44 by de novo synthesis.[28]

An important aspect of CD44 is the regulation of its affinity for its principal ligand, HA. CD44 expressed on the vast majority of primary cells exhibits low affinity for HA while cellular activation is associated with increased affinity of CD44 for HA, reportedly due to one or more mechanisms including increased expression, receptor oligomerization, expression of alternatively spliced variants and post-translational modifications, including changes in glycosylation, sulphation and phosphorylation.[29–38]

The principal ligand implicated in many of the defined functions of CD44 is HA.[12,30] One important function of CD44 is in fact its role in the assembly and turnover of HA-containing matrices.[39,40] However, it is important to note that CD44 also binds other matrix components, including collagen types I and VI and fibrinogen and fibronectin, and osteopontin[12,41–43] that may also be important in the function of CD44 in atherogenesis. In addition, it has recently been demonstrated that docking of matrix metalloproteinases to CD44 may be an important mechanism for the local activation of TGF-β1 and the regulation of inflammation/fibrosis.[44]

CD44 PROMOTES ATHEROSCLEROSIS IN A MURINE MODEL (Figure 2)

Using a genetic approach it was demonstrated that CD44-null mice had markedly reduced atherosclerosis compared with CD44 heterozygote and wild-type littermates.[10]

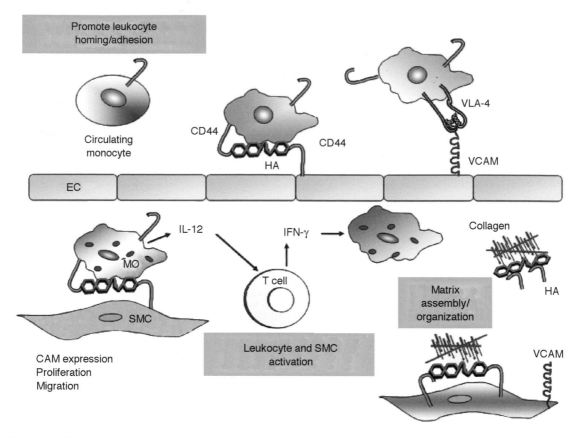

Figure 2 CD44 has the potential to regulate atherogenesis through multiple mechanisms

The extent of atherosclerotic lesions in apoE$^{-/-}$.CD44$^{+/+}$ and apoE$^{-/-}$.CD44$^{-/-}$ mice was compared. The extent of atherosclerosis was markedly reduced in CD44$^{-/-}$.apoE$^{-/-}$ and CD44$^{+/-}$.apoE$^{-/-}$ mice compared to CD44$^{+/+}$.apoE$^{-/-}$ mice maintained on a chow diet without having any effect on plasma cholesterol levels. Further investigation indicated that CD44 can potentiate atherogenesis through several mechanisms involving cells of both the haematopoietic and non-haematopoietic compartments:

1. CD44 mediates the recruitment of monocytes/macrophages to atherosclerotic lesions.[10]
2. The pro-inflammatory low molecular weight form of the CD44 ligand HA (LMW-HA) that accumulates in athero-

sclerotic lesions can induce the production of inflammatory mediators known to promote atherogenesis including the cytokine interleukin-12 (IL-12).[5] IL-12 is critical for the generation of a TH1 type inflammatory response, in part through the induction of interferon-gamma (IFN-γ) production. The IL-12/IFN-γ pathway is an important pro-atherogenic component of the inflammatory response. In studying the signalling pathways that regulate CD44/HA-induced IL-12 production, a novel 12/15-lipoxygenase-dependent pathway that mediates the expression of IL-12 in macrophages and in atherosclerotic lesions was discovered.[45]

3. CD44 is required for the phenotypic dedifferentiation of VSMCs in atherosclerotic lesions to the 'synthetic' state.[10]

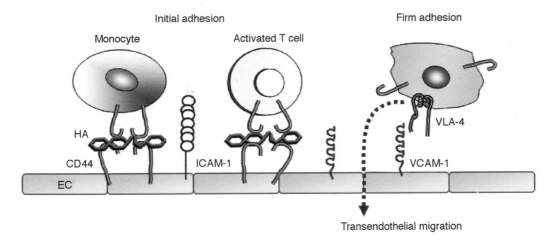

Figure 3 CD44 mediates leukocyte recruitment to atherosclerotic lesions. CD44 mediates the initial binding of circulating monocytes and activated T cells to activated endothelium. CD44 on leukocytes binds to HA produced by activated endothelium and docked to the lumenal surface via CD44 on the endothelial surface. Subsequent engagement of leukocyte integrins such as VLA-4 by endothelial cell adhesion molecules such as VCAM-1 results in firm adhesion leading to transendothelial migration

4. The low molecular weight pro-inflammatory forms of HA that accumulate in atherosclerotic lesions stimulate VCAM-1 expression and proliferation of cultured primary aortic VSMCs, whereas high molecular weight forms of HA (HMW-HA) inhibit VSMC proliferation.

CD44 MEDIATES RECRUITMENT OF MONOCYTES/MACROPHAGES AND T CELLS (Figure 3)

CD44 is expressed on both inflammatory cells and activated endothelial cells and can mediate the adhesion of inflammatory cells to ECs.[4,46] Using a genetic approach it was demonstrated that expression of CD44 on monocytes/macrophages was critical for the recruitment of macrophages to atherosclerotic lesions.[10] Thus, trafficking of monocytes/macrophages from apoE$^{-/-}$.CD44$^{-/-}$ mice to atherosclerotic lesions when adoptively transferred into apoE$^{-/-}$.CD44$^{+/+}$ mice was markedly reduced (by 70–90%) when compared to the trafficking of apoE$^{-/-}$.CD44$^{+/+}$ monocytes/macrophages to atherosclerotic lesions in apoE$^{-/-}$, CD44$^{+/+}$ mice. These results indicate that expression of CD44 on monocytes/macrophages is required for their recruitment to lesions. In addition, it has been reported that recruitment of activated T cells to sites of inflammation is mediated by CD44. The net effect of T cells also appears to be to promote atherogenesis. Therefore it will be of considerable interest to extend the studies of monocyte/macrophage recruitment to atherosclerotic lesions to determine whether CD44-mediated interactions are also important for the recruitment of T cells to atherosclerotic lesions. Activated ECs also upregulate CD44 as well as their production of HA that binds to the EC surface via CD44.[46,47] In studies of T cell homing, it was shown that, in addition to CD44 expressed on T cells, the upregulation of endothelial cell HA production and its docking to EC CD44 also play a role in the recruitment of T cells to sites of inflammation.[48] Therefore, it will also be of interest in future studies to determine whether EC CD44

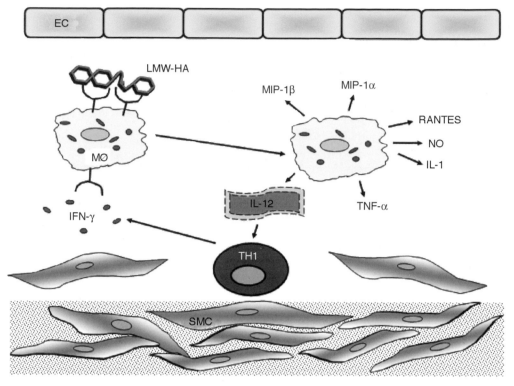

Figure 4 CD44 induces the interleukin-12/interferon-γ (IL-12/IFN-γ) pro-inflammatory axis in atherosclerotic lesions. LMW-HA binding to CD44 induces macrophage release of pro-inflammatory mediators, including IL-12 that promotes a TH1 type inflammatory response. An important function of IL-12 is to induce the production of IFN-γ by several cell types including TH1 T cells and natural killer cells, thus establishing a positive amplification loop by, in turn, inducing enhanced production of IL-12 by macrophages

and HA mediate monocyte/macrophage and T cell recruitment to atherosclerotic lesions, as has been described in the case of other inflammatory lesions.

CD44 REGULATES THE PRODUCTION OF INFLAMMATORY MEDIATORS BY MACROPHAGES AND T CELLS (Figure 4)

CD44 stimulates the production of inflammatory mediators by macrophages (Figure 4) such as MCP-1, TNF and iNOS[5,6,49] that have been implicated in the pathogenesis of atherosclerosis. In addition, the engagement of CD44 by LMW-HA was found to be one of the most potent inducers of IL-12 production in macrophages. Release of IL-12 leads to the generation of a TH1 type inflammatory response, in part through the induction of IFN-γ. The pro-atherogenic effects of IL-12 and IFN-γ are now well established.[50–53]

A potentially very interesting recent finding is that CD44/HA, as well as lipopolysaccharides, can activate a novel 12/15-lipoxygenase-dependent pathway leading to IL-12 gene expression.[45] Importantly, the IL-12 production by macrophages in atherosclerotic lesions was found to be predominantly dependent on this novel 12/15-lipoxygenase-mediated mechanism since the levels of IL-12 and IFN-γ detected in the atherosclerotic lesions of apobec$^{-/-}$.LDLR$^{-/-}$.12/15-LO$^{-/-}$ mice were markedly reduced compared to the levels detected in apobec$^{-/-}$.LDLR$^{-/-}$.12/15-LO$^{+/+}$

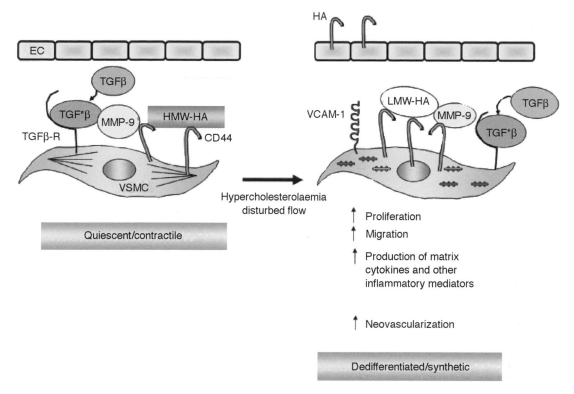

Figure 5   CD44 may play a role in vascular remodelling by regulating vascular smooth muscle cell de-differentiation, proliferation and migration and matrix assembly and organization

mice.[45] In contrast, in the same 12/15-lipoxy-genase-deficient mice, the IL-12 and IFN-γ response to infection with *Toxoplasma gondii* was comparable to that seen in 12/15-LO[+/+] littermate controls. These results indicate that the signalling pathways involved in the production of IL-12 may vary in a cell type and/or stimulus-dependent manner. If this indeed proves to be the case it will open up the possibility of pharmacologically inhibiting the pro-atherogenic IL-12/IFN-γ axis in atherosclerotic lesions without necessarily disrupting the induction of TH1 responses required, for example, to resolve a number of infections. Further understanding of the signalling pathways and transcriptional regulation of IL-12 may therefore provide novel targets for the rational design of therapeutic interventions to modulate the inflammatory response in atherosclerotic lesions.

CD44 HAS THE POTENTIAL TO REGULATE VASCULAR REMODELLING THROUGH MULTIPLE MECHANISMS (Figure 5)

Development of atherosclerotic lesions is associated with vascular remodelling. The proliferation, de-differentiation, activation and migration of VSMC and matrix reorganization are all important aspects of vascular remodelling. The role of CD44 in leukocyte homing to atherosclerotic lesions and leukocyte activation notwithstanding, data indicate that CD44 also plays a critical role in vascular homeostasis and in regulating the function of VSMCs in atherosclerotic lesions. A characteristic feature of atherosclerotic lesions is transition of VSMCs from a contractile to a synthetic phenotype. The synthetic phenotype is characterized by changes in gene expression (increased expression of

CAMs and decreased α-smooth muscle actin),[3] as well as proliferation and migration of medial VSMCs into the neointima.[2,54,55] It appears that CD44 may play an important role in regulating the phenotypic de-differentiation, growth and migration of VSMC. Together with the evidence that both cell-surface and matrix-associated CD44 play important roles in the assembly and organization of extracellular matrix, these data suggest that CD44 may be an important factor in vascular remodelling.

CD44/HA regulates vascular smooth muscle cell growth and de-differentiation

Recent evidence suggests that CD44 mediates signals that maintain quiescence of VSMC in normal vessel, but mediates pro-atherogenic signals in atherosclerotic lesions in hypercholesterolaemic mice.[10] The suggestion that CD44 plays a role in homeostasis is in part based on data that the high molecular weight form of HA (HMW-HA) that predominates in extracellular matrix under homeostatic conditions inhibits VSMC growth. In contrast, interaction of CD44 with the intermediate to low molecular weight forms of HA (LMW-HA) that accumulate in atherosclerotic lesions stimulates the growth and phenotypic de-differentiation of VSMC. CD44 was shown to promote human VSMC proliferation.[7] Furthermore, the expression of high levels of CD44 on cultured murine VSMCs is maintained by the production of endogenous endothelin and an endothelin-converting enzyme inhibitor was shown to block HA-induced VSMC proliferation.[56] LMW-HA also induced increased expression of VCAM-1 on murine VSMCs in vitro, at least in part through the activation of NF-κB.[10] It was also demonstrated that CD44 is required for the upregulation of VCAM-1 on VSMCs in murine atherosclerotic lesions. Similar to the findings in human VSMCs, LMW-HA induced the proliferation of murine VSMCs through a CD44-dependent mechanism.[10] Thus, the ability of HA to stimulate VSMC activation is dependent upon the form of HA. The intermediate to low molecular weight forms of HA that accumulate in atherosclerotic lesions as the result of degra-

dation of HMW-HA, either by hyaluonidases or by oxygen/nitrogen radicals,[57] stimulate the growth and activation of human as well as murine VSMC and do so largely via CD44. In marked contrast, HMW-HA, which is the predominant form found in normal vessels, inhibits growth factor-induced proliferation of VSMC in vitro, also through interaction with CD44. Based on these results it was hypothesized that, rather than a default pathway, the maintenance of VSMCs in a quiescent state may require receptor-mediated interactions with components of extracellular matrix. In addition, ECs in normal vessels produce several factors that contribute to maintaining VSMCs in a quiescent state, including prostacyclin, nitric oxide and TGF-β. Taken together, these findings suggest the HMW-HA may contribute to maintenance of the contractile state of VCSMs, while LMW-HA may promote de-differentiation to the synthetic state.

The role of CD44 in vascular smooth muscle cell adhesion and migration

Cellular adhesion, motility and migration are partially dependent on the integrity of integrin–adhesion complexes and organization of the actin cytoskeleton.[58,59] Cell movement is determined in part by the balance between adhesion and de-adhesion of integrin–adhesion complexes.[60,61] Data are accumulating that implicate CD44 in the regulation of cell adhesion and motility. CD44 plays a role in the homing and migration of leukocytes, and its association with increased invasiveness of certain tumours suggests that it may participate in adhesion and cell motility.[23,62] Its affinity for HA contributes to the potential for CD44 to participate in cellular migration, particularly in HA-rich matrices.[63] Interaction of CD44 with cytoskeletal components provides the basis by which CD44 can regulate adhesion complexes and play a role in tissue remodelling. CD44 interactions with ERM proteins, and the coupling of CD44 to signal transduction pathways involving Rho family GTPases, PI3-kinases and tyrosine kinases, suggest that CD44 may participate in cytoskeletal reorganization and signalling events important for establishing cell polarity.

Actin polymerization is dependent on a variety of factors: formation of integrin-adhesion complexes with stable focal adhesion contacts, activation of src kinases and RhoA GTPases and downstream effectors such as focal adhesion kinase (FAK) and paxillin, and growth factors such as TGF-β.[64–67] Studies have implicated CD44 as a co-receptor for α4β1 integrin in adhesion,[68] and as having a role in α4β1-mediated cell trafficking.[69] However, direct evidence supporting a role for CD44 in integrin-dependent adhesion or signalling is still lacking. A more convincing link exists between CD44 and the cytoskeleton. The cytoplasmic domain of CD44 undergoes post-translational modifications, which impacts on its binding affinity for cytoskeletal-associated proteins such as ankyrin and the ezrin/radixin/moesin (ERM) proteins.[70–72] Furthermore, CD44 can mediate the activation of src kinases and may associate with small GTPases. CD44 may also regulate GTPase activity through its association with Rho GDP-dissociation inhibitor.[73,74] Based on these observations, the potential for CD44 to participate in integrin-dependent adhesion and its impact on leukocyte and vascular cell function in lesions warrants further investigation.

Rho-family GTPases have been implicated in cell polarization, with Cdc42 and Rac contributing to a balanced formation of lamellapodia and filopodia.[75,76] The integrated formation of lamellapodia and filopodia leads to both stable protrusions at the leading edge and detachments in the rear, providing a basis for directional migration.[60,77,78] These observations suggest that regulation of the actin cytoskeleton and adhesion is a critical feature contributing to directional migration. Differentially activated integrins located at the leading edge translate to specific intracellular signalling events, leading to stable lamellapodia formation.

The ERM proteins serve as important membrane cytoskeletal linkers, contributing to the formation of integrin complexes and actin reorganization.[79] Phosphatidylinositol-4,5-bisphosphate (PIP2) has been shown to stabilize binding between CD44 and the ERM proteins and phosphatidylinositol 3,4,5-triphosphate kinase (PI3K) and integrin activation participate in maintaining polarization.[80,81] CD44 localizes to the leading edge following activation of key GTPases, indicating it may play a role in determining cell polarity through stabilization of F-actin.[81–83] Thus CD44 may participate in directional migration of VSMCs through its interaction with intracellular proteins implicated in cell polarity. Furthermore, these observations provide a potential mechanism by which CD44 may participate in cytoskeletal re-organization and signalling events, establishing the cell polarity critical for directional migration and thereby playing an important role in vascular remodelling. Further studies to determine the mechanisms by which CD44 regulates VSMC locomotion, polarity and migration are likely to provide additional potential targets for therapeutic intervention in atherosclerosis.

Matrix composition

CD44 is critical to both the formation and turnover HA-rich peri-cellular matrix that influences adhesion and migration of cells.[23,63] Also, specific proteoglycan forms of CD44 have been shown to exhibit affinity for ECM proteins such as fibronectin, collagen and osteopontin. ECM proteins such as fibronectin contain RGD motifs and, upon binding to integrins, induce activation of RhoA, formation of stress fibres and establishment of focal adhesion complexes that provide a link between the extracellular environment and the cytoskeleton.[58,84] Certain proteoglycans, such as syndecan-4, serve a similar function by exposing integrin-binding sites on fibronectin, facilitating the formation of adhesion complexes and playing a role in the organization of extracellular matrix.[85] This provides a mechanism by which CD44 may impact the composition and organization of ECM and thus affect vascular remodelling.

CD44 may regulate atherogenesis by regulating the activation of TGF-β

VSMCs reside in the media of normal vessels in a quiescent, contractile state. ECs contribute to maintaining VSMC quiescence by the production of prostacyclin, nitric oxide and TGF-β, all of which are downregulated at sites prone to the development of atherosclerotic lesions in response to variations in haemodynamic and mechanical forces. In contrast to the effects of TGF-β in normal vessels, TGF-β serves as a chemotactic, mitogenic and differentiation stimulus for parenchymal cells in areas of tissue injury. However, the role of TGF-β is complex in that it can contribute to inflammation at some stages, but can also play a role in the suppression of inflammation. Cell surface adhesion molecules including $\alpha_v\beta_6$ and proteases such as MMP-9 play a role in activation of latent TGF-β, thereby localizing the effects of active TGF-β in an autocrine/paracrine fashion.[44,86]

Recent studies in a murine model of bleomycin-induced lung fibrosis[87] demonstrated a pivotal role for CD44 in the resolution of lung inflammation and the transition to a reparative fibrotic response. This study revealed that CD44-deficient mice had normal to enhanced levels of latent TGF-β, but reduced levels of active TGF-β in bronchial alveolar lavage fluid, suggesting that CD44 may be critical for regulating TGF-β activity.

The effects of TGF-β may be many, including modification of the integrin repertoire, alteration of ECM components and induction of core protein expression along with associated glycosaminoglycans. Furthermore, there are data to indicate that an intact cytoskeleton is required for $\alpha_v\beta_6$ integrin-mediated activation of latent TGF-β, suggesting that without a stable cytoskeleton, localized activation of TGF-β may be altered.[86] Also intriguing is the notion that CD44 may regulate activation of TGF-β by serving as a docking site for MMP-9 at the cell surface, thereby locally activating latent TGF-β.[44] Previous studies have also suggested that CD44 may interact with the TGF-β receptor 1.[88] TGF-β is an important factor in determining the balance between inflammation and fibrosis. As the balance between the fibrotic and inflammatory responses may be critical in determining the susceptibility of atherosclerotic plaques to rupture, it is important to gain a better understanding of the effects of TGF-β and the role of CD44 in mediating the activation of TGF-β in the vessel wall.

Other potential roles for CD44 in atherogenesis

Atherosclerotic lesions are characterized by neovascularization. CD44 has been implicated in angiogenesis[44,89,90] although the mechanisms involved are not well defined. Regulation of both EC and VSMC growth and migration is critical to angiogenesis and, as discussed above, can be regulated by CD44. Thus, the impact of CD44 on neovascularization of atherosclerotic lesions is another area worthy of further investigation.

Finally, considerable experimental evidence suggests that CD44 promotes cell growth[7,91] and, in some cell types, prevents cell death through apoptosis.[92-94] The influence of CD44 on both expansion and death of macrophages and VSMCs may have profound effects on lesion size and the morphology of atherosclerotic lesions and therefore warrants further investigation.

Potential role of soluble CD44 in atherosclerosis

Soluble CD44 (sCD44) is present at substantial levels in normal mouse and human plasma and further increases are associated with immune activation, while sCD44 levels are reduced in states of immunodeficiency.[17] Although the physiological and pathophysiological significance of soluble CD44 is not yet known, it is evident that sCD44 has affinity for HA.[95] Protease-mediated release of CD44 also leads to further presenilin-dependent gamma-secretase-mediated proteolytic processing of the vestiges of the receptor.[20] This leads to the release of a fragment of the intracellular domain that can translocate to the nucleus, where it regulates gene expression.[21] In view of the need for novel biomarkers of inflammation in cardiovascular disease, the results of ongoing studies to assess whether sCD44 levels are significantly increased in the plasma of patients with confirmed CVD compared to age- and gender-matched controls will be of interest. In addition to its potential as a biomarker, sCD44 is known to have ligand binding capacity and therefore to have the potential to impact on disease progression. Thus, future studies to investigate the impact of sCD44 on atherogenesis in mice may provide useful information regarding targeting of this adhesion receptor with novel therapeutic approaches to CVD.

CONCLUSIONS AND IMPLICATIONS WITH REGARD TO DEVELOPING NOVEL THERAPEUTICS

In spite of the rapid advances in identifying risk factors of CVD and in understanding the cellular and molecular mechanisms underlying atherogenesis, CVD continues to be the leading cause of death in the US. Appreciation of the role of inflammation in atherogenesis suggests new opportunities for developing novel therapeutics that, in combination with lipid-lowering regimens, may enhance pharmacological approaches to attenuate the development and progression of atherosclerotic lesions and/or possibly stabilize or regress pre-existing lesions.

It is worth considering the potential of targeting CD44 in CVD and other inflammatory diseases for several reasons. One important feature of CD44 that makes it a particularly attractive target is that, although CD44 appears to play an important role in inflammation, all evidence to date suggests that this receptor is not critical to any essential homeostatic functions, at least in mice. In addition, CD44 may be particularly amenable to pharmacological intervention in view of the multiple levels at which this receptor is regulated in its function and the multiple mechanisms by which the receptor may

Table 1   Levels of regulation of CD44

- Expression
- Adhesion function
- Signal transduction
- Proteolytic processing

regulate the response of both inflammatory cells and vascular cells in atherosclerotic lesions (Table 1). Specifically, CD44 is regulated at the level of its expression and also in its affinity for its ligand. Furthermore, proteolytic processing of the receptor can modify cell–cell and cell–matrix interactions and generate biologically active fragments of CD44. Additional studies are required to fully delineate the mechanisms by which CD44 regulates gene expression, cell growth and cell migration. Once understood, the underlying mechanisms are likely to provide opportunities for modulating the structure and function of CD44 and/or the pathways downstream of CD44 to selectively interfere with the pro-atherogenic activities of this receptor in the vessel wall.

ACKNOWLEDGEMENTS

The author expresses her sincere gratitude to her many colleagues including Dr Daniel Rader and Dr Richard Assoian, who continuously fuel her interest in the role of inflammation in atherosclerosis. The author also greatly appreciates the opportunity to engage in this research in collaboration with past and present members of her laboratory, especially Dr Carolyn Cuff, Dr Liang Zhao and Melissa Middleton. Ms Adrienne Whitmore provided invaluable assistance in the preparation of this manuscript.

Studies in the author's laboratory have been supported by the PHS through grants from the NHBLI.

References

1. Topper JN, Gimbrone MA Jr. Blood flow and vascular gene expression: fluid shear stress as a modulator of endothelial phenotype. Mol Med Today 1999; 5:40–6
2. Braun M, Pietsch P, Schror K, et al. Cellular adhesion molecules on vascular smooth muscle cells. Cardiovasc Res 1999; 41:395–401
3. Rolfe BE, Muddiman JD, Smith NJ, et al. ICAM-1 expression by vascular smooth muscle is phenotype-dependent. Atherosclerosis 2000; 149:99–110
4. DeGrendele HC, Estess P, Siegelman MH. Requirement for CD44 in activated T cell extravasation into an inflammatory site. Science 1997; 278:672–5
5. Hodge-Dufour J, Noble PW, Horton MR, et al. Induction of IL-12 and chemokines by hyaluronan requires adhesion dependent priming of resident but not elicited macrophages. J Immunol 1997; 159: 2492–500
6. McKee CM, Penno MB, Cowman M, et al. Hyaluronan (HA) fragments induce chemokine gene expression in alveolar macrophages. The role of HA size and CD44. J Clin Invest 1996; 98:2403–13
7. Jain M, He Q, Lee W-S, et al. Role of CD44 in the reaction of vascular smooth muscle cells to arterial wall injury. J Clin Invest 1996; 97:596–603
8. Evanko SP, Raines EW, Ross R, et al. Proteoglycan distribution in lesions of atherosclerosis depends on lesion severity, structural characteristics, and the proximity of platelet-derived growth factor and transforming growth factor-β. Am J Pathol 1998; 152:533–46
9. Riessen R, Wight TN, Pastore C, et al. Distribution of hyaluronan during extracellular matrix remodeling in human restenotic arteries and balloon-injured rat carotid arteries. Circulation 1996; 93:1141–7
10. Cuff CA, Kothapalli D, Azonobi I, et al. The adhesion receptor CD44 promotes atherosclerosis by mediating inflammatory cell recruitment and vascular cell activation. J Clin Invest 2001; 108:1031–40
11. Wang X, Xu L, Wang H, et al. CD44 deficiency in mice protects brain from cerebral ischemia injury. J Neurochem 2002; 83:1172–9
12. Lesley J, Hyman R, Kincade PW. CD44 and its interaction with extracellular matrix. Adv Immunol 1993; 54:271–335
13. Naor D, Sionov RV, Ish-Shalom D. CD44: structure, function, and association with the malignant process. Adv Cancer Res 1997; 71:241–319
14. Ponta H, Sherman L, Herrlich PA. CD44: from adhesion molecules to signalling regulators. Nat Rev Mol Cell Biol 2003; 4:33–45
15. Yang B, Yang BL, Savani RC, et al. Identification of a common hyaluronan binding motif in the hyaluronan binding proteins RHAMM, CD44 and link protein. EMBO J 1994; 13:286–96
16. Kohda D, Morton CJ, Parkar AA, et al. Solution structure of the link module: a hyaluronan-binding domain involved in extracellular matrix stability and cell migration. Cell 1996; 86:767–75
17. Katoh S, McCarthy JB, Kincade PW. Characterization of soluble CD44 in the circulation of mice. Levels are affected by immune activity and tumor growth. J Immunol 1994; 153:3440–9
18. Katoh S, Taniguchi H, Matsubara Y, et al. Overexpression of CD44 on alveolar eosinophils with high concentrations of soluble CD44 in bronchoalveolar lavage fluid in patients with eosinophilic pneumonia. Allergy 1999; 54:1286–92
19. Cichy J, Bals R, Potempa J, et al. Proteinase-mediated release of epithelial cell-associated CD44. Extracellular CD44 complexes with components of cellular matrices. J Biol Chem 2002; 277:44440–7
20. Cichy J, Puré E. The liberation of CD44. J Cell Biol 2003; 161:839–43
21. Lammich S, Okochi M, Takeda M, et al. Presenilin dependent intramembrane proteolysis of CD44 leads to the liberation of its intracellular domain and the secretion of an Abeta-like peptide. J Biol Chem 2002; 277:44754–9
22. Okamoto I, Kawano Y, Murakami D, et al. Proteolytic release of CD44 intracellular domain and its role in the CD44 signaling pathway. J Cell Biol 2001; 255:755–62
23. Camp RL, Scheynius A, Johansson C, et al. CD44 is necessary for optimal contact allergic responses but is not required for normal leukocyte extravasation. J Exp Med 1993; 178:497–508
24. Shi M, Dennis K, Peschon JJ, et al. Antibody-induced shedding of CD44 from adherent cells is linked to the assembly of the cytoskeleton. J Immunol 2001; 167:123–31
25. Nakamura H, Suenaga N, Taniwaki K, et al. Constitutive and induced CD44 shedding by ADAM-like proteases and membrane-type 1 matrix metalloproteinase. Cancer Res 2004; 64:876–82
26. Kajita M, Itoh Y, Chiba T, et al. Membrane-type 1 matrix metalloproteinase cleaves CD44 and promotes cell migration. J Cell Biol 2001; 153:893–904
27. Kawano Y, Okamoto I, Murakami D, et al. Ras oncoprotein induces CD44 cleavage through phosphoinositide 3-OH kinase and the Rho family of small G proteins. J Biol Chem 2000; 275:29628–35
28. Yu Q, Toole BP. A new alternatively spliced exon between v9 and v10 provides a molecular basis for synthesis of soluble CD44. J Biol Chem 1996; 271:20603–7
29. Puré E, Camp RL, Peritt D, et al. Defective phosphorylation and hyaluronate binding of CD44 with point mutations in the cytoplasmic domain. J Exp Med 1995; 181:55–62

30. Lazaar AL, Puré E. CD44: a model for regulated adhesion function. Immunologist 1995; 3:19–25

31. Perschl A, Lesley J, English N, et al. Role of CD44 cytoplasmic domain in hyaluronan binding. Eur J Immunol 1995; 25:495–501

32. Katoh S, Zheng Z, Oritani K, et al. Glycosylation of CD44 negatively regulates its recognition of hyaluronan. J Exp Med 1995; 182:419–29

33. Lesley J, English N, Perschl A, et al. Variant cell lines selected for alterations in the function of the hyaluronan receptor CD44 show differences in glycosylation. J Exp Med 1995; 182:431–7

34. Maiti A, Maki G, Johnson P. TNF-alpha induction of CD44-mediated leukocyte adhesion by sulfation. Science 1998; 282:941–3

35. Cichy J, Puré E. Oncostatin M and transforming growth factor-β1 induce post-translational modification and hyaluronan binding to CD44 in lung-derived epithelial tumor cells. J Biol Chem 2000; 275:18061–9

36. Delcommenne M, Kannagi R, Johnson P. TNF-alpha increases the carbohydrate sulfation of CD44: induction of 6-sulfo N-acetyl lactosamine on N- and O-linked glycans. Glycobiology 2002; 12:613–22

37. Brown KL, Maiti A, Johnson P. Role of sulfation in CD44-mediated hyaluronan binding induced by inflammatory mediators in human CD14(+) peripheral blood monocytes. J Immunol 2001; 167:5367–74

38. Johnson P, Maiti A, Brown KL, et al. A role for the cell adhesion molecule CD44 and sulfation in leukocyte–endothelial cell adhesion during an inflammatory response? Biochem Pharmacol 2000; 59:455–65

39. Knudson W, Bartnik E, Knudson CB. Assembly of pericellular matrices by COS-7 cells transfected with CD44 lymphocyte-homing receptor genes. Proc Natl Acad Sci USA 1993; 90:4003–7

40. Underhill CB, Nguyen HA, Shizari M, et al. CD44 positive macrophages take up hyaluronan during lung development. Devel Biol 1993; 155:324–36

41. Henke CA, Roongta U, Mickelson DJ, et al. CD44-related chondroitin sulfate proteoglycan, a cell surface receptor implicated with tumor cell invasion, mediates endothelial cell migration on fibrinogen and invasion into a fibrin matrix. J Clin Invest 1996; 97:2541–52

42. Jalkanen S, Jalkanen M. Lymphocyte CD44 binds the COOH-terminal heparin-binding domain of fibronectin. J Cell Biol 1992; 116:817–25

43. Weber GF, Ashkar S, Glimcher MJ, et al. Receptor–ligand interaction between CD44 and osteopontin (Eta-1). Science 1996; 271:509–12

44. Yu Q, Stamenkovic I. Cell surface-localized matrix metalloproteinase-9 proteolytically activates TGF-β and promotes tumor invasion and angiogenesis. Genes Devel 2000; 14:163–76

45. Zhao L, Cuff CA, Moss E, et al. Selective interleukin-12 synthesis defect in 12/15-lipoxygenase-deficient macrophages associated with reduced atherosclerosis in a mouse model of familial hypercholesterolemia. J Biol Chem 2002; 277:35350–6

46. DeGrendele HC, Estess P, Picker LJ, et al. CD44 and its ligand hyaluronate mediate rolling under physiologic flow: a novel lymphocyte–endothelial cell primary adhesion pathway. J Exp Med 1996; 183:1119–30

47. Nandi A, Estess P, Siegelman MH. Hyaluronan anchoring and regulation on the surface of vascular endothelial cells is mediated through the functionally active form of CD44. J Biol Chem 2000; 275:14939–48

48. Mohamadzadeh M, DeGrendele H, Arizpe H, et al. Proinflammatory stimuli regulate endothelial hyaluronan expression and CD44/HA-dependent primary adhesion. J Clin Invest 1998; 101:97–108

49. Horton MR, McKee CM, Bao C, et al. Hyaluronan fragments synergize with interferon-γ to induce the C-X-C chemokines mig and interferon-inducible protein-10 in mouse macrophages. J Biol Chem 1998; 273:35088–94

50. Lee T-S, Yen H-C, Pan C-C, et al. The role of interleukin 12 in the development of atherosclerosis in ApoE-deficient mice. Arterioscler Thromb Vasc Biol 1999; 19:734–42

51. Gupta S, Pablo AM, Jiang X, et al. IFN-gamma potentiates atherosclerosis in ApoE knock-out mice. J Clin Invest 1997; 99:2752–61

52. Davenport P, Tipping PG. The role of interleukin-4 and interleukin-12 in the progression of atherosclerosis in apolipoprotein E-deficient mice. Am J Pathol 2003; 163:1117–25

53. Benagiano M, Azzurri A, Ciervo A, et al. T helper type 1 lymphocytes drive inflammation in human atherosclerotic lesions. Proc Natl Acad Sci USA 2003; 100: 6658–63

54. Cybulsky MI, Iiyama K, Li H, et al. A major role for VCAM-1, but not ICAM-1, in early atherosclerosis. J Clin Invest 2001; 107:1255–62

55. Li H, Cybulsky MI, Gimbrone MA, et al. Inducible expression of vascular cell adhesion molecule-1 by vascular smooth muscle cells in vitro and within rabbit atheroma. Am J Pathol 1993; 143:1551–9

56. Tanaka Y, Makiyama Y, Mitsui Y. Endothelin-1 is involved in the growth promotion of vascular smooth cells by hyaluronic acid. Int J Cardiol 2000; 76:39–47

57. Li M, Rosenfeld L, Vilar RE, et al. Degradation of hyaluronan by peroxynitrite. Arch Biochem Biophysics 1997; 341:245–50

58. Hynes RO. Integrins: versatility, modulation and signaling in cell adhesion. Cell 1992; 69:11–25

59. Burridge K, Fath K. Focal contacts: transmembrane links between the extracellular matrix and the cytoskeleton. BioEss 1989; 10:104–8

60. Lauffenburger DA, Horwitz AF. Cell migration: a physically integrated molecular process. Cell 1996; 84:359–69

61. Huttenlocher A, Ginsberg MH, Horwitz AF. Modulation of cell migration by integrin-mediated cytoskeletal linkages and ligand-binding affinity. J Cell Biol 1996; 134:1551–62

62. Bourguignon LY, Gunja-Smith Z, Iida N, et al.

CD44v(3,8-10) is involved in cytoskeleton-mediated tumor cell migration and matrix metalloproteinase (MMP-9) association in metastatic breast cancer cells. J Cell Physiol 1998; 176:206–15

63. Knudson CB. Hyaluronan receptor-directed assembly of chondrocyte pericellular matrix. J Cell Biol 1993; 120:825–34

64. Bhowmick NA, Ghiassi M, Aakre M, et al. TGF-beta-induced RhoA and p160ROCK activation is involved in the inhibition of Cdc25A with resultant cell-cycle arrest. Proc Natl Acad Sci USA 2003; 100:15548–53

65. Ridley AJ, Hall A. The small GTP-binding protein rho regulates the assembly of focal adhesions and actin stress fibers in response to growth factors. Cell 1992; 70:389–99

66. Nobes CD, Hall A. Rho, rac, and cdc42 GTPases regulate the assembly of multimolecular focal complexes associated with actin stress fibers, lamellipodia, and filopodia. Cell 1995; 81:53–62

67. Parsons JT, Martin KH, Slack JK, et al. Focal adhesion kinase: a regulator of focal adhesion dynamics and cell movement. Oncogene 2000; 19:5606–13

68. Verfaillie CM, Benis A, Iida J, et al. Adhesion of committed human hematopoietic progenitors to synthetic peptides from the C-terminal heparin-binding domain of fibronectin: cooperation between the integrin alpha 4 beta 1 and the CD44 adhesion receptor. Blood 1994; 84:1802–11

69. Kawakami N, Nishizawa F, Sakane N, et al. Roles of integrins and CD44 on the adhesion and migration of fetal liver cells to the fetal thymus. J Immunol 1999; 163:3211–16

70. Tsukita S, Oishi K, Sato N, et al. ERM family members as molecular linkers between the cell surface glycoprotein CD44 and actin-based cytoskeletons. J Cell Biol 1994; 126:391–401

71. Legg JW, Lewis CA, Parsons M, et al. A novel PKC-regulated mechanism controls CD44 ezrin association and directional cell motility. Nat Cell Biol 2002; 4:399–407

72. Zhu D, Bourguignon LY. Interaction between CD44 and the repeat domain of ankyrin promotes hyaluronic acid-mediated ovarian tumor cell migration. J Cell Physiol 2000; 183:182–95

73. Bourguignon LY, Zhu H, Shao L, et al. Rho-kinase (ROK) promotes CD44v(3,8-10)-ankyrin interaction and tumor cell migration in metastatic breast cancer cells. Cell Motil Cytoskel 1999; 43:269–87

74. Takahashi K, Sasaki T, Mammoto A, et al. Direct interaction of the Rho GDP dissociation inhibitor with ezrin/radixin/moesin initiates the activation of the Rho small G protein. J Biol Chem 1997; 272: 23371–5

75. Hall A. Rho GTPases and the actin cytoskeleton. Science 1998; 279:509–14

76. Hall A, Nobes CD. Rho GTPases: molecular switches that control the organization and dynamics of the actin cytoskeleton. Phil Trans R Soc Lond B Biol Sci 2000; 355:965–70

77. Etienne-Manneville S, Hall A. Integrin-mediated activation of Cdc42 controls cell polarity in migrating astrocytes through PKCzeta. Cell 2001; 106:489–98

78. Webb DJ, Parsons JT, Horwitz AF. Adhesion assembly, disassembly and turnover in migrating cells – over and over and over again. Nat Cell Biol 2002; 4:E97–E100

79. Mackay DJ, Esch F, Furthmayr H, et al. Rho- and Rac-dependent assembly of focal adhesion complexes and actin filaments in permeabilized fibroblasts: an essential role for ezrin/radixin/moesin proteins. J Cell Biol 1997; 138:927–38

80. Hirao M, Sato N, Kondo T, et al. Regulation mechanism of ERM (Ezrin/Radixin/Moesin) protein/plasma membrane association: possible involvement of phosphatidylinositol turnover and Rho-dependent signaling pathway. J Cell Biol 1996; 135:37–51

81. Katagiri K, Shimonaka M, Kinashi T. Rap1-mediated lymphocyte function-associated antigen-1 activation by the T cell antigen receptor is dependent on phospholipase C-gamma1. J Biol Chem 2004; 279: 11875–81

82. Seveau S, Eddy RJ, Pierini MFR, et al. Cytoskeleton-dependent membrane domain segregation during neutrophil polarization. Mol Biol Cell 2001; 12:3550–62

83. del Pozo MA, Vicente-Manzanares M, Tejedor R, et al. Rho GTPases control migration and polarization of adhesion molecules and cytoskeletal ERM components in T lymphocytes. Eur J Immunol 1999; 29:3609–20

84. Clark EA, Brugge JS. Integrins and signal transduction pathways: the road taken. Science 1995; 268:233–9

85. Saoncella S, Echtermeyer F, Denhez F, et al. Syndecan-4 signals cooperatively with integrins in a Rho-dependent manner in the assembly of focal adhesions and actin stress fibers. Proc Natl Acad Sci USA 1999; 96:2805–10

86. Munger JS, Huang X, Kawakatsu H, et al. The integrin alpha v beta 6 binds and activates latent TGF beta 1: a mechanism for regulating pulmonary inflammation and fibrosis. Cell 1996; 96:319–28

87. Teder P, Vandivier RW, Jiang D, et al. Resolution of lung inflammation by CD44. Science 2002; 296:155–8

88. Bourguignon LYW, Singleton PA, Zhu H, et al. Hyaluronan promotes signaling interaction between CD44 and transforming growth factor β receptor I in metastatic breast tumor cells. J Biol Chem 2002; 277:39703–12

89. Trochon V, Mabilat C, Bertrand P, et al. Evidence of involvement of CD44 in endothelial cell proliferation, migration and angiogenesis in vitro. Int J Cancer 1996; 66:664–8

90. Savani RC, Cao G, Pooler PM, et al. Differential involvement of the hyaluronan (HA) receptors CD44 and receptor for HA mediated motility in endothelial cell function and angiogenesis. J Biol Chem 2001; 276:36770–8

91. Khaldoyanidi S, Denzel A, Zoller M. Requirement for CD44 in proliferation and homing of hematopoietic precursor cells. J Leukocyte Biol 1996; 60:579–92

92. Ayroldi E, Cannarile L, Migliorati G, et al. CD44 (Pgp-1) inhibits CD3 and dexamethasone-induced apoptosis. Blood 1995; 86:2672–8

93. Gunthert AR, Strater J, Von Reyher U, et al. Early detachment of colon carcinoma cells during CD95 (APO-1/Fas)-mediated apoptosis. I. De-adhesion from hyaluronate by shedding of CD44. J Cell Biol 1996; 134:1089–96

94. Yu Q, Toole BP, Stamenkovic I. Induction of apoptosis of metastatic mammary carcinoma cells in vivo by disruption of tumor cell surface CD44 function. J Exp Med 1997; 186:1985–96

95. Skelton TP, Zeng C, Nocks A, et al. Glycosylation provides both stimulatory and inhibitory effects on cell surface and soluble CD44 binding to hyaluronan. Cell Biol 1998; 140:431–46

Lipoxygenases: potential therapeutic target in atherosclerosis

18

L. Zhao and C.D. Funk

LIPOXYGENASES: BACKGROUND INFORMATION

The lipoxygenases (LOs) constitute a family of non-haem iron dioxygenase enzymes that stereospecifically insert molecular oxygen into polyunsaturated fatty acids.[1–4] Based on the specific position where arachidonic acid (AA) is oxidized, they are divided into 5-, 8-, 12-, 15- or 12/15-LO. There are seven functional lipoxygenases in mice and six in humans and the first genetic defects in human LO pathways were reported recently.[5] Both plants and animals express lipoxygenases and, in the case of mammals, the preferred substrate is often AA and the product a hydro(pero)xy-eicosa-tetraenoic acid (H(P)ETE). In this chapter, we will consider two members, 12/15-LO and 5-LO.

We use the collective term 12/15-LO to cover the 'leukocyte type' 12-lipoxygenase (L-12LO) of mice (also present in pigs and rats but not present in the human genome[6,7]) and 15-LO-1 of humans (also present in rabbits, but a distinct 15-LO-1 gene does not appear to be in the published mouse genome[8]).[9] 12/15-LO from different species produces variable ratios of 12-HETE to 15-HETE. However, such species differences are not observed with 5-LO since there is conversion of AA strictly to 5-HPETE and then to leukotriene (LT)A$_4$[10–14] (Figure 1).

BASIC SCIENCE OF 12/15-LO AND 5-LO: MOLECULAR STRUCTURE AND EXPRESSION

The mouse/human 12/15-LO genes span 7.8/10.7 kb including 14 exons and 13 introns on mouse chromosome 11/human chromosome 17. The primary sequences share 74% identity between species. The three-dimensional crystal structure of the rabbit enzyme has been elucidated. The 75 kDa protein possesses an N-terminal β barrel domain[15] related to the C-terminal domain in lipases and is probably involved in membrane binding for proper

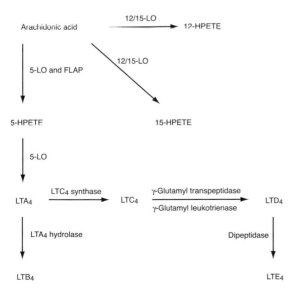

Figure 1 12/15-LO and 5-LO pathways

acquisition of substrate. The C-terminal catalytic domain contains the iron atom involved in catalysis that is bound by three strictly conserved histidines and the carboxyl moiety of the C-terminal isoleucine residue.

Mouse 12/15-LO is distributed in several tissues with the highest expression in peritoneal macrophages, and lesser expression in adipose tissue, pancreatic islet cells and a variety of brain regions (cortex, hippocampus, striatum, brainstem, cerebellum, pituitary and pineal glands).[16,17] 12/15-LO resides in the cytosol of resting macrophages. When macrophages are incubated with apoptotic cells, this enzyme translocates from cytosol to the plasma membrane and is more extensively concentrated at sites where macrophages bind apoptotic cells, co-localizing with polymerized actin of emerging filopodia.[18] The enzyme appears to translocate to the plasma membrane in a cultured macrophage cell line (J774.1), overexpressing 12/15-LO when incubated with LDL in a LRP-dependent fashion,[19] but peritoneal macrophage 12/15-LO does not translocate in the presence of oxidized LDL.[20]

12/15-LO$^{-/-}$ mice, in which expression of 12/15-LO is abolished and subsequent formation of 12-HETE/15-HETE is absent, have been created.[21] This mouse model has become an essential tool in unravelling biological and pathophysiological functions of 12/15-LO. So far, growing evidence has suggested roles of 12/15-LO in various pathological processes, including atherosclerosis,[22–26] drug addiction responses,[17] prostate carcinoma[27] and ischaemic preconditioning-induced cardioprotection.[28] In the current chapter, our discussion will focus on the importance of this enzyme in atherosclerosis and related mechanisms.

The human 5-LO gene contains 14 exons spread out over 72 kb on human chromosome 10q11.2 in a CpG-rich DNA segment. It encodes a 673-amino-acid protein with a calculated molecular mass of 78 kDa.[29,30] The mouse 5-LO gene maps to the central region of chromosome 6 with a similar exon/intron format.[31] The crystal structure of 5-LO has not been elucidated. However, a number of important features have been inferred from homol-

ogy modelling and verified by biochemical data.[32–38] Like 12/15-LO, 5-LO is predicted to contain two domains. The N-terminal domain appears to resemble a C2 domain, a Ca^{++}-dependent membrane targeting module, found in several signalling molecules like protein kinase C and cytosolic phospholipase A$_2$. Two bound Ca^{++} ions are present in this domain and, together with conserved tryptophan residues, they govern subcellular localization to phosphatidylcholine-rich membranes like the nuclear envelope upon cellular activation.[32–34] The catalytic domain with the essential iron atom may resemble the elucidated 15-LO structure, but in addition contains sites for phosphorylation not present in 15-LO, as well as an SH3-binding domain and nuclear localization sequences.[35–37]

In resting bone-marrow-derived mast cell and some macrophage populations, 5-LO is found within the nucleus. Recent data suggest that the positioning of 5-LO within the nucleus of resting cells is a powerful determinant of the capacity to generate LTB$_4$ upon subsequent activation.[38] Studies using 5-LO$^{-/-}$ mice have provided extensive evidence for the importance of 5-LO in multiple disease models such as inflammation,[39] arthritis,[40] pulmonary fibrosis,[41] autoimmune disease,[42] pancreatitis,[43] asthma,[44] microbial infection,[45,46] atherosclerosis[47] and renal transplant rejection.[48] Current understanding of the action of 5-LO in atherosclerosis is discussed in this chapter.

MODEL SYSTEMS: ROLE OF 12/15-LO IN ATHEROSCLEROSIS

Atherosclerosis, a chronic inflammatory disorder of the vascular wall, is characterized by the progressive formation of fatty streak lesions, stable plaques and unstable or ruptured plaques which triggers acute clinical complications such as infarction and stroke. Although considerable experimental and clinical studies have provided evidence in understanding the pathogenesis of this disease, the mechanisms of atherogenesis still remain to be investigated further.

Mouse models of atherosclerosis have become the key research tools to explore the pathogenesis of atherosclerosis.[49–52] Studies of 12/15-LO deficiency and human 15-LO-1 overexpression in mouse models of atherosclerosis have provided considerable evidence revealing the functional importance of 12/15-LO in atherogenesis. The apolipoprotein E (apoE)-deficient mouse is the hallmark model since it develops typical lesions on a normal chow diet that faithfully mimic human disease progression, including monocyte adhesion, foamy macrophages, fatty streaks and advanced fibrosis.[49,50] Disruption of 12/15-LO in apoE$^{-/-}$ mice reduced atherosclerotic lesion progression in aortic vasculature throughout the lifespan of the mice, despite no differences in cholesterol, triglyceride levels and lipoprotein levels.[22,23] Recent data demonstrate that deficiency of 12/15-LO in bone marrow-derived cells protects apoE$^{-/-}$ mice fed a Western diet from atherosclerosis to the same extent as complete absence of 12/15-LO. Consistent with this observation, reconstitution of apoE$^{-/-}$, 12/15-LO$^{-/-}$ mice with bone marrow of apoE$^{-/-}$ mice fully restores lesion burden to the levels of apoE$^{-/-}$ mice, suggesting that 12/15-LO in bone-marrow-derived cells accounts for the pro-atherogenic activity of this enzyme.[52a] These data suggest an essential role of 12/15-LO in atherosclerotic lesion development in the apoE$^{-/-}$ mouse model.

The low-density lipoprotein receptor (LDL-R)-deficient mouse model is also well established, but requires fat feeding to induce lesion development and elevated LDL cholesterol levels.[51] Collective studies by two independent groups have demonstrated significantly reduced atherosclerotic lesions at both the aortic root and the entire aorta in LDL-R$^{-/-}$, 12/15-LO$^{-/-}$ mice on a high-fat, high-cholesterol diet for 3, 9, 12 and 18 weeks, in the absence of alterations in plasma lipids.[24] In a separate study, overexpression of human 15-LO-1 using the preproendothelin-1 promoter led to enhanced lesion development in LDL-R$^{-/-}$ mice on an atherogenic diet for 3 and 6 weeks.[25] Thus, the pro-atherogenic role of mouse 12/15-LO or human 15-LO-1 was verified in a second mouse model of atherosclerosis.

The apobec-1/LDL-R double knockout model is perhaps one of the best models of atherosclerosis that mimics human familial hypercholesterolaemia.[52] In order to further confirm the role of 12/15-LO in atherogenesis, we crossed the 12/15-LO$^{-/-}$ mice to this third mouse model of atherosclerosis. Significantly reduced (~50%) lesion size throughout the aorta was observed in both male and female apobec-1/LDL-R, 12/15-LO triple knockout 8-month-old mice compared to apobec-1, LDL-R double knockout mice, despite no differences in plasma total cholesterol levels.[26] Thus, studies in mice consistently support a role of 12/15-LO in promoting atherogenesis in three different mouse models of atherosclerosis.

In hypercholesterolaemic rabbit models, modulation of 15-LO activity appears to play an important role in atherogenesis. Two studies with a putatively selective 15-LO inhibitor (the compound PD146176) lacking significant antioxidant properties have shown a significant reduction in diet-induced atherosclerosis and monocyte/macrophage accumulation in lesions.[53,54] However, conflicting data with overexpression of 15-LO from the lysozyme promoter or anaemia-induced 15-LO expression leading to a paradoxical reduction of lesion formation have been reported.[55,56] The pro- and anti-atherogenic possibilities of 15-LO involvement in atherogenesis in rabbits remain to be further determined.

The role of 12/15-LO in restenosis has been examined in a rat model. One study demonstrated increased 12/15-LO mRNA and protein expression in the neointima of balloon-injured rat carotid arteries.[57] Specific 12/15-LO inactivation using a ribozyme significantly reduced the intima-to-media thickness ratio in the left common carotid arteries of rats 12 days after balloon catheter injury.[58] Another line of evidence supporting the pro-atherogenic role of 12/15-LO arises from a pig model. Accelerated atherosclerosis in hyperlipaemic groups was associated with enhanced expression of 12-LO, both at the mRNA and protein levels.[59]

MECHANISMS INVOLVED IN THE PRO-ATHEROGENIC ROLE OF 12/15-LO

LDL oxidation

Considerable evidence has accumulated over the years supporting the hypothesis that LDL oxidation plays an important role in atherogenesis.[60–68] 12/15-LO catalyses the oxygenation of AA or linoleic acid in free form or when esterified to cholesterol or phospholipids to generate predominantly the 12/15-H(P)ETE or 13-H(P)ODE forms (free or esterified), respectively.[69,70] Recent data suggest that low-density lipoprotein receptor-related protein (LRP)-mediated membrane translocation of 12/15-LO is required for oxidation of LDL in macrophages.[19,71] 12/15-LO represents one of the many pathways to generate oxidized LDL (oxLDL) in vivo,[67,72–75] although some in vitro studies challenge lipoxygenase involvement.[76,77] 15-LO-1 co-localizes with epitopes of oxLDL in human and rabbit atherosclerotic lesions, and stereospecific products of the lipoxygenase reaction have been demonstrated in atherosclerotic lesions of rabbits and humans.[78–80] Retroviral transfer of the 15-LO gene into rabbit iliac arteries of rabbits fed a high-fat diet led to accumulation of oxLDL-like epitopes.[81] In the apoE$^{-/-}$ mouse model, disruption of 12/15-LO resulted in decreased urinary and plasma levels of oxidant stress markers (isoprostane 8,12–iso-iPF$_{2\alpha}$-VI and IgG antibodies directed against malondialdehyde-modified LDL epitopes) in parallel with decreased atherosclerosis.[22,23] We also provided evidence that anti-oxidant vitamin E reduced lesion size and urinary 8,12–iso-iPF$_{2\alpha}$-VI levels in apoE$^{-/-}$ mice, but had no further effect in apoE$^{-/-}$,12/15-LO$^{-/-}$ mice, which verified that the pro-atherogenic effect of 12/15-LO could be attributed to its action on lipid peroxidation (unpublished data). Decreased isoprostane levels associated with reduced atherosclerosis progression were further confirmed in the apobec-1/LDL-R$^{-/-}$,12/15-LO$^{-/-}$ mouse model.[26] In the apoE$^{-/-}$ bone marrow transplantation (BMT) model, reduced atherosclerotic lesion size in apoE$^{-/-}$ mice receiving apoE$^{-/-}$, 12/15-LO$^{-/-}$ bone marrow cells correlated with decreased plasma level of autoantibodies to oxLDL.[52a] Enhanced atherosclerotic lesion development was associated with greater susceptibility of LDL oxidation in LDL-R$^{-/-}$, 15-LO-1 transgenic mice than in LDL-R$^{-/-}$ mice.[25] These combined data are strongly suggestive of a 12/15-LO component to LDL oxidation and atherogenesis.

Inflammatory response

The importance of inflammation and the underlying molecular and cellular mechanisms contributing to atherogenesis is clearly recognized.[82,83] Hypercholesterolaemia and inflammation should be considered different aspects of a single, shared pathogenetic pathway in atherosclerosis.[84] Monocytes/macrophages, endothelial cells, lymphocytes and smooth muscle cells are essential cellular components of the inflammatory response in different stages of atherosclerosis progression, from development of the fatty streak to processes that ultimately contribute to plaque rupture and myocardial infarction.[85–88] The initial adhesion of monocytes to the endothelium is mediated by several adhesion molecules, such as vascular cell adhesion molecule-1 (VCAM-1), P-selectin and integrin $\alpha_4\beta_1$ (VLA4).[89–96] Recent data demonstrated that deficient 12/15-LO activity in mouse peritoneal macrophages led to reduced endothelial activation (in terms of VCAM-1 expression) in the presence of LDL.[52a] In contrast, transgenic 12/15-LO overexpressing mice have enhanced monocyte/endothelial cell interactions through molecular regulation of endothelial adhesion molecules.[97] Inhibition of 12/15-LO (with either an adenovirus expressing a ribozyme to 12/15-LO or the 12/15-LO inhibitor cinnamyl-3,4-dihydroxy-alpha-cyano-cinnamate) also reduced monocyte/endothelial interactions in db/db mice, possibly through interactions of $\alpha_4\beta_1$ integrins on monocytes with endothelial VCAM-1 and connecting segment 1 fibronectin and interactions of β_2 integrins with endothelial intercellular adhesion molecule 1.[98]

Lesional T cells appear to be activated and produce Th1 (such as interleukin-12 (IL-12) and interferon-γ (IFN-γ)) and Th2 cytokines (such as IL-4 and IL-13). IL-12 is a key factor in the induction of T-cell dependent activation of macrophages and plays an active role in regulating the immune response of atherosclerosis in apoE-deficient mice.[99,100] Peritoneal macrophages from 12/15-LO[-/-] mice exhibit a prominent defect of IL-12p40 production compared to wild-type mice. Significant decreases in IL-12p40 and IFN-γ mRNA as well as IL-12p40 protein expression in apobec-1/LDL-R, 12/15-LO triple knockout mice aortas were observed. These data provide a means whereby 12/15-LO influences atherogenesis via altered synthesis of Th1 cytokines.[26] 13-HPODE, a product of 12/15-LO, activates nuclear factor-κB (NF-κB), as well as Ras, mitogen-activated protein kinases (MAPK1/2), p38 and c-Jun amino-terminal kinase in porcine VSMCs.[101] In mouse vascular smooth muscle cells, 12/15-LO deficiency resulted in significantly reduced growth-factor-induced cell migration, proliferation, AP-1-, p38- and cAMP-response element binding protein activation, as well as diminished superoxide and fibronectin production.[102] These results suggest that 12/15-LO is responsible for modulation of multiple key inflammatory responses in atherosclerosis.

MODEL SYSTEMS: ROLE OF 5-LO IN ATHEROSCLEROSIS

Leukotrienes, products of the 5-LO pathway, are known to exert pro-inflammatory effects in vivo.[103,104] LTB_4, an inflammatory cell (especially neutrophils) chemoattractant, and LTE_4 have been detected in human and rabbit atherosclerotic lesions.[105,106] However, the role of 5-LO in animal models of atherosclerosis has not been appreciated until recently, when Mehrabian et al[47] reported that 5-LO expression is detected in mouse atherosclerotic lesions. A recent study demonstrated that deficiency of B-LT_1, the high-affinity chemoattractant LTB_4 receptor, significantly reduced atherosclerotic lesion size

in apoE[-/-] mice on Western diet for 4 weeks.[107] Aiello et al[108] provided evidence that an LTB_4 antagonist (CP-105,696), via pharmacological blockade of its receptor B-LT_1, contributes to reduced monocyte infiltration in developing atherosclerotic lesions in apoE[-/-] mice. Further study in LDL-R[-/-] mice revealed that LTB_4 may exert its pro-atherogenic effect through an MCP-1 pathway.[108]

Genetic studies[47,109,110] with the atherosclerosis-susceptible strain C57BL/6 (B6) and either the resistant strain CAST/Ei or MOLF/Ei led to the conclusion that one or more genes on mouse chromosome 6 centred over the 63 cM (40–89 cM) interval is/are responsible for atherosclerosis susceptibility. The mouse 5-LO gene resides within this locus (53 cM, 117 Mb from telomere[31]). Interestingly, reduced levels of 5-LO expression and LT production were found in a congenic strain (CON6) in which the CAST/Ei chromosome 6 segment was integrated onto the B6 background,[47] suggesting that the 5-LO locus in this strain might be responsible for atherosclerosis resistance. Sequence analysis of the CAST/Ei 5-LO sequence revealed two amino acid differences with the B6 strain (Val645/Ile646 vs Ile645/Val646, respectively) and these substitutions, when introduced into human 5-LO (also Ile645/Val646), led to impaired 5-LO activity.[111] It should be noted, however, that the original determined sequence in a hybrid B6x129 strain of mice has the sequence Ile645/Ile646[31] and displays completely normal 5-LO activity.

Striking results indicated that the 5-LO locus was responsible for atherosclerosis susceptibility on an LDL-R knockout background, revealing a profound effect much greater than any other genes to date.[47] Two important caveats with these studies include limited numbers of animals examined in the atherosclerotic lesion analysis and the effect of 5-LO being observed at the heterozygous level; i.e. not with LDL-R,5-LO double knockouts.[47,112] Based on these concerns, we examined the role of 5-LO in the apoE[-/-] mouse model. Our data do not support a role of 5-LO in spontaneous lesion development in apoE[-/-] mice, however, on a pro-

Table 1   Modulation of 12/15-LO (or 15-LO-1) and 5-LO pathways in animal models of atherosclerosis

Pathway	Species	Animal model	Major observation	Reference
12/15-LO 15-LO-1	Mouse	apoE$^{-/-}$	Significant reduction of aortic lesion size in 12/15-LO$^{-/-}$ mice at 10 w, 15 w, 8 m, 12 m and 15 m on chow diet	22, 23
		apoE$^{-/-}$	Significant reduction of aortic lesion size in apoE$^{-/-}$ mice receiving apoE$^{-/-}$, 12/15-LO$^{-/-}$ mice bone marrow cells on Western diet	Unpublished data
		LDL-R$^{-/-}$	Significant reduction of aortic lesion size in 12/15–LO$^{-/-}$ mice at 3, 9, 12 and 18 weeks on high-fat, high-cholesterol diet	24
		LDL-R$^{-/-}$	15–LO-1 overexpression in endothelial cells enhances lesion development on high-fat, high-cholesterol diet for 3 and 6 weeks	25
		apobec-1/LDL-R$^{-/-}$	Significant decrease of aortic lesion percentage in 12/15-LO$^{-/-}$ mice on chow diet at 8 months	26
	Rabbit	Diet-induced hypercholesterolaemic model	PD146176 significantly reduces atherosclerotic lesion size and monocyte/macrophage accumulation	53, 54
		Diet-induced hypercholesterolaemic model	15-LO-1 overexpression or anaemia-induced 15-LO-1 expression significantly decreases atherosclerotic lesion size	55, 56
5-LO	Mouse	apoE$^{-/-}$	B-LT$_1$ deficiency significantly reduces atherosclerotic lesion size on Western diet for 4 weeks	107
		apoE$^{-/-}$	LTB$_4$ antagonist, CP-105,696, significantly reduces atherosclerotic lesion size and monocye infiltration	108
		apoE$^{-/-}$	Significant reduction of aneurysm formation in 5-LO$^{-/-}$ mice fed high-fat, high-cholesterol diet for 8 weeks	113
		LDL-R$^{-/-}$	Atherosclerotic lesion development significantly reduced in 5-LO$^{+/-}$ mice	47

atherogenic, pro-inflammatory diet effects on and aneurysm formation become apparent.[113]

Recently, 5-LO expression has been documented in advanced human atherosclerotic lesions, localized to macrophages, dendritic cells, foam cells, mast cells and neutrophilic granulocytes.[114] The number of 5-LO-expressing cells markedly increased in advanced lesions, suggesting an association between 5-LO and lesion development. A preliminary study claims a role of 5-LO in human plaque instability.[115] Thus, enhanced 5-LO expression was observed in plaques characterized as 'unstable' vs 'stable' and was associated with increased LTB$_4$ production,

increased matrix metalloproteinase-2 (MMP-2) and MMP-9 activity and decreased collagen content in the former samples.[115] A genetic study in humans has attempted to link 5-LO to cardiovascular disease (CVD) susceptibility.[116] Carotid intima-media thickness (IMT) was determined bilaterally with B-mode ultrasound, evaluating the risk of atherosclerosis and CVD, and a polymorphism in the transcription-factor-binding region of the 5-LO promoter was genotyped in 470 samples. The findings suggest that carriers of two variant alleles of the repeat GC-box/Sp1 region (< or >5 copies) in the 5-LO gene place about 6% of the population at markedly increased risk for atherosclerosis and CVD. This 5-LO polymorphism-dependent atherogenic effect is enhanced by dietary intake of arachidonic acid, blunted by n-3 fatty acids and associated with increased plasma level of C-reactive protein.[116] However, it must be stressed here that no biochemical parameters of the 5-LO pathway correlating the variant alleles with disease propensity have been measured, so the data remain highly speculative.

POTENTIAL MECHANISMS INVOLVED IN THE ROLE OF 5-LO IN ATHEROSCLEROSIS

The studies mentioned above are beginning to reveal potential mechanisms for 5-LO involvement in multiple stages of atherosclerosis progression, including adhesion of monocytes to endothelial cells, chemotaxis and migration of monocytes/macrophages and plaque instability. The participation of 5-LO in these processes could be mediated through biosynthesis of pro-inflammatory leukotrienes, 5-oxo-6,8,11,14-eicosatetraenoic acid (5-oxo-ETE) and/or 5-HETE. Pre-treatment of human endothelial cells with a 5-LO inhibitor blocked IL-1β-induced VCAM-1 expression.[117] A recent study by Friedrich et al[118] demonstrated that LTB$_4$, a major product of the 5-LO pathway, is an agonist of monocyte adhesion, possibly through triggering β$_1$- and β$_2$-integrin-dependent adhesion in vascular models. Monocyte chemoattractant protein-1 (MCP-1), a prototype of CC chemokines, through its receptor CCR2, plays an important role in the pathogenesis of atherosclerosis.[119,120] A specific LTB$_4$ receptor antagonist (CP-105,696) inhibited caecal ligation and puncture-induced recruitment of both neutrophils and macrophages, which was accompanied by a reduced level of MCP-1 in a murine model of septic peritonitis.[121] A similar pattern of cross-talk between LTB$_4$ and MCP-1 may also occur in the artery wall.[122] In fact, evidence of LTB$_4$/MCP-1 interaction has been reported, whereby LTB$_4$ promotes atherogenesis in LDL-R$^{-/-}$ mice via MCP-1.[108] In addition, 5-oxo-ETE and 5-HETE

induce directional migration and actin polymerization of human monocytes in vitro.[123] Matrix metalloproteinases (MMPs) are key modulators of plaque stability in atherosclerosis.[124,125] 5-LO activity has been shown to mediate CD147-induced generation of pro-MMP-2 from fibroblasts.[126] LTB$_4$ induces MMP-2, MMP-3 and MMP-9 secretion in cultured Tsup-1 cells (T lymphoblastoma cell line).[127] These data suggest a potential role of 5-LO in plaque vulnerability.

THERAPEUTIC POTENTIAL OF 15-LO AND 5-LO INHIBITORS IN ATHEROGENESIS

15-LO has been recognized as a potential target in human atherogenesis since at least 1990[78] and therapeutic strategies have been proposed.[128] Evidence from several experimental animal models (mice and rabbits) presented above supports the rationale for such an approach. Plausible mechanisms involved in 15-LO inhibition include reduction of lipid peroxidation, diminished inflammatory responses and prevention of monocyte–endothelial cell interactions. Although several 15-LO inhibitors have been developed,[53,54,129,130] none of them has been applied beyond animal studies.

A considerable controversy erupted in the past year with respect to human lipoxygenase expression patterns in atherosclerotic tissue. The dogma in the field since 1990 has been that 15-LO-1 expression is high in macrophages of atherosclerotic lesions and that 5-LO expression is absent or negligible.[78] A study by Spanbroek et al[114] has come to the opposite conclusions: 5-LO/leukotriene pathway biosynthetic and signalling components are abundantly expressed, whereas 15-LO-1 expression is negligible. Who is right? Are there explanations for the divergent results? Do the solid mouse 12/15-LO atherosclerosis data with atherosclerotic models provide accurate predictors for human disease intervention? Perhaps the development of novel 15-LO specific inhibitors and the evaluation of their efficacy in clinical trials will have to wait until a firm consensus is reached on human lipoxygenase expression patterns in atherosclerotic disease samples and resolving the answers to these questions.

5-LO inhibition in preventing inflammatory disease has been established for two decades.[103] The premise that this pathway is relevant to the inflammatory component of atherosclerosis only gained momentum in the last year or two, based on the recent studies in mice and humans.[47,108,114] Some of the reasons for this long delay since inception of 5-LO inhibitors include:

- The long-known fact that LTB$_4$ is predominantly a neutrophil chemoattractant (a minor player in atherosclerosis), with much lesser effects on monocytes/macrophages (key cell type in atherogenesis);
- The relatively recent recognition of atherosclerosis as an inflammatory disease rather than a vascular injury disorder;
- The apparent absence of 5-LO expression in lesional macrophages.[78]

Numerous 5-LO pathway inhibitors (leukotriene modifiers) have been developed over the past two decades.[131–134] Zileuton is the only 5-LO inhibitor currently approved for use in humans.[133,134] While it has demonstrated therapeutic benefits in asthma symptom management, its application in the clinics has been limited due to requirements for liver function testing and poor pharmacokinetics.[135] The recent exciting data in humans and mice in coronary disease samples and atherosclerotic models should encourage the pharmaceutical industry to renew efforts at developing better specific 5-LO inhibitors with excellent pharmacodynamics for testing in people at risk for cardiovascular disease.

ACKNOWLEDGEMENTS

This work was supported by NIH grant HL53558 and CIHR grant MOP-67146 to CD Funk, and American Heart Association Postdoctoral Fellowship 0225369U to L Zhao.

References

1. Funk CD. Prostaglandins and leukotrienes: advances in eicosanoid biology. Science 2001; 294:1871–5
2. Brash AR. Lipoxygenases: occurrence, functions, catalysis, and acquisition of substrate. J Biol Chem 1999; 274:23679–82
3. Funk CD. The molecular biology of mammalian lipoxygenases and the quest for eicosanoid functions using lipoxygenase-deficient mice. Biochim Biophys Acta 1996; 1304:65–84
4. Yamamoto S. 'Enzymatic' lipid peroxidation: reactions of mammalian lipoxygenases. Free Radic Biol Med 1991; 10:149–59
5. Jobard F, Lefevre C, Karaduman A, et al. Lipoxygenase-3 (ALOXE3) and 12(R)-lipoxygenase (ALOX12B) are mutated in non-bullous congenital ichthyosiform erythroderma (NCIE) linked to chromosome 17p13.1. Hum Mol Genet 2002; 11:107–13
6. Lander ES, Linton LM, Birren B, et al. Initial sequencing and analysis of the human genome. Nature 2001; 409:860–921
7. Venter JC, Adams MD, Myers EW, et al. The sequence of the human genome. Science 2001; 291:1304–51
8. Waterston RH, Lindblad-Toh K, Birney E, et al. Initial sequencing and comparative analysis of the mouse genome. Nature 2002; 420:520–62
9. Kuhn H, Walther M, Kuban RJ. Mammalian arachidonate 15-lipoxygenases: structure, function, and biological implications. Prost Other Lipid Mediat 2002; 68/69:263–90
10. Shimizu T, Radmark O, Samuelsson B. Enzyme with dual lipoxygenase activities catalyzes leukotriene A4 synthesis from arachidonic acid. Proc Natl Acad Sci USA 1984; 81:689–93
11. Rouzer CA, Matsumoto T, Samuelsson B. Single protein from human leukocytes possesses 5-lipoxygenase and leukotriene A4 synthase activities. Proc Natl Acad Sci USA 1986; 83:857–61
12. Ueda N, Kaneko S, Yoshimoto T, et al. Purification of arachidonate 5-lipoxygenase from porcine leukocytes and its reactivity with hydroperoxyeicosatetraenoic acids. J Biol Chem 1986; 261: 7982–8
13. Shimizu T, Izumi T, Seyama Y, et al. Characterization of leukotriene A$_4$ synthase from murine mast cells:

evidence for its identity to arachidonate 5-lipoxygenase. Proc Natl Acad Sci USA 1986; 83:4175–9

14. Hogaboom GK, Cook M, Newton JF et al. Purification, characterization and structural properties of a single protein from rat basophilic leukemia (RBL-1) cells possessing 5-lipoxygenase and leukotriene A₄ synthetase activities. Mol Pharmacol 1986; 30:510–19

15. Gillmor SA, Villasenor A, Fletterick R, et al. The structure of mammalian 15-lipoxygenase reveals similarity to the lipases and the determinants of substrate specificity. Nat Struct Biol 1997; 4:1003–9

16. Chen XS, Kurre U, Jenkins NA, et al. cDNA cloning, expression, mutagenesis of C-terminal isoleucine, genomic structure, and chromosomal localizations of murine 12-lipoxygenases. J Biol Chem 1994; 269:13979–87

17. Walters CL, Wang BC, Godfrey M, et al. Augmented responses to morphine and cocaine in mice with a 12-lipoxygenase gene disruption. Psychopharmacology (Berl) 2003; 170:124–31

18. Miller YI, Chang MK, Funk CD, et al. 12/15-lipoxygenase translocation enhances site-specific actin polymerization in macrophages phagocytosing apoptotic cells. J Biol Chem 2001; 276:19431–9

19. Zhu H, Takahashi Y, Xu W, et al. Low density lipoprotein receptor-related protein-mediated membrane translocation of 12/15-lipoxygenase is required for oxidation of low density lipoprotein by macrophages. J Biol Chem 2003; 278:13350–5

20. Miller YI, Worrall DS, Funk CD, et al. Actin polymerization in macrophages in response to oxidized LDL and apoptotic cells: role of 12/15-lipoxygenase and phosphoinositide 3-kinase. Mol Biol Cell 2003; 14:4196–206.

21. Sun D, Funk CD. Disruption of 12/15-lipoxygenase expression in peritoneal macrophages. Enhanced utilization of the 5-lipoxygenase pathway and diminished oxidation of low density lipoprotein. J Biol Chem 1996; 271:24055–62

22. Cyrus T, Witztum JL, Rader DJ, et al. Disruption of 12/15-lipoxygenase results in inhibition of atherosclerotic lesion development in mice lacking apolipoprotein E. J Clin Invest 1999; 103:1597–604

23. Cyrus T, Pratico D, Zhao L, et al. Absence of 12/15-lipoxygenase expression decreases lipid peroxidation and atherogenesis in apolipoprotein E-deficient mice. Circulation 2001; 103:2277–82

24. George J, Afek A, Shaish A, et al. 12/15-Lipoxygenase gene disruption attenuates atherogenesis in LDL-receptor deficient mice. Circulation 2001; 104:1646–50

25. Harats D, Shaish A, George J, et al. Overexpression of 15-lipoxygenase in vascular endothelium accelerates early atherosclerosis in LDL receptor-deficient mice. Arterioscler Thromb Vasc Biol 2000; 20:2100–5

26. Zhao L, Cuff CA, Moss E, et al. Selective interleukin-12 synthesis defect in 12/15-lipoxygenase deficient macrophages associated with reduced atherosclerosis in mouse model of familial hypercholesterolemia. J Biol Chem 2002; 277:35350–6

27. Shappell SB, Olson SJ, Hannah SE, et al. Elevated expression of 12/15-lipoxygenase and cyclooxygenase-2 in a transgenic mouse model of prostate carcinoma. Cancer Res 2003; 63:2256–67.

28. Gabel SA, London RE, Funk CD, et al. Leukocyte-type 12-lipoxygenase-deficient mice show impaired ischemic preconditioning-induced cardioprotection. Am J Physiol Heart Circ Physiol 2001; 280:H1963–9

29. Funk CD, Matsumoto T, Hoshiko S, et al. Characterization of the human 5-lipoxygenase gene. Proc Natl Acad Sci USA 1989; 86:2587–91

30. Matsumoto T, Funk CD, Radmark O, et al. Molecular cloning and amino acid sequence of human 5-lipoxygenase. Proc Natl Acad Sci USA 1988; 85:26–30

31. Chen XS, Naumann T, Kurre U, et al. cDNA cloning, expression, mutagenesis, intracellular localization and gene chromosomal assignment of mouse 5-lipoxygenase. J Biol Chem 1995; 270:17993–9

32. Hammarberg T, Provost P, Persson B, et al. The N-terminal domain of 5-lipoxygenase binds calcium and mediates calcium stimulation of enzyme activity. J Biol Chem 2000; 275:38787–93.

33. Kulkarni S, Das S, Funk CD, et al. Molecular basis of the specific subcellular localization of the C2-like domain of 5-lipoxygenase. J Biol Chem 2002; 277:13167–74

34. Chen XS, Funk CD. The N-terminal 'beta-barrel' domain of 5-lipoxygenase is essential for nuclear membrane translocation. J Biol Chem 2001; 276: 811–18

35. Werz O, Szellas D, Steinhilber D, et al. Arachidonic acid promotes phosphorylation of 5-lipoxygenase at Ser-271 by MAPK-activated protein kinase 2 (MK2). J Biol Chem 2002; 277:14793–800.

36. Lepley RA, Fitzpatrick FA. 5-lipoxygenase contains a functional Src homology 3-binding motif that interacts with the Src homology 3 domain of Grb2 and cytoskeletal proteins. J Biol Chem 1994; 269:24163–8.

37. Jones SM, Luo M, Peters-Golden M, et al. Identification of two novel nuclear import sequences on the 5-lipoxygenase protein. J Biol Chem 2003; 278:10257–63.

38. Luo M, Jones SM, Peters-Golden M, et al. Nuclear localization of 5-lipoxygenase as a determinant of leukotriene B₄ synthetic capacity. Proc Natl Acad Sci USA 2003; 100:12165–70

39. Chen XS, Sheller JR, Johnson EN, et al. Role of leukotrienes revealed by targeted disruption of the 5-lipoxygenase gene. Nature 1994; 372:179–82

40. Griffiths RJ, Smith MA, Roach ML, et al. Collagen-induced arthritis is reduced in 5-lipoxygenase-activating protein-deficient mice. J Exp Med 1997; 185:1123–9

41. Peters-Golden M, Bailie M, Marshall T, et al. Protection from pulmonary fibrosis in leukotriene-deficient mice. Am J Respir Crit Care Med 2002; 165:229–35

42. Goulet JL, Griffiths RC, Ruiz P, et al. Deficiency of 5-lipoxygenase abolishes sex-related survival differences in MRL-lpr/lpr mice. J Immunol 1999; 163:359–66

43. Cuzzocrea S, Rossi A, Serraino I, et al. 5-lipoxygenase knockout mice exhibit a resistance to acute pancreatitis induced by cerulein. Immunology 2003; 110:120–30

44. Coffey M, Peters-Golden M. Extending the understanding of leukotrienes in asthma. Curr Opin Allergy Clin Immunol 2003; 3:57–63

45. Aliberti J, Serhan C, Sher A. Parasite-induced lipoxin A$_4$ is an endogenous regulator of IL-12 production and immunopathology in *Toxoplasma gondii* infection. J Exp Med 2002; 196:1253–62

46. Bailie MB, Standiford TJ, Laichalk LL, et al. Leukotriene-deficient mice manifest enhanced lethality from Klebsiella pneumonia in association with decreased alveolar macrophage phagocytic and bactericidal activities. J Immunol 1996; 157:5221–4.

47. Mehrabian M, Allayee H, Wong J, et al. Identification of 5-lipoxygenase as a major gene contributing to atherosclerosis susceptibility in mice. Circ Res 2002; 91:120–6

48. Goulet JL, Griffiths RC, Ruiz P, et al. Deficiency of 5-lipoxygenase accelerates renal allograft rejection in mice. J Immunol 2001; 167:6631–6

49. Reddick RL, Zhang SH, Maeda N. Atherosclerosis in mice lacking apo E. Evaluation of lesional development and progression. Arterioscler Thromb 1994; 14:141–7

50. Nakashima Y, Plump AS, Raines EW, et al. ApoE-deficient mice develop lesions of all phases of atherosclerosis throughout the arterial tree. Arterioscler Thromb 1994; 14:133–40

51. Ishibashi S, Goldstein JL, Brown MS, et al. Massive xanthomatosis and atherosclerosis in cholesterol-fed low density lipoprotein receptor-negative mice. J Clin Invest 1994; 93:1885–93

52. Powell-Braxton L, Veniant M, Latvala RD, et al. A mouse model of human familial hypercholesterolemia: markedly elevated low density lipoprotein cholesterol levels and severe atherosclerosis on a low-fat chow diet. Nat Med 1998; 4:934–8

52a. Huo Y, Zhao L, Hyman MC, et al. Critical role of macrophage 12/15-lipoxygenase for atherosclerosis in apolipoprotein E-deficient mice. Circulation 2004; 110:2024–31

53. Bocan TM, Rosebury WS, Mueller SB, et al. A specific 15-lipoxygenase inhibitor limits the progression and monocyte-macrophage enrichment of hypercholesterolemia-induced atherosclerosis in the rabbit. Atherosclerosis 1998; 136:203–16

54. Sendobry SM, Cornicelli JA, Welch K, et al. Attenuation of diet-induced atherosclerosis in rabbits with a highly selective 15-lipoxygenase inhibitor lacking significant antioxidant properties. Br J Pharm 1997; 120:1199–206.

55. Shen J, Herderick E, Cornhill JF, et al. Macrophage-mediated 15-lipoxygenase expression protects against atherosclerosis development. J Clin Invest 1996; 98:2201–8

56. Trebus F, Heydeck D, Schimke I, et al. Transient experimental anemia in cholesterol-fed rabbits induces systemic overexpression of the reticulocyte-type 15-lipoxygenase and protects from aortic lipid deposition. Prost Leuk Ess Fatty Acids 2002; 67:419–28

57. Natarajan R, Pei H, Gu JL, et al. Evidence of 12-lipoxygenase expression in balloon injured rat carotid arteries. Cardiovasc Res 1999; 41:481–99

58. Gu JL, Pei H, Thomas L, et al. Ribozyme-mediated inhibition of rat leukocyte-type 12-lipoxygenase prevents intimal hyperplasia in balloon-injured rat carotid arteries. Circulation 2001; 103:1446–52.

59. Natarajan R, Gerrity RG, Gu JL, et al. Role of 12-lipoxygenase and oxidant stress in hyperglycaemia-induced acceleration of atherosclerosis in a diabetic pig model. Diabetologia 2002; 45:125–33

60. Funk CD, Cyrus T. 12/15-Lipoxygenase, oxidative modification of LDL and atherogenesis. Trends Cardiovasc Med 2001; 11:116–24

61. Cathcart MK, Folcik VA. Lipoxygenases and atherosclerosis: protection versus pathogenesis. Free Radic Biol Med 2000; 28:1726–34

62. Kuhn H, Chan L. The role of 15-lipoxygenase in atherogenesis: pro- and antiatherogenic actions. Curr Opin Lipidol 1997; 8:111–17

63. Steinberg D, Parthasarathy S, Carew TE, et al. Beyond cholesterol. Modifications of low-density lipoprotein that increase its atherogenicity. New Engl J Med 1989; 320:915–24

64. Yla-Herttuala S, Palinski W, Rosenfeld ME, et al. Evidence for the presence of oxidatively modified low density lipoprotein in atherosclerotic lesions of rabbit and man. J Clin Invest 1989; 84:1086–95

65. Parthasarathy S, Rankin SM. Role of oxidized low density lipoprotein in atherogenesis. Prog Lipid Res 1992; 31:127–43

66. Berliner JA, Navab M, Fogelman AM, et al. Atherosclerosis: basic mechanisms. Oxidation, inflammation, and genetics. Circulation 1995; 91:2488–96

67. Berliner JA, Heinecke JW. The role of oxidized lipoproteins in atherogenesis. Free Rad Biol Med 1996; 20:707–27

68. Steinberg D. Oxidative modification of LDL and atherogenesis. Circulation 1997; 95:1062–71

69. Belkner J, Wiesner R, Rathman J, et al. Oxygenation of lipoproteins by mammalian lipoxygenases. Eur J Biochem 1993; 213:251–61

70. Belkner J, Stender H, Kuhn H. The rabbit 15-lipoxygenase preferentially oxygenates LDL cholesterol esters, and this reaction does not require vitamin E. J Biol Chem 1998; 273:23225–32

71. Xu W, Takahashi Y, Sakashita T, et al. Low density lipoprotein receptor-related protein is required for macrophage-mediated oxidation of low density lipoprotein by 12/15-lipoxygenase. J Biol Chem 2001; 276:36454–9

72. Kuhn H, Belkner J, Zaiss S, et al. Involvement of 15-

lipoxygenase in early stages of atherogenesis. J Exp Med 1994; 179:1903–11

73. Rankin SM, Parthasarathy S, Steinberg D. Evidence for a dominant role of lipoxygenase(s) in the oxidation of LDL by mouse peritoneal macrophages. J Lipid Res 1991; 32:449–56

74. Parthasarathy S, Wieland E, Steinberg D. A role for endothelial cell lipoxygenase in the oxidative modification of low density lipoprotein. Proc Natl Acad Sci USA 1989; 86:1046–50

75. Sigari F, Lee C, Witztum JL, et al. Fibroblasts that overexpress 15-lipoxygenase generate bioactive and minimally modified LDL. Arterioscler Thromb Vasc Biol 1997; 17:3639–45

76. Sparrow CP, Olszewski J. Cellular oxidative modification of low density lipoprotein does not require lipoxygenases. Proc Natl Acad Sci USA 1992; 89:128–31

77. Jessup W, Darley-Usmar V, O'Leary V. et al. 5-lipoxygenase is not essential in macrophage-mediated oxidation of low-density lipoprotein. Biochem J 1991; 278 (Pt 1): 163–9

78. Yla-Herttuala S, Rosenfeld ME, Parthasarathy S, et al. Colocalization of 15-lipoxygenase mRNA and protein with epitopes of oxidized low density lipoprotein in macrophage-rich areas of atherosclerotic lesions. Proc Natl Acad Sci USA 1990; 87:6959–63

79. Folcik VA, Nivar-Aristy RA, Krajewski LP, et al. Lipoxygenase contributes to the oxidation of lipids in human atherosclerotic plaques. J Clin Invest 1995; 96:504–10

80. Kuhn H, Heydeck D, Hugou I, et al. In vivo action of 15-lipoxygenase in early stages of human atherogenesis. J Clin Invest 1997; 99:888–93

81. Yla-Herttuala S, Luoma J, Viita H, et al. Transfer of 15-lipoxygenase gene into rabbit iliac arteries results in the appearance of oxidation-specific lipid–protein adducts characteristic of oxidized low density lipoprotein. J Clin Invest 1995; 95: 2692–8

82. Libby P. Inflammation in atherosclerosis. Nature 2002; 420:868–74

83. Libby P, Ridker PM, Maseri A. Inflammation and atherosclerosis. Circulation 2002; 105:1135–43

84. Steinberg D. Atherogenesis in perspective: hypercholesterolemia and inflammation as partners in crime. Nat Med 2002; 8:1211–17

85. Li AC, Glass CK. The macrophage foam cell as a target for therapeutic intervention. Nat Med 2002; 8:1235–42

86. Hansson GK. Regulation of immune mechanisms in atherosclerosis. Ann NY Acad Sci 2001; 947:157–65; discussion 165–6

87. Hansson GK. Inflammation and immune response in atherosclerosis. Curr Atheroscler Rep 1999; 1:150–5

88. Gouni-Berthold I, Sachinidis A. Does the coronary risk factor low density lipoprotein alter growth and signaling in vascular smooth muscle cells? FASEB J 2002; 16:1477–87

89. Huo Y, Hafezi-Moghadam A, Ley K. Role of vascular cell adhesion molecule-1 and fibronectin connecting segment-1 in monocyte rolling and adhesion on early atherosclerotic lesions. Circ Res 2000; 87:153–9

90. Nageh MF, Sandberg ET, Marotti KR. Deficiency of inflammatory cell adhesion molecules protects against atherosclerosis in mice. Arterioscler Thromb Vasc Biol 1997; 17:1517–20

91. Collins RG, Velji R, Guevara NV, et al. P-selectin or ICAM-1 deficiency substantially protects against atherosclerosis in apo E deficient mice. J Exp Med 2000; 191:189–94

92. Dong ZM, Chapman SM, Brown AA, et al. The combined role of P- and E-selectins in atherosclerosis. J Clin Invest 1998; 102:145–52

93. Dong ZM, Brown AA, Wagner DD. Prominent role of P-selectin in the development of advanced atherosclerosis in ApoE-deficient mice. Circulation 2000; 101:2290–5

94. Shih PT, Brennan ML, Vora DK. Blocking very late antigen-4 integrin decreases leukocyte entry and fatty streak formation in mice fed an atherogenic diet. Circ Res 1999; 84:345–51

95. Shih PT, Elices MJ, Fang ZT. Minimally modified low-density lipoprotein induces monocyte adhesion to endothelial connecting segment-1 by activating beta 1 integrin. J Clin Invest 1999; 103:613–25

96. Huo Y, Ley K. Adhesion molecules and atherogenesis. Acta Physiol Scand 2001; 173:35–43

97. Reilly KB, Srinivasan S, Hatley ME, et al. 12/15 lipoxygenase activity mediates inflammatory monocyte: endothelial interactions and atherosclerosis in vivo. J Biol Chem 2004; 279:9440–50

98. Hatley ME, Srinivasan S, Reilly KB, et al. Increased production of 12/15 lipoxygenase eicosanoids accelerates monocyte/endothelial interactions in diabetic db/db mice. J Biol Chem 2003; 278:25369–75

99. Lee TS, Yenm HC, Pan CC, et al. The role of interleukin 12 in the development of atherosclerosis in apoE-deficient mice. Arterioscler Thromb Vasc Biol 1999; 9: 734–42

100. Uyemura K, Demer LL, Castle SC, et al. Cross-regulatory roles of interleukin (IL)-12 and IL-10 in atherosclerosis. J Clin Invest 1996; 97:2130–8

101. Natarajan R, Reddy MA, Malik KU, et al. Signaling mechanism of nuclear factor-kappa B-mediated activation of inflammatory genes by 13-hydroperoxyoctadecadienoic acid in cultured vascular smooth muscle cells. Arterioscler Thromb Vasc Biol 2001; 21:1408–13

102. Reddy MA, Kim YS, Lanting L, et al. Reduced growth factor responses in vascular smooth muscle cells derived from 12/15-lipoxygenase-deficient mice. Hypertension 2003; 41:1294–300

103. Samuelsson B. Leukotrienes: mediators of immediate hypersensitivity actions and inflammation. Science 1983; 220:568–75

104. Lewis RA, Austen KF, Soberan RJ. Leukotrienes and other products of 5-lipoxygenase pathway. Biochemistry and relation to pathobiology in human diseases. N Engl J Med 1990; 323:645–55

105. De Caterina R, Mazzone A, Giannessi D, et al. Leukotriene B$_4$ production in human atherosclerotic plaques. Biomed Biochim Acta 1988; 47:S182–5

106. Patrignani P, Daffonchio L, Hernandez A, et al. Release of contracting autacoids by aortae of normal and atherosclerotic rabbits. J Cardiovasc Pharmacol 1992; 20(Suppl 12):S208–10

107. Subbarao K, Jala VR, Mathis S, et al. Role of leukotriene B$_4$ receptor in the development of atherosclerosis: potential mechanisms. Arterioscler Thromb Vasc Biol 2004; 24:369–75

108. Aiello RJ, Bourassa PA, Lindsey S, et al. Leukotriene B$_4$ receptor antagonism reduces monocytic foam cells in mice. Arterioscler Thromb Vasc Biol 2002; 22:443–9

109. Mehrabian M, Wong J, Wang X, et al. Genetic locus in mice that blocks development of atherosclerosis despite extreme hyperlipidemia. Circ Res 2001; 89:125–30

110. Welch CL, Bretschger S, Latib N, et al. Localization of atherosclerosis susceptibility loci to chromosomes 4 and 6 using the Ldlr knockout mouse model. Proc Natl Acad Sci USA 2001; 98:7946–51

111. Kuhn H, Anton M, Gerth C, et al. Amino acid differences in the deduced 5-lipoxygenase sequence of CAST atherosclerosis-resistance mice confer impaired activity when introduced into the human ortholog. Arterioscler Thromb Vasc Biol 2003; 23:1072–6

112. Mehrabian M, Allayee H. 5-lipoxygenase and atherosclerosis. Curr Opin Lipidol 2003; 14:447–57

113. Zhao L, Moos MP, Gräbner R, et al. The 5-lipoxygenase pathway promotes pathogenesis of hyperlipidemia-dependent aortic aneurysm. Nat Med 2004; 10: 966–73

114. Spanbroek R, Gräbner R, Lotzer K, et al. Expanding expression of the 5-lipoxygenase pathway within the arterial wall during human atherogenesis. Proc Natl Acad Sci USA 2003; 100:1238–43

115. Cipollone F, Mezzetti A, Fazia M, et al. Identification of 5-lipoxygenase as a major gene contributing to atherosclerotic plaque instability in humans. Circulation 2003; 108:IV–223

116. Dwyer JH, Allayee H, Dwyer KM, et al. Arachidonate 5-lipoxygenase promoter genotype, dietary arachidonic acid, and atherosclerosis. N Engl J Med 2004; 350:29–37

117. Lee S, Felts KA, Parry GC, et al. Inhibition of 5-lipoxygenase blocks IL-1 beta-induced vascular adhesion molecule-1 gene expression in human endothelial cells. J Immunol 1997; 158:3401–7

118. Friedrich EB, Tager AM, Liu E, et al. Mechanisms of leukotriene B4-triggered monocyte adhesion. Arterioscler Thromb Vasc Biol 2003; 23:1761–7

119. Gu L, Okada Y, Clinton SK, et al. Absence of monocyte chemoattractant protein-1 reduces atherosclerosis in low density lipoprotein receptor-deficient mice. Mol Cell 1998; 2:275–81

120. Boring L, Gosling J, Cleary M, et al. Decreased lesion formation in CCR2–/– mice reveals a role for chemokines in the initiation of atherosclerosis. Nature 1998; 394:894–7

121. Matsukawa A, Hogaboam CM, Lukacs NW, et al. Endogenous monocyte chemoattractant protein-1 (MCP-1) protects mice in a model of acute septic peritonitis: cross-talk between MCP-1 and leukotriene B$_4$. J Immunol 1999; 163:6148–54

122. Rosenfeld ME. Leukocyte recruitment into developing atherosclerotic lesions: the complex interaction between multiple molecules keeps getting more complex. Arterioscler Thromb Vasc Biol 2002; 22:361–3

123. Sozzani S, Zhou D, Locati M, et al. Stimulating properties of 5-oxo-eicosanoids for human monocytes: synergism with monocyte chemotactic protein-1 and -3. J Immunol 1996; 157:4664–71

124. Fabunmi RP, Sukhova GK, Sugiyama S, et al. Expression of tissue inhibitor of metalloproteinases-3 in human atheroma and regulation in lesion-associated cells: a potential protective mechanism in plaque stability. Circ Res 1998; 83:270–8

125. Rajagopalan S, Meng XP, Ramasamy S, et al. Reactive oxygen species produced by macrophage-derived foam cells regulate the activity of vascular matrix metalloproteinases in vitro. Implications for atherosclerotic plaque stability. J Clin Invest 1996; 98:2572–9

126. Taylor PM, Woodfield RJ, Hodgkin MN, et al. Breast cancer cell-derived EMMPRIN stimulates fibroblast MMP2 release through a phospholipase A(2) and 5-lipoxygenase catalyzed pathway. Oncogene 2002; 21:5765–72

127. Leppert D, Hauser SL, Kishiyama JL, et al. Stimulation of matrix metalloproteinase-dependent migration of T cells by eicosanoids. FASEB J 1995; 9:1473–81

128. Cornicelli JA, Trivedi BK. 15-Lipoxygenase and its inhibition: a novel therapeutic target for vascular disease. Curr Pharm Des 1999; 5:11–20

129. Schewe T, Sadik C, Klotz LO, et al. Polyphenols of cocoa: inhibition of mammalian 15-lipoxygenase. Biol Chem 2001; 382:1687–96

130. Sadik CD, Sies H, Schewe T. Inhibition of 15-lipoxygenases by flavonoids: structure–activity relations and mode of action. Biochem Pharmacol 2003; 65:773–81

131. Koshihara Y, Neichi T, Murota S, et al. Caffeic acid is a selective inhibitor for leukotriene biosynthesis. Biochim Biophys Acta 1984; 792: 92–7

132. Evans JF, Leville C, Mancini JA, et al. 5-Lipoxygenase-activating protein is the target of a quinoline class of leukotriene synthesis inhibitors. Mol Pharmacol 1991; 40:22–7

133. Dupont R, Goossens JF, Cotelle N, et al. New bis-catechols 5-lipoxygenase inhibitors. Bioorg Med Chem 2001; 9:229–35

134. Israel E, Rubin P, Kemp JP, et al. The effect of inhibition of 5-lipoxygenase by zileuton in mild-to-moderate asthma. Ann Intern Med 1993; 119:1059–66

135. Busse WW, McGill KA, Horwitz RJ. Leukotriene pathway inhibitors in asthma and chronic obstructive pulmonary disease. Clin Exp Allergy 1999; 29(Suppl 2):110–15

Role of secretory phospholipase A₂ isozymes (Lp-PLA₂)

19

C.H. Macphee

INTRODUCTION

Atherosclerosis, the major cause of coronary heart disease (CHD), has been proposed to begin during early childhood and to progress in a non-linear fashion throughout adulthood. The aetiology of atherogenesis can be best described as a chronic inflammatory disease of the arterial intima, dominated by a leukocyte infiltrate comprising predominately T-lymphocytes and monocyte-derived macrophages. This chapter will focus on the putative role of secreted phospholipase A₂ (sPLA₂) isozymes[1,2] in atherosclerosis, with a particular emphasis on lipoprotein-associated phospholipase A₂ (Lp-PLA₂), also known as plasma platelet-activating factor acetylhydrolase (PAF-AH) or type VIIA PLA₂.

BACKGROUND

Although both secreted and cytosolic enzymes comprise the growing PLA₂ superfamily,[1,2] only the sPLA₂ sub-group will be considered in this chapter because an acknowledged critical process in the pathophysiology of atherosclerosis is the extracellular metabolism of lipoproteins. In order to evaluate fully the potential role of the sPLA₂ family in atherogenesis it is first necessary to summarize the current concepts concerning the pathogenesis of atherosclerosis as well as list the cell types involved.

Epidemiological, clinical and genetic studies indicate that elevated plasma levels of low density lipoprotein (LDL) greatly increase the risk for atherosclerosis.[3] Furthermore, it is generally accepted that a key pathogenic event is the retention[4] and subsequent oxidation[5,6] of apoB-rich lipoproteins (in particular, LDL) within the arterial wall. Whilst proteoglycans[7] appear to play an important role in promoting lipoprotein retention, the precise mechanisms by which LDL becomes oxidatively modified remain rather unclear. Evidence, however, is accumulating that supports a major role for myeloperoxidase in promoting lipid oxidation in human, but not mouse, atherosclerotic lesion development.[8,9] Suffice it to say that vascular cells, including all constituents of the atherosclerotic plaque, can produce and use reactive oxygen species (ROS)[10,11] which ultimately can oxidize LDL. Furthermore, there is mounting epidemiological evidence that lesion development, as well as lesion stability, may be significantly influenced by infection.[12] Induction of inflammation is an important component in the defence against micro-organisms and bacterial lipopolysaccharides are well known stimuli for enhanced ROS generation, as is any type of systemic inflammation[13] regardless of cause. Thus, the precise processes which modulate lipid peroxidation of LDL may vary according to the stage of lesion development as well as the presence or absence of an underlying infection or systemic inflammation.

Once modified, oxidized LDL (oxLDL) can promote a plethora of pro-inflammatory atherogenic effects, influencing all cell types that comprise the plaque, i.e. monocyte-derived macrophages, T lymphocytes, endothelial and smooth muscle cells.[5,6,14–16] Oxidized

LDL, for example, has been demonstrated to induce diverse effects including endothelial dysfunction[17] and cell death,[18,19] two clinically relevant activities that could help develop a pro-thrombotic state and promote plaque instability, respectively. One of the earliest events following LDL oxidation is the PLA$_2$-dependent hydrolysis of the oxidized phospholipids generating lysophosphatidylcholine (lyso-PC) and oxidized fatty acids,[20,21] both of which have been shown to be causal agents in inflammation. Indeed, it has been demonstrated that the concentration of lyso-PC is significantly elevated in atherosclerotic arteries.[22,23] With this albeit brief and somewhat simplified overview of atherogenesis we can now assess which, if any, of the various isozymes of sPLA$_2$ could be causative factors in influencing human disease progression and giving rise to major adverse coronary events. Specific attention, therefore, will be focused on which sPLA$_2$s fit the following biological profile: participate in lipoprotein metabolism (especially oxLDL), are upregulated in atherosclerotic lesions, contribute to inflammation/host defence and are positively associated with cardiovascular disease and/or events.

sPLA$_2$ ISOZYMES AND ATHEROGENESIS

PLA$_2$s are an ubiquitous class of enzymes that hydrolyse the *sn*-2 acyl bond of phospholipids of cell membranes and lipoproteins to yield free fatty acids (FFAs) and lysophospholipids.[1,2] Both of these products are themselves pro-inflammatory but are also precursors of other pro-inflammatory lipid mediators such as leukotrienes, eicosanoids, prostaglandins and platelet-activating factor.[24] In general, the mammalian sPLA$_2$s (groups IB, IIA,C–F, II, V, X, XII) have low molecular masses (13–19 kDa), require calcium for activity and lack specificity for arachidonate-containing phospholipids. Whilst the biological functions of these sPLA$_2$s are still under investigation, it appears that a primary action is to mediate the second larger wave of arachidonic acid release for subsequent eicosanoid forma-

tion, which is somewhat surprising considering that they are not arachidonyl-sensitive enzymes.[24] These phospholipases contain a His/Asp dyad active site and act optimally on aggregated substrates such as micelles or membranes, a phenomenon termed 'interfacial activation.' Lp-PLA$_2$ (i.e. type VIIA), a 45 kDa calcium-independent sPLA$_2$, on the other hand, is not an interfacial enzyme but utilizes a distinct Ser/His/Asp triad active site that accesses its substrates from the aqueous phase.[25] This property of Lp-PLA$_2$ enables a broad substrate specificity that is governed primarily by aqueous phase solubility.[26] Although Lp-PLA$_2$ was discovered due to its ability to hydrolyse platelet-activating factor,[27] its mechanism of action raises the distinct possibility that it can hydrolyse a wide variety of physiological substrates, including phospholipids containing non-truncated oxidatively modified (i.e. polar) polyunsaturated fatty acids.

Table 1 summarizes key functions of the 11 known mammalian extracellular sPLA$_2$s as they pertain to atherogenesis, namely involvement in LDL oxidation, expression in disease and whether evidence exists for any to be a positive risk factor for coronary heart disease in humans. Although data for some of the sPLA$_2$s are incomplete, Table 1 clearly shows that two of these extracellular enzymes, Lp-PLA$_2$ and type IIA, qualify as potential causative factors in the promotion of atherosclerosis. Thus, the rest of this chapter will focus entirely on discussing and comparing the evidence for these two enzymes. It must be noted that, although sPLA$_2$-V and -X are not yet sufficiently characterized to include in a full analysis, both hold some potential to be linked with atherosclerosis due to their leukocyte expression and ability to hydrolyse anionic phospholipids.[28]

Lp-PLA$_2$ (PAF-AH) AND sPLA$_2$-IIA

Plaque expression and oxidation of LDL

Lp-PLA$_2$

Leukocytes,[29] and in particular monocytes, macrophages and T-cells,[30–32] appear to be the

Table 1 Secreted mammalian PLA₂ enzymes

sPLA₂ type	Other name	Catalytic site	Involved during LDL oxidation	Upregulated in human atherosclerotic plaque	Levels associated with risk for CHD
IB	Pancreatic	His/Asp dyad	No	No	No
IIA	Synovial	His/Asp dyad	Yes	Yes	Yes
IIC		His/Asp dyad	No	No	No
IID		His/Asp dyad	No	No	No
IIE		His/Asp dyad	No	No	No
IIF		His/Asp dyad	No	No	No
III		His/Asp dyad	No	No	No
V		His/Asp dyad	?	?	?
VIIA	Lp-PLA₂ PAF-AH	Ser/His/Asp triad	Yes	Yes (macrophages and T-cells)	Yes
X		His/Asp dyad	?	Yes (macrophages)	?
XII		His/Asp dyad	No	No	No

only source of circulating Lp-PLA₂. Given that these cells represent the exact same leukocyte population that is intimately involved in atherogenesis,[6] it comes as no surprise to note that the enzyme is greatly upregulated in atherosclerotic lesions.[32] The observation that lipopolysaccharide (LPS) represents the most powerful natural stimulus for enhanced expression and secretion implies a major role of Lp-PLA₂ for this enzyme in host defence and the acute phase response.[31,33] Tumour necrosis factor and interleukin-1 are key cytokines in bacterial infection and, interestingly, both have been reported to increase plasma Lp-PLA₂ activity, but only modestly when compared with LPS, suggesting that they may partly mediate the effect of LPS.[33] Thus, Lp-PLA₂ can be viewed as one of the acute-phase proteins.

Lp-PLA₂ is associated predominantly with LDL in human plasma, with the remainder (~20%) distributed across high density lipoprotein (HDL) and very low density lipoprotein (VLDL).[34] It has been reported that Lp-PLA₂ binds preferentially to the highly atherogenic small dense LDL[35] and is found enriched in pro-inflammatory electronegative LDL particles[36] as well as lipoprotein(a).[37] The critical determinant in lipoprotein binding appears to be a specific interaction between two domains on human Lp-PLA₂ and the carboxy terminus of apolipoprotein B-100 on LDL.[38] Moreover, it has been suggested that the catalytic properties

of Lp-PLA₂ are influenced by its lipoprotein environment.[39,40] Since Lp-PLA₂ accesses its substrate from the aqueous phase,[26] caution is advised when only activity measurements are utilized to determine the contribution of Lp-PLA₂ across various lipoprotein fractions. This is because the catalytic rate will vary with changes in the concentrations of components, such as lipids and proteins, that can bind substrate and alter its aqueous phase concentration. Thus, both Lp-PLA₂ activity and mass measurements are required before a definitive conclusion can be made on the contributions of this enzyme across different lipoprotein fractions.

The association of the majority of plasma Lp-PLA₂ with apoB-containing lipoproteins in human plasma is highly significant because Lp-PLA₂ remains latent until LDL undergoes oxidative modification. Lp-PLA₂ is solely responsible for a well-known consequence of LDL oxidation, the rapid hydrolysis of oxidized phosphatidylcholine moieties within modified LDL.[41–43] This generates biologically relevant quantities of lyso-PC and oxidized free fatty acids (ox-FFAs). Both of these lipid products have been demonstrated to be causal agents in inflammation and atherosclerosis.[43] This is especially true for lyso-PC, whose concentration is significantly elevated in plaques.[23] For example, in vitro studies of lyso-PC demonstrate that it has the following pro-atherogenic activities: chemoattractant for monocytes and T-cells, induces the elaboration of chemokines and adhesion molecules, upregulates the release of MPO, stimulates superoxide production, impairs endothelial-dependent relaxation, inhibits endothelial migration after injury and can cause cell death.[43–49] It therefore follows that inhibition of Lp-PLA$_2$ could provide a novel approach in the treatment of atherosclerosis through prevention of the generation of two bioactive lipid mediators.

Support for this concept comes from the observation that inhibition of Lp-PLA$_2$ not only abolished the increase in lyso-PC during oxidation of LDL, but prevented the generation of oxidized non-esterified fatty acid moieties that were very effective human monocyte chemo-attractants.[43] In addition, related experiments have demonstrated that inhibition of Lp-PLA$_2$ can significantly diminish the cytotoxic and apoptosis-inducing effects of oxidized LDL on human macrophages.[50] This finding may be relevant to the death of macrophage foam cells and smooth muscle cells known to occur in atherosclerotic lesions and associated with progression to a state vulnerable to rupture.[51]

Although these findings support a pro-inflammatory role for Lp-PLA$_2$ in athero-genesis, a body of evidence suggests the opposite.[52–54] This view arose primarily because of the ability of Lp-PLA$_2$ (i.e. PAF-AH) to degrade and inactivate exogenously added PAF, a molecule attributed with pro-inflammatory and pro-thrombotic properties. While the role of PAF in inflammation has been intensively studied by numerous researchers for many years, the demonstration of its role in pathological conditions remains elusive. For instance, although PAF was thought to have a potential significant role in the pathogenesis of asthma, this has been questioned due to lack of clinical efficacy of a variety of structurally diverse PAF receptor antagonists.[55] Furthermore, it remains to be determined whether Lp-PLA$_2$ actually plays a significant role in the metabolism of endogenously generated PAF.

This proposed anti-inflammatory role for Lp-PLA$_2$ was subsequently used to explain, at least in part, the anti-atherogenic properties of HDL, even though the majority (~80%) of the enzyme in human plasma is located on another lipoprotein, LDL.[34] The situation is very different in rodents and rabbits, where the vast majority of plasma Lp-PLA$_2$ is found associated with HDL.[52] The hypothesis in this instance is based upon the premise that the oxidized phospholipids represent the inflammatory mediators and not the two aqueous-phase soluble products, lyso-PC and oxidized fatty acids.[52,56] This concept raises several paradoxes, even excluding the fact that the enzyme is found primarily on LDL in humans. First, although it is generally accepted that Lp-PLA$_2$ is solely responsible for the generation of lyso-PC during the oxidation of LDL, the same enzyme appears to play only a minor role in the generation of lyso-PC that occurs during the oxidation of human HDL.[43] Second, whereas other sPLA$_2$s are consistently viewed as pro-inflammatory due to their ability to generate lyso-PC and FFAs, this link is somehow ignored or forgotten for Lp-PLA$_2$. Third, recent studies have demonstrated that oxidized phosphatidyl-cholines can inhibit ligand activation of toll-like receptors[57,58] and upregulate the expression of haem oxygenase-1,[59] both of which provide protection against inflammation. The authors propose that these lipid oxidation products can function as a feedback mechanism to limit inflammation and associated tissue damage, especially when in conjunction with oxidative stress. Interestingly, a polymorphism in the toll-like receptor 4 known to attenuate receptor signalling has been associated with a decreased risk of atherosclerosis.[60,61]

Support for an anti-inflammatory role for Lp-PLA$_2$ does exist from various pre-clinical studies which showed that recombinant human Lp-PLA$_2$ could prevent or attenuate pathological inflammation in a number of animal models.[52] Similar efficacy, however, could not be replicated in the clinic, the last study being in individuals with sepsis.[62] The consistent lack of clinical efficacy has resulted in the termination of this particular approach.

sPLA₂-IIA

The plasma concentration of group IIA PLA₂ can increase many fold during the acute phase so, like Lp-PLA₂, it can be viewed as another member of the acute-phase proteins. It follows, therefore, that large amounts of sPLA₂-IIA are detected in the exudating fluids and plasma of patients with various systemic and local inflammatory diseases.[2] This particular sPLA₂ has a broad cellular distribution and, unlike Lp-PLA₂, its expression is not limited to leukocytes. Inflammatory effector cells do, however, store sPLA₂-IIA in their secretory granules and release it promptly following cell activation.[2,63] In normal arteries sPLA₂-IIA is mainly found with smooth muscle cells of the media, whereas in human atherosclerotic plaques it has been detected in some, but not all, macrophage-derived foam cells.[63,64] A similar finding was observed in intimal lesions from WHHL rabbits, where sPLA₂-IIA was expressed in a small population of foam cells.[65]

It has been demonstrated that the phospholipids of native LDL as well as high density lipoprotein (HDL) can be hydrolysed by human sPLA₂-IIA.[63,66,67] Thus, unlike Lp-PLA₂, sPLA₂-IIA is not dependent upon LDL becoming oxidized to enable cleavage of phospholipids. Moreover, sPLA₂-IIA-modified LDL shows increased affinity for proteoglycans, an increased propensity to aggregate and an enhanced ability to deliver cholesterol to cells.[66] Interestingly, the modification of HDL by sPLA₂-IIA treatment also resulted in enhanced lipid deposition following incubation with macrophages, endothelial and hepatoma cells. The experimental data indicate that all sPLA₂-IIA-treated lipoproteins possess an enhanced ability to transfer cholesterol to both vascular and non-vascular tissues. Thus, sPLA₂-IIA clearly has the potential to alter lipoprotein metabolism in a broad sense, but its ability to influence the hydrolysis of apoB-containing lipoproteins within the arterial intima is highly questionable. This is due to its apparent inability to act on phosphatidylcholine,[67,68] the major phospholipid of both lipoproteins and cell membranes. Recall that the concentration of lyso-PC is greatly elevated in atherosclerotic plaques.[23]

Thus, it would appear that Lp-PLA₂ is better placed to contribute to the hydrolysis of oxidized LDL within the developing atherosclerotic lesion, whilst sPLA₂-IIA may still play a part by enhancing the intimal retention of apoB-containing lipoproteins. As noted earlier, the group V and X secretory PLA₂s may ultimately evolve into stronger candidates since both are efficient in binding and hydrolysing phosphatidylcholines.[28] They, like sPLA₂-IIA, are not dependent upon oxidative modification for substrate generation, a characteristic that remains unique to Lp-PLA₂. Both, however, are very efficient in the hydrolysis of both LDL and HDL.[65,67] Recent findings, for example, suggest that the lipolytic modification of HDL by both group V and X sPLA₂s can lead to a reduction of its anti-atherogenic functions, including an impaired ability to mediate cellular cholesterol efflux.[65]

Association with coronary heart disease

Lp-PLA₂

This section will be split into two parts, the first dealing with plasma levels of Lp-PLA₂ and the second concentrating on known genetic polymorphisms. Since Lp-PLA₂ is responsible for approximately 95% of the hydrolysis of exogenously added PAF (when used at around 50 μM) in human plasma, this method represents a straightforward means of comparing circulating levels in controls versus patients. The first studies to use this method during the late 1980s consistently demonstrated a positive association with cardiovascular disease. Documented elevations in plasma Lp-PLA₂ levels were noted in individuals with atherosclerosis,[69–71] diabetes,[72] stroke[73,74] and even essential hypertension.[75] More recently, these observations have been confirmed and extended using both Lp-PLA₂ activity and mass (determined via a specific immunoassay) measurements.

Blankenberg et al showed increasing plasma Lp-PLA₂ activity levels in both male and female patients with stable and unstable coronary artery disease as compared with those without angiographically confirmed coronary artery disease (CAD).[76] Interestingly, no correlation could be demonstrated between Lp-PLA$_2$ activity and inflammatory markers, including other acute-phase reactants such as C-reactive protein (CRP). This latter observation confirmed the findings of Packard et al, who earlier used the Lp-PLA$_2$ immunoassay for the first time to show a strong positive association with the risk of CAD (defined as myocardial infarction, revascularization or death) in a nested case-control study involving individuals who participated in the West of Scotland Coronary Prevention Study (WOSCOPS).[77] Lp-PLA$_2$ mass was found to be an independent risk marker, with a 2-fold increased risk associated with Lp-PLA$_2$ levels in the highest quintile compared with the lowest quintile. This relationship was not influenced by markers of inflammation such as CRP and white cell count, or other traditional risk factors such as fibrinogen and lipid parameters including LDL cholesterol. An earlier study by the same group had demonstrated significantly higher Lp-PLA$_2$ levels in men with angiographically proven CAD compared with age-matched controls, independent of LDL- and HDL-cholesterol, smoking and systolic blood pressure.[78] The independence of Lp-PLA$_2$ when compared with CRP is of note because both are acute-phase proteins, but each apparently represents different inflammatory pathways. Based on the weight of scientific evidence, the American Heart Association recently stated that measurement of CRP could be used to help further evaluation and therapy in the primary prevention of cardiovascular disease in patients at intermediate risk.[79]

The idea that Lp-PLA$_2$ and CRP could be complementary in identifying individuals at high CAD risk found further support from a very recent case-control analysis of men and women who participated in the Atherosclerosis Risk in Communities (ARIC) study. For individuals in ARIC with LDL-cholesterol below 130 mg/dl, Lp-PLA$_2$ and CRP were both significantly and independently associated with

CAD in fully adjusted models.[80] As in WOSCOPS, Lp-PLA$_2$ mass was not correlated with CRP levels. However, although Lp-PLA$_2$ levels were significantly higher in cases than non-cases in the complete cohort, in a model adjusted for traditional risk factors, and in particular LDL-cholesterol, the association was attenuated. A similar attenuation was also demonstrated in another, albeit much smaller, prospective study of apparently healthy middle-aged women.[81] Thus, although Lp-PLA$_2$ levels are consistently elevated in patients at risk of CHD, many more studies are needed to confirm that Lp-PLA$_2$ levels represent a strong independent predictor of future cardiovascular risk. The studies do acknowledge that there is a significant positive correlation of Lp-PLA$_2$ with LDL cholesterol (its main carrier in human plasma), a significant inverse correlation with HDL-cholesterol and a lack of any correlation between Lp-PLA$_2$ and CRP.

Whilst there is growing evidence that plasma levels of Lp-PLA$_2$ may represent an independent predictor of coronary heart disease, a quite different picture emerges from studies of a loss of function mutation in Lp-PLA$_2$, which exists primarily in the Japanese population.[52,82] This single nucleotide polymorphism (V279F) is found in around 30% of the Japanese population (4% homozygous, 27% heterozygous), with plasma from homozygotes demonstrating a complete inability to hydrolyse exogenously added PAF. The inactivating missense mutation was first reported in 1988 by Miwa,[83] who stated that there were no significant differences between the Lp-PLA$_2$ enzyme activities of patients with and without asthmatic attacks. The next group to comment on the mutation concluded that none of the subjects with the enzyme deficiency had a history of allergy, circulatory shock or chronic inflammatory diseases.[84] A similar observation was made by others who showed that the mutant allele did not correlate with asthma prevalence, type or severity.[85] Another manuscript published in the same year, however, concluded that the mutation was a modulating locus for the severity of asthma.[86] A similarly confusing picture emerges when considering the association of the mutation with CAD risk, because the findings tend to be completely the opposite to what the growing epidemiology around plasma Lp-PLA$_2$ levels is indicating.

The first CAD association study, and largest to-date, reported a positive association with the Lp-PLA$_2$ missense mutation in male, but not female, patients with diagnosed myocardial infarction.[87,88] A later study by the same group, however, failed to confirm the previously observed association between genotype and CAD.[89] Another publication showed a statistically significant link with the Lp-PLA$_2$ mutation and stroke patient.[90] Intriguingly, the same group had previously demonstrated that plasma Lp-PLA$_2$ activities were significantly elevated in stroke.[73,74] However, there is some consistency to this apparent paradox because, in the genetic association paper, it was shown that in normal and heterozygous subjects, Lp-PLA$_2$ activity was higher in stroke cases as compared to controls. In three other studies, with various cardiovascular phenotypes, this paradoxical pattern was also observed.[91–93] Moreover, in the three publications by Yamada and colleagues which showed the frequency of the 279F allele to be significantly higher in CAD cases as compared to controls, the Lp-PLA$_2$ activity in non- or heterozygous carriers was comparable.[88,94,95]

If low or absent Lp-PLA$_2$ levels are truly predisposing for an increased risk for cardiovascular disease, then subjects with disease who do not carry the 279F allele should also have significantly lower Lp-PLA$_2$ activity as compared to controls. Furthermore, it is noteworthy that the generation of lyso-PC and water-soluble products (i.e. oxidized fatty acids) from oxidized phospholipids was similar in plasma samples from both normals and individuals heterozygous for the null mutation.[96] Homozygote subjects, on the other hand, demonstrated a significant reduction in these Lp-PLA$_2$ products. These findings indicate that functional differences can only be observed between homozygotes and normals, which is not consistent with the published disease associations in heterozygotes.

Thus, the data generated in Japanese subjects are conflicting and more comprehensive studies are needed to resolve these discrepancies. This need was further highlighted by a recent investigation of another Lp-PLA$_2$ polymorphism (Val379) that is also associated with reduced enzyme activity, which demonstrated a reduced risk of myocardial infarction in a Caucasian population.[97]

sPLA$_2$-IIA

Only one study has investigated the association of sPLA$_2$-IIA and CAD risk and found that it was a significant risk marker for the presence of CAD and was able to predict clinical coronary events independently of other risk factors.[98] Unlike Lp-PLA$_2$, sPLA$_2$-IIA levels were significantly correlated with CRP levels, suggesting they are common components of the same inflammatory pathway. In a multivariate analysis, sPLA$_2$-IIA, but not CRP, remained a significant predictor of future coronary events, although this requires confirmation in many additional studies covering diverse population groups. Currently no data exist linking an sPLA$_2$-IIA polymorphism with CAD risk.

SUMMARY

The weight of biochemical evidence indicates that Lp-PLA$_2$, rather than sPLA$_2$-IIA, has the greater potential to be a causal player in atherogenesis. Although further research is obviously required, especially to address queries around genetic associations, the real test will be to demonstrate clinical benefit through the use of a small-molecule inhibitor of the enzyme. To this end, a highly potent and selective inhibitor of Lp-PLA$_2$[99] is currently in phase II clinical studies. If effective, this therapeutic approach of directly modifying plaque inflammatory processes will complement LDL and HDL interventions for reduction of cardiovascular risk associated with atherosclerotic vascular disease.

References

1. Six DA, Dennis EA. The expanding superfamily of phospholipase A_2 enzymes, classification and characterisation. Biochim Biophys Acta 2000; 1488:1–19

2. Kudo I, Murakami M. Phospholipase A_2 enzymes. Prost Other Lipid Mediat 2002; 68–69:3–58

3. Brown MS, Goldstein JL. Koch's postulates for cholesterol. Cell 1992; 71:187–8

4. Williams KJ, Tabas I. The response-to-retention hypothesis of early atherogenesis. Arteriol Thromb Vasc Biol 1995; 15:551–61

5. Berliner JA, Heinecke JW. The role of oxidised lipoproteins in atherogenesis. Free Radic Biol Med 1996; 20:707–27

6. Ross R. Atherosclerosis – an inflammatory disease. N Engl J Med 1999; 340:115–26

7. Skalen K, Gustafsson M, Rydberg EK, et al. Subendothelial retention of atherogenic lipoproteins in early atherosclerosis. Nature 2002; 417:750–4

8. Heinecke JW. Oxidised amino acids: culprits in human atherosclerosis and indicators of oxidative stress. Free Rad Biol Med 2002; 32:1090–1101

9. Brennan ML, Penn MS, Van Lente F, et al. Prognostic value of myeloperoxidase in patients with chest pain. N Engl J Med 2003; 349:1595–604.

10. Harrison D, Griendling KK, Landmesser U, et al Role of oxidative stress in atherosclerosis. Am J Cardiol 2003; 91:7A–11A

11. Griendling KK, FitzGerald GA. Oxidative stress and cardiovascular injury: animal and human studies. Circulation 2003; 108:2034–40

12. Kiechl S, Egger G, Mayr M, et al. Chronic infections and the risk of carotid atherosclerosis. Circulation 2001; 103:1064–70

13. Buffon A, Biasucci LM, Liuzzo G, et al. Widespread coronary inflammation in unstable angina. N Engl J Med 2002; 347:5–12

14. Holvoet P. Oxidation of low density lipoproteins in atherosclerosis and thrombosis: inhibitory effects of antioxidants, estrogen and high density lipoproteins. Vasc Dis 1997; 2:499–509

15. Dart AM, Chin-Dusting JPF. Lipids and the endothelium. Cardiovasc Res 1999; 43:308–22

16. Leitinger N. Oxidised phospholipids as modulators of inflammation in atherosclerosis. Curr Opin Lipidol 2003; 14:421–30

17. Cai H, Harrison DG. Endothelial dysfunction in cardiovascular diseases: the role of oxidant stress. Circ Res 2000; 87:840–4

18. Martinet W, Kockx MM. Apoptosis in atherosclerosis: focus on oxidised lipids and inflammation. Curr Opin Lipidol 2001; 12: 535–41

19. Littlewood TD, Bennett MR. Apoptotic cell death in atherosclerosis. Curr Opin Lipidol 2003; 14:469–75

20. Parthasarathy S, Steinbrecher UP, Barnett J, et al. Essential role of a phospholipase A_2 activity in endothelial cell-induced modification of low density lipoprotein. Proc Natl Acad Sci USA 1985; 82:3000–4

21. Quinn MT, Parthasarathy S, Steinberg D. Lysophosphatidylcholine: a chemotactic factor for human monocytes and its potential role in atherogenesis. Proc Natl Acad Sci USA 1988; 85:2805–9

22. Keaney JF, Xu A, Cunningham D, et al. Dietary probucol preserves endothelial function in cholesterol-fed rabbits by limiting vascular oxidative stress and superoxide generation. J Clin Invest 1995; 95:2520–9

23. Thukkani AK, McHowat J, Hsu FF, et al. Identification of α-chloro fatty aldehydes and unsaturated lysophosphatidylcholine molecular species in human atherosclerotic lesions. Circulation 2003; 108:3128–33

24. Balsinde J, Winstead MV, Dennis EA. Phospholipase A_2 regulation of arachidonic acid mobilisation. FEBS Lett 2002; 531:2–6

25. Min JH, Jain MK, Wilder C, et al. Membrane-bound plasma platelet activating factor acetylhydrolase acts on substrate in the aqueous phase. Biochemistry 1999; 38:12935–42

26. Min JH, Wilder C, Aoki J, et al. Platelet-activating factor acetylhydrolase: broad substrate specificity and lipoprotein binding does not modulate the catalytic properties of the plasma enzyme. Biochemistry 2001; 40:4539–49

27. Farr RS, Cox CP, Wardlow ML, et al. Preliminary studies of an acid-labile factor in human sera that inactivates platelet-activating factor. Clin Immunol Immunopathol 1980; 15:318–30

28. Murakami M, Kudo I. New phospholipase A_2 isozymes with a potential role in atherosclerosis. Curr Opin Lipidol 2003; 14: 431–6

29. Asano K, Okamoto S, Fukunaga K, et al. Cellular source(s) of platelet-activating factor acetylhydrolase activity in plasma. Biochem Biophys Res Commun 1999; 261:511–14

30. Elstad MR, Stafforini DM, McIntyre TM, et al. Platelet-activating factor acetylhydrolase increases during macrophage differentiation. J Biol Chem 1989; 264: 8467–70

31. Howard KM, Olson MS. The expression and localization of plasma platelet-activating factor acetylhydrolase in endotoxemic rats. J Biol Chem 2000; 275: 19891–6

32. Hakkinen T, Luoma J, Macphee CH, et al. Lipoprotein-associated phospholipase A_2 is expressed by macrophages in human and rabbit atherosclerotic lesions. Arterioscler Thromb Vasc Biol 1999; 19: 2909–17

33. Memon RA, Fuller J, Moser AH, et al. In vivo regulation of plasma platelet-activating factor acetylhydrolase during the acute phase response. Am J Physiol 1999; 277:R94–R103

34. Caslake MJ, Packard CJ, Suckling KE, et al. Lipoprotein-associated phospholipase A$_2$, platelet-activating factor acetylhydrolase: a potential new risk factor for coronary artery disease. Atherosclerosis 2000; 150:413–19

35. Tselepis AD, Dentan C, Karabina S-AP, et al. PAF-degrading acetylhydrolase is preferentially associated with dense LDL and VHDL-1 in human plasma. Catalytic characteristics and relation to the monocyte-derived enzyme. Arterioscler Thromb Vasc Biol 1995; 15:1764–73

36. Benitez S, Sanchez-Quesada JL, Ribas V, et al. Platelet-activating factor acetylhydrolase is mainly associated with electronegative low-density lipoprotein subfraction. Circulation 2003; 108:92–6

37. Blencowe C, Hermetter A, Kostner GM, et al. Enhanced association of platelet-activating factor acetylhydrolase with lipoprotein (a) in comparison with low density lipoprotein. J Biol Chem 1995; 270:31151–7

38. Stafforini DM, Tjoelker LW, McCormick SPA, et al. Molecular basis of the interaction between platelet-activating factor acetylhydrolase and low density lipoprotein. J Biol Chem 1999; 274:7018–24

39. Stafforini DM, McIntyre TM, Carter ME, et al. Human plasma platelet-activating factor acetylhydrolase: association with lipoprotein particles and role in the degradation of platelet-activating factor. J Biol Chem 1987; 262:4215–22

40. McCall MR, La Belle M, Forte TM, et al. Dissociable and nondissociable forms of platelet-activating factor acetylhydrolase in human plasma LDL: implications for LDL oxidative susceptibility. Biochim Biophys Acta 1999; 1437:23–36

41. Steinbrecher UP, Pritchard PH. Hydrolysis of phosphatidylcholine during LDL oxidation is mediated by platelet-activating factor acetylhydrolase. J Lipid Res 1989; 30:305–15

42. Tew DG, Southan C, Rice SQJ, et al. Purification, properties, sequencing and cloning of a lipoprotein-associated, serine-dependent phospholipase involved in the oxidative modification of low density lipoproteins. Arterioscler Thromb Vasc Biol 1996; 16:591–9

43. Macphee CH, Moores KE, Boyd HF, et al. Lipoprotein-associated phospholipase A$_2$, platelet-activating factor acetylhydrolase, generates two bioactive products during the oxidation of low density lipoprotein: use of a novel inhibitor. Biochem J 1999; 338:479–87

44. Kabarowski JHS, Xu Y, Witte ON. Lysophosphatidylcholine as a ligand for immunoregulation. Biochem Pharmacol 2002; 64:161–7

45. Murugesan G, Rani MRS, Gerber CE, et al. Lyso-phosphatidylcholine regulates human microvascular endothelial cell expression of chemokines. J Mol Cell Cardiol 2003; 35:1375–84

46. Rong JX, Berman JW, Taubman MB, et al. Lysophosphatidylcholine stimulates monocyte chemoattractant protein-1 gene expression in rat

47. Silliman CC, Elzi DJ, Ambruso DR, et al. Lysophosphatidylcholines prime the NADPH oxidase and stimulate multiple neutrophil functions through changes in cytosolic calcium. J Leukocyte Biol 2003; 73:511–24

48. Lum H, Qiao J, Walter RJ, et al. Inflammatory stress increases receptor for lysophosphatidylcholine in human microvascular endothelial cells. Am J Physiol Circ Physiol 2003; 285:H1786–9

49. Macphee CH. Lipoprotein-associated phospholipase A$_2$: a potential new risk factor for coronary artery disease and a therapeutic target. Curr Opin Pharmacol 2001; 1:121–5

50. Carpenter KL, Dennis IF, Challis IR, et al. Inhibition of lipoprotein-associated phospholipase A$_2$ diminishes the death-inducing effects of oxidised LDL on human monocyte-macrophages. FEBS Lett 2001; 505:357–63

51. Okura Y, Brink M, Itabe H, et al. Oxidized low-density lipoprotein is associated with apoptosis of vascular smooth muscle cells in human atherosclerotic plaques. Circulation 2000; 102:2680–6

52. Tjoelker LW, Stafforini DM. Platelet-activating factor acetylhydrolase in health and disease. Biochim Biophys Acta 2000; 1488:102–23

53. Tselepis AD, Chapman MJ. Inflammation, bioactive lipids and atherosclerosis: potential roles of lipoprotein-associated phospholipase A$_2$, platelet activating factor-acetylhydrolase. Atheroscler Suppl 2002; 3:57–68

54. Caslake MJ, Packard CJ. Lipoprotein-associated phospholipase A$_2$ (platelet activating factor-acetylhydrolase) and cardiovascular disease. Curr Opin Lipidol 2003; 14:347–52

55. Gomez FP, Rodriguez-Roisin R. Platelet-activating factor antagonists: current status in asthma. BioDrugs 2000; 14:21–30

56. Berliner JA, Subbanagounder G, Leitinger N, et al. Evidence for a role of phospholipid oxidation products in atherogenesis. Trends Cardiovasc Med 2001; 11:142–7

57. Bochkov VN, Kadl A, Huber J, et al. Protective role of phospholipid oxidation products in endotoxin-induced tissue damage. Nature 2002; 419:77–81

58. Walton KA, Cole AL, Yeh M, et al. Specific phospholipid oxidation products inhibit ligand activation of toll-like receptors 4 and 2. Arterioscler Thromb Vasc Biol 2003; 23:1197–203

59. Kronke G, Bochkov VN, Huber J, et al. Oxidized phospholipids induce expression of human heme oxygenase-1 involving activation of cAMP-responsive element-binding protein. J Biol Chem 2003; 278: 51006–14

60. Kiechl S, Lorenz E, Reindl M, et al. Toll-like receptor 4 polymorphisms and atherogenesis. N Engl J Med 2002; 347:185–92

61. Ameziane N, Beillat T, Verpillat P, et al. Association of the Toll-like receptor 4 gene Asp299Gly polymor-

phism with acute coronary events. Arterioscler Thromb Vasc Biol 2003; 23:61–4

62. Opal S, Laterre P-F, Abraham E, et al. Recombinant human platelet-activating factor acetylhydrolase for treatment of severe sepsis: results of a phase III, multicenter, randomized, double-blind, placebo-controlled, clinical trial. Crit Care Med 2004; 32:332–41

63. Hurt-Camejo E, Camejo G, Peilot H, et al. Phospholipase A_2 in vascular disease. Circ Res 2001; 89:298–304

64. Menschikowski M, Kasper M, Lattke P, et al. Secretory group II phospholipase A_2 in human atherosclerotic plaques. Atherosclerosis 1995; 118:173–81

65. Ishimoto Y, Yamada K, Yamamoto S, et al. Group V and X secretory phospholipase A_2s-induced modification of high-density lipoprotein linked to the reduction of its antiatherogenic functions. Biochim Biophys Acta 2003; 1642:129–38

66. Jaross W, Eckey R, Menschikowski M. Biological effects of secretory phospholipase A_2 group IIA on lipoproteins and in atherogenesis. Eur J Clin Invest 2002; 32:383–93

67. Gesquiere L, Cho W, Subbaiah PV. Role of group IIa and group V secretory phospholipase A_2 in the metabolism of lipoproteins. Substrate specificities of the enzymes and the regulation of their activities by sphingomyelin. Biochemistry 2002; 41:4911–20

68. Kim KP, Han SK, Hong M, et al. The molecular basis of phosphatidylcholine preference of human group-V phospholipase A_2. Biochem J 2000; 348:643–7

69. Ostermann G, Ruhling K, Zabel-Langhennig R, et al. Plasma from atherosclerotic patients exerts an increased degradation of platelet-activating factor. Thromb Res 1987; 47:279–85

70. Ostermann G, Lang A, Holtz H, et al. The degradation of platelet-activating factor in serum and its discriminative value in atherosclerotic patients. Thromb Res 1988; 52:529–40

71. Graham RM, Stephens CJ, Sturm MJ, et al. Plasma platelet-activating factor degradation in patients with severe coronary artery disease. Clin Sci 1992; 82:535–41

72. Hofmann B, Ruhling K, Spangenberg P, et al. Enhanced degradation of platelet-activating factor in serum from diabetic patients. Haemostasis 1989; 19:180–4

73. Satoh K, Imaizumi T, Kawamura Y, et al. Activity of platelet-activating factor (PAF) acetylhydrolase in plasma from patients with ischemic cerebrovascular disease. Prostaglandins 1988; 35:685–98

74. Satoh K, Yoshida H, Imaizumi T, et al. Platelet-activating factor acetylhydrolase in plasma lipoproteins from patients with ischemic stroke. Stroke 1992; 23:1090–2

75. Satoh K, Imaizumi T, Kawamura Y, et al. Increased activity of the platelet-activating factor acetylhydrolase in plasma low density lipoprotein from patients with essential hypertension. Prostaglandins 1989; 37:673–82.

76. Blankenberg S, Stengel D, Rupprecht HJ, et al. Plasma PAF-acetylhydrolase in patients with coronary artery disease: results of a cross-sectional analysis. J Lipid Res 2003; 44:1381–6

77. Packard CJ, O'Reilly DS, Caslake MJ, et al. Lipoprotein-associated phospholipase A_2 as an independent predictor of coronary heart disease. West of Scotland Coronary Prevention Study Group. N Engl J Med 2000; 343:1148–55

78. Caslake MJ, Packard CJ, Suckling KE, et al. Lipoprotein-associated phospholipase A_2, platelet-activating factor acetylhydrolase: a potential new risk factor for coronary artery disease. Atherosclerosis 2000; 150:413–19

79. Pearson TA, Mensah GA, Alexander RW, et al. Markers of inflammation and cardiovascular disease: application to clinical and public health practice. Circulation 2003; 107:499–511

80. Ballantyne CM, Hoogeveen RC, Bang H, et al. Lipoprotein-associated phospholipase A_2, high-sensitivity C-reactive protein, and risk for incident coronary heart disease in middle-aged men and women in the Atherosclerosis Risk in Communities (ARIC) study. Circulation 2004; 109:837–42.

81. Blake GJ, Dada N, Fox JC, et al. A prospective evaluation of lipoprotein-associated phospholipase A_2 levels and the risk of future cardiovascular events in women. J Am Coll Cardiol 2001; 38:1302–6.

82. Karasawa K, Harada A, Satoh N, et al. Plasma platelet-activating factor acetylhydrolase. Progress Lipid Res 2003; 42:93–114

83. Miwa M, Miyake T, Yamanaka T, et al. Characterization of serum platelet-activating factor (PAF) acetylhydrolase. Correlation between deficiency of serum PAF acetylhydrolase and respiratory symptoms in asthmatic children. J Clin Invest 1988; 82:1983–91.

84. Yoshida H, Satoh K, Koyama M, et al. Deficiency of plasma platelet-activating factor acetylhydrolase: roles of blood cells. Am J Hematol 1996; 53:158–64

85. Satoh N, Asano K, Naoki K, et al. Plasma platelet-activating factor acetylhydrolase deficiency in Japanese patients with asthma. Am J Respir Crit Care Med 1999; 159:974–9

86. Stafforini DM, Numao T, Tsodikov A, et al. Deficiency of platelet-activating factor acetylhydrolase is a severity factor for asthma. J Clin Invest 1999; 103:989–97.

87. Yamada Y, Ichihara S, Fujimura T, et al. Identification of the G994→ T missense in exon 9 of the plasma platelet-activating factor acetylhydrolase gene as an independent risk factor for coronary artery disease in Japanese men. Metabolism 1998; 47:177–81

88. Yamada Y, Yoshida H, Ichihara S, et al. Correlations between plasma platelet-activating factor acetylhydrolase (PAF-AH) activity and PAF-AH genotype, age, and atherosclerosis in a Japanese population. Atherosclerosis 2000; 150:209–16

89. Yamada Y, Izawa H, Ichihara S, et al. Prediction of the

risk of myocardial infarction from polymorphisms in candidate genes. N Engl J Med 2002; 347:1916–23

90. Hiramoto M, Yoshida H, Imaizumi T, et al. A mutation in plasma platelet-activating factor acetyl-hydrolase (Val279→Phe) is a genetic risk factor for stroke. Stroke 1997; 28:2417–20

91. Yoshida H, Imaizumi T, Fujimoto K, et al. A mutation in plasma platelet-activating factor acetylhydrolase (Val279Phe) is a genetic risk factor for cerebral hemorrhage but not for hypertension. Thromb Haemost 1998; 80:372–5

92. Unno N, Nakamura T, Kaneko H, et al. Plasma platelet-activating factor acetylhydrolase deficiency is associated with atherosclerotic occlusive disease in Japan. J Vasc Surg 2000; 32:263–7

93. Unno N, Nakamura T, Mitsuoka H, et al. Single nucleotide polymorphism (G994→T) in the plasma platelet-activating factor-acetylhydrolase gene is associated with graft patency of femoropopliteal bypass. Surgery 2002; 132:66–71

94. Ichihara S, Yamada Y, Yokota M. Association of a G994→T missense mutation in the plasma platelet-activating factor acetylhydrolase gene with genetic susceptibility to nonfamilial dilated cardiomyopathy in Japanese. Circulation 1998; 98:1881–5

95. Yamada Y, Ichihara S, Izawa H, et al. Association of a G994 → T (Val279 → Phe) polymorphism of the plasma platelet-activating factor acetylhydrolase gene with myocardial damage in Japanese patients with nonfamilial hypertrophic cardiomyopathy. J Hum Genet 2001; 46:436–41

96. Subramanian VS, Goyal J, Miwa M, et al. Role of lecithin-cholesterol acyltransferase in the metabolism of oxidized phospholipids in plasma: studies with platelet-activating factor-acetyl hydrolase-deficient plasma. Biochim Biophys Acta 1999; 1439:95–109

97. Abuzeid AM, Hawe E, Humphries SE, et al. Association between the Ala379Val variant of the lipoprotein associated phospholipase A$_2$ and risk of myocardial infarction in the north and south of Europe. Atherosclerosis 2003; 168:283–8

98. Kugiyama K, Ota Y, Takazoe K, et al. Circulating levels of secretory type II phospholipase A$_2$ predict coronary events in patients with coronary artery disease. Circulation 1999; 100:1280–4

99. Blackie JA, Bloomer JC, Brown MJ, et al. The identification of clinical candidate SB-480848: a potent inhibitor of lipoprotein-associated phospholipase A$_2$. Bioorg Med Chem Lett 2003; 13:1067–70.

Index